EXPERIENCING MOTIVATIONAL INTERVIEWING FROM THE INSIDE OUT

SELF-PRACTICE/SELF-REFLECTION GUIDES FOR PSYCHOTHERAPISTS

James Bennett-Levy, Series Editor

This series invites therapists to enhance their effectiveness "from the inside out" using self-practice/self-reflection (SP/SR). Books in the series lead therapists through a structured three-stage process of focusing on a personal or professional issue they want to change, practicing therapeutic techniques on themselves (self-practice), and reflecting on the experience (self-reflection). Research supports the unique benefits of SP/SR for providing insights and skills not readily available through more conventional training procedures. The approach is suitable for therapists at all levels of experience, from trainees to experienced supervisors. Series volumes have a large-size format for ease of use and feature reproducible worksheets and forms that purchasers can download and print.

Experiencing CBT from the Inside Out: A Self-Practice/Self-Reflection Workbook for Therapists
James Bennett-Levy, Richard Thwaites, Beverly Haarhoff, and Helen Perry

Experiencing Schema Therapy from the Inside Out: A Self-Practice/Self-Reflection Workbook for Therapists
Joan M. Farrell and Ida A. Shaw

Experiencing Compassion-Focused Therapy from the Inside Out: A Self-Practice/Self-Reflection Workbook for Therapists
Russell L. Kolts, Tobyn Bell, James Bennett-Levy, and Chris Irons

Experiencing ACT from the Inside Out: A Self-Practice/Self-Reflection Workbook for Therapists
Dennis Tirch, Laura R. Silberstein-Tirch, R. Trent Codd, III, Martin J. Brock, and M. Joann Wright

Experiencing Motivational Interviewing from the Inside Out: A Self-Practice/Self-Reflection Workbook for Practitioners
David B. Rosengren, Lynne H. Johnston, and Charlotte E. Hilton

Experiencing Motivational Interviewing from the Inside Out

A Self-Practice/Self-Reflection Workbook for Practitioners

David B. Rosengren
Lynne H. Johnston
Charlotte E. Hilton

Series Editor's Note by James Bennett-Levy

THE GUILFORD PRESS
New York London

A Division of Guilford Publications, Inc.
www.guilford.com

Printed in the United States of America

This book is printed on acid-free paper.

Last digit is print number: 9 8 7 6 5 4 3 2 1

Library of Congress Cataloging-in-Publication Data

Names: Rosengren, David B., author. | Johnston, Lynne H., author. | Hilton, Charlotte E., author.
Title: Experiencing motivational interviewing from the inside out : a self-practice/self-reflection workbook for practitioners / David B. Rosengren, Lynne H. Johnston, and Charlotte E. Hilton.
Description: New York : The Guilford Press, [2025] | Series: Self-practice/self-reflection guides for psychotherapists | Includes bibliographical references and index. |
Identifiers: LCCN 2024035203 | ISBN 9781462556298 (paperback) | ISBN 9781462556304 (cloth)
Subjects: LCSH: Motivational interviewing. | Counseling. | Interviewing in mental health.
Classification: LCC BF637.I5 R673 2024 | DDC 158.3—dc23/eng/20241104
LC record available at *https://lccn.loc.gov/2024035203*

About the Authors

David B. Rosengren, PhD, is President and CEO of the Prevention Research Institute, a private nonprofit organization in Lexington, Kentucky. He is a clinical psychologist with a broad background in treatment, research, training, and administration. Previously, he was a research scientist and consultant at the University of Washington's Alcohol and Drug Abuse Institute, and worked as a motivational interviewing (MI) consultant and trainer. Dr. Rosengren helped to establish the Motivational Interviewing Network of Trainers (MINT), an international association representing more than 1,500 MI trainers spread across 40 countries and six continents. His research interests include mechanisms of change for clients and practitioners, training methods, and implementation and dissemination science. He has written journal articles and book chapters on addictions, MI, training, and the change process.

Lynne H. Johnston, PhD, DClin Psych, is a consultant clinical psychologist in the National Health Service and in private practice in the United Kingdom. Dr. Johnston has significant clinical, research, training, and consultancy experience. She is a member of MINT and a founding member of MINT UK and Ireland. She has worked as an MI consultant, trainer, and supervisor since 2001 and delivers training to professional groups across the United Kingdom and internationally. Dr. Johnston is Honorary Associate Professor at the University of Glasgow and Visiting Professor at the University of Sunderland, United Kingdom. She is currently supervising doctoral research in training, supervision, and practitioner skill development. She has authored journal articles and book chapters on clinical formulation, MI, training, supervision, and program evaluation.

Charlotte E. Hilton, PhD, is a Chartered Psychologist in the United Kingdom with expertise across health, social care, and high-performance sport settings. She is an active member of MINT and MINT UK and Ireland, and is passionate about supporting people through change and growth. Dr. Hilton regularly delivers MI training to people who work in a diverse range of professions, and has a history of working within mental and public health settings and primary care. She practices and writes from an evidence-driven perspective, with the intention of having practical utility and an applied focus. Dr. Hilton is a Visiting Fellow at the University of Derby, United Kingdom, and Associate Professor at the University of Florida.

Series Editor's Note

In the ever-evolving field of counseling and psychotherapy, personal practice and self-reflection are two of the cornerstones of practitioners' professional development. It is therefore a great pleasure to be writing the Series Editor's Note for *Experiencing Motivational Interviewing from the Inside Out: A Self-Practice/Self-Reflection Workbook for Practitioners*, the fifth book in Guilford's Self-Practice/Self-Reflection Guides for Psychotherapists series.

As the series editor, I have had the privilege of overseeing a collection of SP/SR works that delve deeply into various therapeutic modalities, each with a unique emphasis on the practitioner's own journey of self-exploration and professional development. David Rosengren, Lynne Johnston, and Charlotte Hilton's MI SP/SR workbook embodies the core principles of the SP/SR series: it fosters a profound understanding of the therapeutic techniques through personal engagement and reflection.

The expertise of these authors in both MI and SP/SR shines through on every page. It takes absolute mastery to explain therapeutic strategies in such a simple, understandable way; to provide such vivid client examples; and to craft SP/SR exercises that take practitioners deeply into the heart of MI. Rosengren, Johnston, and Hilton admirably accomplish each of these tasks. I confess to having known relatively little about MI before experiencing this book. For a long time, I've been aware that MI, with its empathetic, client-centered approach, has played a transformative role in the landscape of behavior change interventions. Yet, it was one of those methods I've always wanted to know more about, but never quite got to. *Experiencing Motivational Interviewing from the Inside Out* has been a fast-track way for me to recognize what I'd been missing. This workbook provides a real sense of the value of MI—and the opportunity to embody MI skills from firsthand experience. In particular, I've come to recognise that MI's effectiveness lies not just in its techniques, but also in the spirit of collaboration and empathy that underpins it. *Experiencing Motivational Interviewing from the Inside Out* offers practitioners a rare opportunity to immerse themselves in this approach, not as passive learners, but as active participants in their own development.

What sets this workbook apart from most other counseling books for practitioners is its dual focus on practical skill building and personal growth. It provides a structured yet flexible framework that guides practitioners through the intricacies of MI techniques, while also encouraging a reflective practice that fosters personal insight and professional resilience. *Experiencing Motivational Interviewing from the Inside Out* invites practitioners to engage in self-practice exercises that mirror real-life helping scenarios, allowing them to experience firsthand the challenges and triumphs their clients face. The combination of these elements ensures that practitioners not only learn the mechanics of MI but also internalize its spirit, making them more effective and compassionate practitioners.

As you embark on this journey through *Experiencing Motivational Interviewing from the Inside Out*, I encourage you to fully engage with the exercises and reflections. Allow yourself the space to explore your own motivations and challenges, and to celebrate your growth and achievements. This workbook is more than a guide; it is a companion on your path to becoming a more self-aware, skilled, and empathetic MI practitioner.

In closing, I commend the authors for their dedication to advancing the field of MI and for their commitment to fostering the personal and professional development of practitioners. I'm very confident that you will find this workbook to be a valuable resource in your practice and that it will inspire you to continue growing both as a practitioner and as an individual.

James Bennett-Levy, PhD
University of Sydney

Acknowledgments

We owe thanks to many. James Bennett-Levy, who articulated and advanced understanding of how the *inside-out* process works for practitioners, invited us to create this work. His resources and guidance strengthened and sharpened our thinking as we worked to create a book that was a worthy companion to the others in this series.

Many members of the Motivational Interviewing Network of Trainers (MINT) deepened our understanding of MI concepts, training, and research over the years. You number almost as many as the stars in the sky. For this volume, we would like to thank a particular group of MINT members within the United Kingdom and Ireland who contributed to early thinking about the pedagogy of training, as well as the SP/SR method. Casey Bohrman and Frankie Dempsey provided just-in-time reviews to keep this book moving and make sure we were on the right path. Our thanks to Bill Miller and Steve Rollnick for their generosity of spirit, their humility in their work, and their friendship over these many years. You are the spark that created a wildfire.

Staff at The Guilford Press were excellent partners in this process. More than 20 years ago, Senior Editor Kitty Moore invited D. B. R. into this writing process for Guilford and once again extended a hand for this book. A lovely person and even better editor, she provided enthusiasm, encouragement, and wise counsel, as we moved from initial idea to final touches on this book. Behind Kitty are teams of folks doing production editing, copyediting, marketing, permissions, and so on. We would like to thank all of the people who were a part of this process, including Liz Geller, Carolyn Graham, Katherine Lieber, Smadar Levy, Katie Leonard, and Samantha Grossman. We reserve special thanks to Jeannie Tang and Patti Brecht who shepherded us through the process of raw manuscript to finished product and for patience around all our hyphenation and capitalization questions. Any errors in that department are strictly our own.

David B. Rosengren: *Curiosity* and *discovery* are interesting traveling companions, though they require a fickle third, *willingness*, to have the full experience. What delight they chose to accompany us to this work, and I am certainly at my best when they are around. Lynne and Charli have taken me on a remarkable journey, one that I could not have predicted when we first met to talk about this book. I am better for it and in the process have grown deep connections to these two remarkable women. They think deeply, challenge thoughtfully, work diligently, until it's right, and leaven it all with laughter and light. What a joy you made this process—or to put it in Scottish terms, Lynne, it wasn't half-bad. Thank you. As always, my deep appreciation and gratitude to friends and family. I feel fortunate to have your gifts of friendship, love, and forgiveness in my life. A special note to Stephanie, my brave, fierce companion, and partner, who at a critical juncture asked me, *What do you dream of?* That question changed everything. Thank you.

Lynne H. Johnston: I hope this book does justice to the groundbreaking work of James Bennett-Levy in helping practitioners to apply SP/SR to their skill development. I would like to express my gratitude and respect to David Rosengren. His generosity, humility, humor, and work ethic have made this process safe, seamless, and well coordinated. I appreciate Charli Hilton's support in helping me to outline some of my early conceptual ideas, and in stepping away from the detail. Lots of people have helped me, over many years, in my thinking about therapist skill development, training, and supervision across a range of therapeutic approaches. I am grateful for the many hours spent discussing and reflecting with fellow MINTies in the United Kingdom and internationally. Inevitably, time spent in my office has taken me away from my family and friends. I would like to thank them all for their acceptance, compassion, and understanding. Two women in my life have been more of an inspiration, and support, than either of them could ever imagine: my mum, Jean, and finally my life partner, Karen. Thank you.

Charlotte E. Hilton: I am delighted to have been part of the process of formulating and writing this book. My best hope is that it supports people to develop their interest and skills in MI and that this, in some way, helps more people to help others. For me, the process of writing has been influenced by many sources, and I'd like to acknowledge those here. First, to some of the key contributors to thinking and the development of the SP/SR approach who have also helped to influence my own: James Bennett-Levy, Mark Freeston, Richard Thwaites, Anna Chaddock, Beverly Haarhoff, Amy Finlay-Jones, and Melanie Davies. To my coauthors, for their constant curiosity, good humor, and invitations for critical reflection. To the people who have attended my trainings, for their inspirational appetite for learning and willingness to explore SP/SR as part of their MI skill development journey. To my friends, family, and MINT members, for their support and kindness. Finally, to my beloved Labrador, Harvey (who sadly died while I was writing this book), and French bulldog, Bert. Special thanks to my furry companions for being the best teachers of curiosity, genuineness, acceptance, and unconditional love.

Contents

Purchasers can access supplementary materials and a reproducible form at the companion website, *www.guilford.com/rosengren2-materials*.

Module Self-Practice Exercises/Activities

Module	Content focus	Exercise	Type of activity
1	Formulating an area for growth: the evolving focus within MI	Identifying a work or life challenge	Self/partner
2	Four tasks of MI	Engaging as part of initial discussion about a limited partner practice and identification of a challenge focus	Partner
3	Partnership	Examining an important relationship where you're struggling: Batman and Robin questions	Self/partner
4	Acceptance	Recalling my favorite teacher	Self/partner
5	Compassion	Loving-kindness meditation	Self
6	Envisioning	Visualization: looking backward	Self
7	Creating safety	*In vivo*/visualization: looking at my space from a client's perspective	Self
8	Seeing the big picture: engaging	Autobiography in five chapters	Self/partner
9	Being understood: engaging	Engaging in a conversation with someone who challenges us	Other

Module	Content focus	Exercise	Type of activity
10	Opening possibility	Focusing on a change you were not sure you either could or wanted to embrace, but somehow were able to persevere and make	Partner
11	Exploring values	Describing a day off when you get to decide what you want to do, while listening for the underlying values	Partner
12	Routes of travel: open questions and being directional	Your challenge and a day when something different happened:focusing on an exception	Partner
13	Discovering strengths and capacities: affirmation	Exploring a large failure you made, took responsibility for, and asked for help to address: finding your strengths	Partner/self
14	Pulling the pieces together: summaries	Telling three important stories from your life: focus on creating strong summaries—organized, juxtaposed, intentional, and brief	Partner/self
15	Beyond tipping the balance: ambivalence	Exploring ambivalence	Partner/self
16	Sharing information	Moving toward a decision point	Partner/self
17	Evolving focus	Review of evolving focus over the course of this book	Partner/self
18	Reasons for changing: change talk	Review of change talk in working through this book	Self/partner
19	Staying where we are: sustain talk	Two truths: grain of truth and the balancing thought	Partner/self
20	Strengthening our reasons	Looking forward 3 years using information from Modules 17 and 18	Partner/self
21	Committing (or not)	Discussing where you are in relationship to making a change	Partner/self
22	Building *my* plan	Planning worksheet	Partner/self

EXPERIENCING MOTIVATIONAL INTERVIEWING FROM THE INSIDE OUT

PART I

The Journey Ahead

CHAPTER 1

Introducing *Experiencing Motivational Interviewing from the Inside Out*

Background and Context

In this chapter, we provide an overview of why we created this book and how it might add something to the learning process for motivational interviewing (MI) practitioners. Specifically, this chapter aims to help the reader understand why *self-practice and self-reflection* might add meaningfully to their learning process, beyond other approaches, and to offer them a general framework for understanding how this book is organized and written.

Key Questions Discussed in This Chapter

- Why was this book created?
- Why might it be valuable to me as a learner?
- What do I need to understand about how the book is organized?
- Why do I need to engage in work on a real challenge or growth area of my own?
- What language conventions do I need to be aware of?

Why write a book on self-practice and self-reflection for MI, and what is this book's goal?

We had a concern. MI is fundamentally an interpersonal enterprise. It requires us to engage in certain technical skills, as well as have and maintain specific ***heart sets*** and ***mindsets*** about this work. As practitioners in the field, we learned a great deal about what it takes to be technically proficient in MI—to recognize ***change talk*** and produce a high-quality ***reflective listening statement*** in response, for example—and we can teach and train those processes well. But what we kept hearing from our trainees and mentees was their uncertainty even as their skills progressed: *Why am I doing this now and not that?* Those questions, along with our own research and observations, started us down this path.

There were other impetuses as well. William Miller, who along with Steve Rollnick articulated the elements of MI (Miller & Rollnick, 2023), likes to quip that before we begin training people in MI, we should seek their informed consent, as they are likely to emerge from the training with a fundamentally different perspective. MI can and does change the people we are, the way we view and work with people. Why does this happen? We knew from many years of training, supervising, and mentoring people in MI that when they *get* MI, it somehow connects on a more fundamental, personal, and human level. Each of us remembers our own personal MI epiphany in this way—whether that be as clinical psychologists, supervisors, trainers, and researchers (D. B. R./L. H. J.) or as a psychologist working in an academic, health and high-performance, research, or training contexts (C. E. H.). What happens when people understand and experience MI at a deeper, personal, and more fundamental level? To us, it seemed there was a *felt sense of experiencing MI from the inside out* that was important.

As a field, MI grew more proficient in training MI skills, and in training MI trainers, and with this coding instruments began to appear and to be used regularly. We understood that practitioners within a research intervention trial needed to reach a point of *competency* in MI. We could appreciate the benefit of coding tools developed for this purpose. We also saw benefit in receiving feedback on skill development. However, we were also acutely aware of the potential *unintended consequences* of using coding tools as a sole, or primary, method of ongoing practitioner skill development and the risks associated with training a learner to one specific coding instrument. That is, the trainee may simply learn how to *jump through the hoops* of a specific coding tool to demonstrate fidelity to a method, and/or simply become better at scoring more favorably, rather than engaging and reflecting in a meaningful way with the experiential aspects of the learning. We saw limitations associated with this approach to learning MI both from a client (treatment receipt) perspective and as a practitioner (delivery and enactment of treatment skills) perspective. Others identified similar concerns in the use of checklists and coding instruments across areas when complex interpersonal dynamics were at play (e.g., assessment of the quality of qualitative research, Barbour, 2001; cognitive-behavioral therapy, Blackburn et al., 2001). As we got better at measuring and quantifying perhaps, we were focusing on what we could measure and not what was most important—*the tail was wagging the dog*. At the same time, increasing attention was paid to other methods, such as reflective questions, as an alternative to checklist and coding approaches in other treatment approaches (e.g., Bennett-Levy et al., 2015) that intrigued us.

We were also interested in deliberate practice as a method to deepen knowledge and skills (Rousmaniere, 2017). It was clear to us that this type of practice had value in improving skills. It also became evident that a practitioner's reflection on their deliberate practice is, by definition, viewing the experience through only the lens of the practitioner. In our experience as trainers, we have spent many years engaging people in *deliberate practice, real play* exercises (i.e., participants discuss real matters from their lives rather than role-playing a client) whereby trainees work in dyads or triads to experience the various skills associated with an MI-consistent conversation. Crucially, we observed that trainees who engage in the role of a *client*, as well as the practitioner role, connect with, experience, and learn MI in a deeper and more comprehensive way. Our further reflection and discussion with trainees over many years taught us there was significant added value in experiencing MI as a real client in that it enables a deeper ***interoceptive*** level of awareness and appreciation, a *felt sense* of understanding, and learning that was different than the learning in the MI practitioner role. Interoceptive refers to "the process of how the nervous system senses, interprets, and integrates signals originating from within the body" (Quigley et al., 2021, p. 29). We wondered why? What was going on? In what way might this be important? How do we enhance that experience?

In 2003, Bennett-Levy discussed *reflection* as a blind spot in clinical psychology training. By 2015, we questioned a similar blind spot within the MI training and skill development literature. Without self-reflection, it seemed practitioner development could be thwarted. We become technically proficient, but the deeper wisdom of how, what, and most importantly why we do things can elude us. We believed the growing literature, outside the MI world of research, writing, and training, could help us as practitioners, trainers, supervisors, and mentors to think more deeply at a conceptual and practical level, and eventually to develop a different type of approach for how best to gain proficiency in MI. Research on *self-practice and self-reflection (SP/SR)* (e.g., Bennett-Levy et al., 2015) demonstrated that when practitioners had a *felt experience* of the intervention from their *real-life* client role and then spent time thinking deeply about that experience, and applying their insights to their work systematically, it created a foundation for learners to develop skills at a more profound level. This led us to think practically about how we could bring these ideas to the world of MI.

We began discussing our concerns and ideas for a new form of book in 2015, in Berlin, at an international forum for the *Motivational Interviewing Network of Trainers* (MINT). L. H. J. and C. E. H. delivered a workshop presentation to explore the role of *reflection* in developing proficiency in both the conceptual (knowledge) development and implementation of the procedural skills of MI (Johnston et al., 2015). Further discussion with D. B. R. ignited deeper creative and conceptual sparks, and more questions emerged from our early musings:

- How can trainers help practitioners to move beyond an introductory level of knowledge and skill development in MI?
- Are deliberate practice, coding, and supervision enough to help people develop proficiency in MI skills?
- What role do self-coding and self-reflection play in the development of proficiency in MI?
- Where does reflection "in" (in the moment) and "on action" (after the moment) fit in when learning the complexities and nuances in MI, and how can we as trainers help to scaffold this?
- How much attention does a deliberate practice approach pay to reflection on interpersonal process skills in MI? Might a lack of sufficient attention thwart the development of skills in MI?
- How much attention has the MI literature given to the experiential aspects of receiving a good-quality MI-consistent consultation as a key learning method?
- How does feeling/experiencing an MI-consistent conversation impact on the receiver as a learner? What role does self-reflection have in this process?
- Does coding their *own* recordings of practice help a learner to reflect more fully on their practice? In what way?
- Do coding instruments shine a light on a particular corner of MI? What might be missed

if we look only in that direction? What happens to the aspects that remain uncoded, and are they important parts of the variance in practitioner skill development?

- Are coding instruments better at assessing the technical aspects of MI skills, perhaps at the expense of the relational and experiential aspects of MI? If "yes," is this a problem?
- What do coding instruments miss in terms of the unobservable aspects of the interpersonal interaction, and are these aspects important?
- Does the experience of being in an MI-consistent quality conversation impact the recipient differently if it is done as a "real-play" versus a "role-play" and, if yes," why?

Our discussions and reflections on these questions led us to write this book.

The current text is not designed as an introduction to MI or as a general book on MI for a specific context. There are already lots of good introductory texts on MI, and several books that have been written with a specific context in mind, which serve these needs well. The current text aims to help people who already have either a basic, intermediate, or even advanced understanding of MI to move beyond their current skill level to connect with a deeper understanding of MI and to further enhance their skill development as a practitioner in MI by working from the *inside out*. This book does presuppose knowledge of basic conceptual elements, as well as skills associated with MI. It is not the best book for someone completely new to MI. We recommend one of the other seminal texts in that case (e.g., Miller & Rollnick, 2023; Rosengren, 2017). Still, we intend this book for people across the career range, from new to the field to experienced mentor and trainer eager to understand the *why* of MI.

Similarly, we did not want to write another book on *deliberate practice* because there is already a good book published on this by experienced and well-respected MI trainers (Manuel et al., 2022). In addition, we knew that, as noted above, a deliberate MI practice approach focuses on the perspective of the *practitioner-self*, and this stance tends to miss the opportunity to experience the *felt interoceptive awareness* of being in receipt of an MI-consistent conversation from the perspective of the *personal-self*, which we also refer as the *client-self perspective*.

This book invites us to engage in targeted SP exercises that are designed to facilitate our own deeper level of understanding and appreciation of MI. SP does not involve role-play; it involves real-play. That is, the SP process asks us to engage with our real-life challenges to experience personally and deeply the MI approach. Each exercise is designed in a way that builds on our current understanding of and present skill level in MI. We then invite reflection on the experience, first from the perspective of *our self as a client*. That is, from the lens of the person on the receiving end of the MI skill or practice while working on a personal issue. The second set of reflective questions explore and probe further from the perspective of *our self as a practitioner*. It is this deliberate focus on self-practice as a *client* and then self-reflection (*first as a client, then as a practitioner*) that helps us move beyond deliberate practice and into developing our own unique practitioner relationship with MI. One of the functions of the current text is to move *reflection* as an experiential process to the front and center of discussions in practitioner training in MI.

In sum, this text is not designed as a replacement to other helpful practitioner skill development texts, but rather to complement them. As such, you may well find it useful to cross-refer to other texts as part of the iterative learning and ongoing knowledge and skill development process (e.g., Frey & Hall, 2021; Manuel et al., 2022; Rosengren, 2017). We will also highlight at key points in this text some of the other helpful books in the *Inside Out* series that have been published by Guilford Press.

How are the chapters in this book organized and structured, and why?

This book is structured in two parts. Part I offers six chapters, including this one, that discuss the conceptual background and theory of this text. Part II offers 22 practical modules that walk the reader through the application of SP/SR to further their understanding of key concepts and skills within MI.

Part I: Chapters 2–6

In Chapter 2, we introduce the *conceptual framework*; this includes an overview of MI, with attention given to Miller and Rollnick's (2023) recent changes in terminology in the move from the third to fourth edition of *Motivational Interviewing*. We provide a brief overview of key theoretical perspectives on motivational theory and MI. A discussion follows of the ways in which learners have tended to develop their practice in MI, including a critical review of the role of coding tools in this process. The chapter concludes with a review of some theoretical influences in learning and an introduction to a structure used within the book to organize our thinking within each of the SP/SR modules in Part II: *Why, What, How, What If.*

In Chapter 3, we introduce the reader to self-practice and self-reflection, and discuss why an SP/SR approach deepens our understanding, and application, of key concepts and practitioner skills within a therapeutic approach. Next, we explore what is already known about how people learn MI and review the eight tasks that have been proposed in learning MI. We then explore the conceptual background to SP/SR and discuss an earlier model outlining declarative and procedural knowledge systems and the crucial role of reflection within it. We provide a rationale for the use of SP/SR in MI based on the existing application of SP/SR within other approaches (e.g., *cognitive-behavioral therapy* or *CBT*). Finally, the chapter concludes with the introduction of a proposed *personal practice model (PPM)* for MI specifically and a diagram to illustrate the PPM.

In Chapter 4, we introduce the reader to the practical elements of SP/SR and provide an overview of the *guiding principles*, including *how* to engage in the process of SP/SR. We do this by giving specific attention to process, content, and structure in SP/SR. We include a discussion on the importance of self-reflective writing and the various forms that SP/SR can take (e.g., self-study; in pairs [limited partner practice]; in small groups; and with a coach or supervisor).

Chapter 5 builds further on guidelines but does so from the perspective of the facilitator of an SP/SR approach. We discuss the importance of modeling the method and review important considerations in forming and maintaining an SP/SR group for follow-up discussion on reflections and experiences, as well as caring for the individual participants.

Chapter 6 introduces the *traveling companions*. These practitioners represent people across the spectrum of their careers and in their MI knowledge and skills; they reflect amalgams of our trainees and mentees across our training careers. They will help illustrate the self-practice and, at times, self-reflection process through the modules.

Part II: Modules 1–22

We designed the modules to walk learners through a process of experiencing the concepts and skills of MI. Module 1 guides selection of a focus for the self-practice work. Modules 2–6 introduce the ***four tasks of MI*** and the ***MI spirit***, and provide self-practice experiences of the ideas articulated. Modules 7–22 integrate the four tasks, MI spirit, and skills and strategies across experiences of receiving MI. The modules do follow a sequence and are designed to be worked through in a logical order.

Within each module, we have built a learning structure to provide a repetitive pattern of Vygotskian scaffolding that we hope is both predictable and helpful. This has been influenced by learning theories that we discuss in Chapter 2 (e.g., Kolb, 1983; McCarthy & McCarthy, 2005). The generic sample outline below illustrates how these elements fit together in terms of form and function. However, greater detail is provided in Chapter 2

Module Outline

The *Why* (Meaning): Why am I doing this?

- This describes the main conceptual elements of the module.
- This is not meant to be a complete conceptual review.
- Rather, it addresses important ideas and why they're important.

The *What* (Skills): What is it that I am learning here?

- This section describes tools for enacting these important elements.
- It describes the skills.
- It provides scaffolding for some skills or links, including a companion website, for building MI skill proficiency.

The *How* (Experience of the Skills Using SP/SR): How do I do this?

- Overview of exercise.
- Traveling companion: An example.
- Self-practice.
- Self-reflections to personal-self/client-self.

The *What If* (Applying Skills to My Context): How might I adapt this to different situations, contexts, and possibilities in my professional practice?

- Bridging questions to practitioner-self.
- Applying these skills and ideas in broader applications, including my setting.
- Final ideas.

The traveling companions (see Chapter 6) appear throughout the modules and act as an additional scaffold by modeling one way of working on a personal issue in self-practice, reflecting on personal-self or client-self, and then reflecting on professional-self. We want to emphasize that the companion responses are simply examples and are not meant as *right* or *wrong* ways to answer the reflective questions. We want to caution against being unduly influenced by the demonstration responses. Again, we get more from this if we develop our own personal relationship with real-life self-practice exercises and personal–professional reflections. Further information and examples can be found on the companion website, *www.guilford.com/rosengren2-materials.*

What is the difference between this book on SP/SR and other titles in the series?

Several other books have now been published in the Inside Out series across a range of therapeutic approaches, including *acceptance and commitment therapy (ACT)*, *CBT*, *compassion-focused therapy (CFT)*, and *schema therapy* (Bennett-Levy et al., 2015; Farrell & Shaw, 2018; Kolts et al., 2018; Tirch et al., 2019). The current workbook is different in that the application of MI is broader than a therapeutic context per se. We therefore anticipate that the current text will have a broader appeal. In view of this difference, we have made some alterations to language use to reflect a broader application. One example of this is the predominant use of the term *practitioner* throughout rather than *therapist.* The language shifts on occasion to therapy/therapists because of the origins of the development of SP/SR. However, when we introduce SP/SR for MI specifically, you will notice a shift in language back to practitioner. Furthermore, in the final section within each module, we have included a brief section called "What If." The aim of this section is to help practitioners consider a wider focus and application where change conversations take place beyond the therapeutic context alone. We thus include thoughts about extending and modifying these ideas into realms beyond therapy.

We are also aware the term *practitioner* is a protected title in some locations, where it denotes that certain educational and training requirements have been completed. We are not using this term in that respect. See Box 1.1 for information about use of the term *practitioners* in the United Kingdom, for example. Instead, we use this term to reflect that peer counselors, physical therapists, physiatrists, pastors, personal trainers, probation officers, and psychologists—just to name a few p's—have very different educational and training backgrounds, but all use and endeavor to learn more about MI. It is to this broader application that we apply practitioner.

The word "reflection" is used in two main ways in this book, and we therefore want to provide clarity to avoid confusion. Within this text, we use reflection to both describe a *learning process* for the reader, as well as to refer to a *particular form of listening statement* made by the practitioner. While we try to be clear about the context, this is what we have done to help the reader. We use the term *self-reflection* when referring to reflection as a learning process and the term *reflective listening* instead of reflections in discussing practitioner techniques. However, the latter is more cumbersome and we're aware that "reflections" may still sneak through on occasion.

Throughout the book, we opt for inclusive language, using either "I" or "we." This is a writing style that acknowledges we are all learners on a journey in this method. On occasion, we use "you," especially when giving instructions in the self-practice/self-reflection activities. However, we have worked to keep this practice to a minimum. We also use the third-person plural "they" rather than "he" or "she."

BOX 1.1. Use of the Term *Practitioner* in the United Kingdom

In the United Kingdom, the term *practitioner status* is used to denote those *practitioners* who have the relevant training and qualifications to be registered with the Health and Care Professions Council (HCPC). The HCPC maintains an online register (*www.hcpc-uk.org/check-the-register*) including ***all health and care professionals who meet their standards for their training, professional skills, behavior, and health.*** Anyone can check this register to ensure individuals claiming to be practitioners are appropriately qualified and registered. The HCPC register covers a range of professions including arts therapists, biomedical scientists, chiropodists/podiatrists, clinical scientists, dietitians, practitioner psychologist, and the like. There are also specific protected titles within categories. For example, psychologists in the United Kingdom are categorized as practitioner psychologist, registered psychologist, clinical psychologist, forensic psychologist, counseling psychologist, health psychologist, educational psychologist, occupational psychologist, and sport and exercise psychologist. Anyone who claims to be working as a *practitioner psychologist* but who is not registered with HCPC is inappropriately using a restricted title and can be reported to the British Psychological Society (BPS). This approach offers public protection against people who do not hold the necessary qualifications to be working in practice as a psychologist (i.e., they are not working within a regulatory body). To be clear, ***MINT is not a regulatory body*** and therefore any UK readers should be mindful they cannot call themselves MI practitioners because of completion of this book or a MINT training course and should check against the HCPC register and with the BPS if they are uncertain about another individual's qualifications and fitness to practice.

You've undoubtedly noticed that some words have been bolded in the text. We apply this convention when we first introduce an important concept or term in a chapter or module. We use italics when we wish to emphasize a word or phrase.

Finally, as was mentioned earlier, there is a companion website. It is meant to complement the practice materials in this book. At times, there are transcripts of an interaction to provide models of how an interaction might look, including what a limited-practice partner might do in the practitioner role. Other completed forms are offered, as well as additional forms. We encourage the use of these as supplements to learning from this book.

CHAPTER 2

The Conceptual Framework

Background and Context

In this chapter, we provide an overview of key MI concepts, review theoretical models that may help us broaden and deepen our understanding of how MI helps people change, consider methods for learning MI and their limitations, and introduce a learning model we will use throughout the book to aid in the learning process.

Key Questions Discussed in This Chapter

- What are the key concepts in MI?
- How might other theoretical models help us understand MI more deeply?
- What are some of the resources for learning MI, and what might their strengths and limitations be?
- What are Kolb's learning model and Vgotsky's concepts of zone of proximal development and scaffolding, and how might these help us in the learning process?

What Is MI: A 10,000-Foot View

In their fourth edition of *Motivational Interviewing* (MI-4), Miller and Rollnick (2023) offer a simpler definition of MI: "a particular way of talking with people about change and growth to strengthen their own motivation and commitment" (p. 3). This reflects the broader appeal of MI across a range of contexts and *professional helpers*, where conversations about change take place. Although the original topic of change conversation in MI often had a behavioral focus, there is now a greater appreciation that the change focus may be in relation to a belief, attitude, or value, and in areas where a specific block may be preventing a person from engaging more fully with certain aspects of their life (e.g., acceptance and/or forgiveness within relationships or within them) or may simply be a matter of growth. This widening application of MI can be noted across a range of contexts (e.g., vaccine hesitancy, veterinary medicine, or organizational leadership) as well as a continued broadening and integration of MI with other established therapeutic approaches (e.g., CBT).

In MI-4, there has been a clear aim to achieve *simplicity from complexity*, perhaps best exemplified by an increasing simplicity in language. Table 2.1 summarizes some of the key changes in terminology between the third and fourth editions of the MI core text (Miller & Rollnick, 2013, 2023).

In their fourth edition, Miller and Rollnick (2023) have retained the foundation skills of ***OARS+I*** (open-ended questions, affirmations, reflective listening, summaries, and information exchange); an emphasis on the importance of *cultivating change talk*, *softening sustain talk*, *counseling with neutrality*, *evoking hope*, and *confidence*; and their position that *resistance* can be subdivided into ***sustain talk*** and ***discord***. However, a distinction was made between ***simple*** and ***complex affirmations*** to address the confusion that can occur regarding the role of praise in MI. The core processes in MI stand, but have been renamed as *tasks*: ***engaging***, ***focusing***, ***evoking***, and ***planning***. ***MI spirit*** also remains, though the concept of *evoking* was widened to ***empowerment*** as an important conceptual acknowledgment of an individual's own strengths, resources, and autonomy. The importance of ***partnership***, ***acceptance***, and ***compassion*** was preserved from Miller and Rollnick's previous (2013) text (MI-3).

The enduring importance of the ***spirit*** in MI is unsurprising given the links between low therapist empathy and poorer outcomes in MI (e.g., Moyers & Miller, 2013). Yet, it is perhaps no accident the aspects of MI that are more difficult to distill, and accurately measure, are increasingly recognized for their importance (Miller & Moyers, 2021). This mirrors other approaches within psychotherapy where the relational base or alliance has been consistently shown to be of fundamental importance (Flückiger et al., 2018). As long-standing and established trainers in MI, we have noticed over the course of many years that often the MI spirit is a little more challenging to teach, yet it is often so glaringly obvious when that spirit is lacking in the practitioner. Perhaps a key strength of the SP/SR approach in MI is helping practitioners to feel, from an experiential perspective, the difference between being on the receiving end of a practitioner who embodies high or low MI spirit. We believe these experiential aspects of SP/SR reach the components of MI spirit in a deeper way than a deliberate practice approach can achieve alone.

These conceptual components of MI will be discussed in more detail in Modules 2–22.

TABLE 2.1. Key Changes in Terminology between MI-3 and MI-4

Previous term	New term
Agenda mapping	Choosing a path
Developing discrepancy	Planting seeds
Elicit–provide–elicit	Ask–offer–ask
Formulation	Clarifying
Righting reflex	Fixing reflex
Running head start	Pendulum technique

Note. From Miller and Rollnick (2013, 2023).

Theoretical Perspectives and MI

MI has evolved both conceptually and practically. As a person-centered approach, Carl Rogers's work underpins MI and specifically the core conditions of empathy, genuineness (or congruence), and acceptance (or unconditional positive regard). It is these three core conditions that have influenced the conception and practice of MI spirit and the foundational skills used. The development of MI has been organic and iterative, born from direct clinical practice and the reflective experience of William Miller as he supported people through changes in problem drinking (Miller, 2023), and research demonstrating the impact of these methods on people's behaviors and outcomes. The first description of the "MI approach" was published in 1983. As such, MI was atheoretical to begin with, and while models have been suggested (e.g., Miller & Rose, 2009), there is no unified and agreed upon theory of MI at present.

Transtheoretical Model

Around the same time as MI appeared, James Prochaska published his transtheoretical analysis of systems of psychotherapy (Prochaska, 1979) that developed into an integrated model of change called the transtheoretical model of therapy (Prochaska & DiClemente, 1983) and later shortened to the *transtheoretical model (TTM)*. Throughout the 1980s and 1990s, elements of the TTM became somewhat synonymous with MI.

The TTM is often commonly, and incorrectly, referred to as the *stages of change model* (see Hutchison et al., 2009, for a further critique). However, this is simply one of four dimensions in the TTM, which include *processes of change*, *contexts of change*, and *markers of change* (DiClemente, 2018). These are integrated elements that describe how a person progresses down the path of an intentional change in human behavior. The stages of change are a useful heuristic for understanding where someone may be in the change process, but the processes of change describe elements within the individual we seek to engage to assist them in moving through the stages. Contexts describe the social and psychological factors that can influence progression along this path, and although having been well researched outside of the TTM, their role within it has not been as heavily studied. Markers describe things like temptation and self-efficacy, as well as decisional balance (pros and cons). Table 2.2 outlines the four dimensions of the TTM.

The TTM articulated the central role of ***ambivalence*** in the change process if the change is difficult to accomplish. Moreover, ambivalence is not simply about difficulty, but also about how important it is, how confident the person is, how strong the link is to underlying values, and the person's ability to work through the uncertainty. The TTM normalized ambivalence and remains firmly embedded in how MI researchers and trainers think about the change process.

From a practice perspective, a person's stage of readiness to change in TTM is perhaps better understood more completely when we consider their progression through the TTM's 10 *processes of change*: *consciousness raising*; *emotional arousal*; *self-reevaluation*; *environmental reevaluation*; *social liberation*; *self-liberation*; *helping relationships*; *counterconditioning*; *reinforcement management*; and *stimulus control*. In contrast to the overemphasis on the stages of change component, the 10 processes of change are rarely explicitly affiliated with behavior change research and practice, and this includes MI. Perhaps because MI and TTM emerged together, and they made intuitive sense as a good conceptual-practical fit, research studies citing the TTM as a theoretical underpinning to help explain the observed outcomes of MI

TABLE 2.2. The Four Dimensions of the Transtheoretical Model of Intentional Behavior Change

Stages of Change

Precontemplation–Contemplation—Preparation—Action—Maintenance

Processes of Change

Cognitive/experiential	*Behavioral*
• Consciousness raising	• Self-liberation
• Self-reevaluation	• Conditioning/counterconditioning
• Environmental reevaluation	• Stimulus generalization/control
• Emotional arousal/dramatic relief	• Reinforcement management
• Social liberation	• Helping relationships

Markers of Change

Decisional balance	Self-efficacy/temptation

Contexts of Change

Areas of functioning that complement or complicate change.

1. Current life situation
2. Beliefs and attitudes
3. Interpersonal relationships
4. Social systems
5. Enduring personal characteristics

Note. From DiClemente (2018, p. 26). Copyright © 2018 The Guilford Press. Reprinted by permission.

interventions increased dramatically. Miller and Rollnick (2009, 2013) identified the TTM as one of 10 things MI is not. However, there is a reproachment in Miller and Rollnick's latest writing (2023) and the TTM continues to provide important ideas to MI practitioners about *how* change occurs, including readiness to change, the role of ambivalence in the change process, and how understanding the kinship between the two can be helpful to the provider (e.g., recognizing that emotional arousal and consciousness raising are important processes of change, which MI can help to ignite within the individual). Velasquez and colleagues (2016) provide an excellent overview of how these elements can complement each other. Velasquez can also be heard on the *Talking to Change* podcast (Hinds & Kaplan, 2022).

Self-Determination Theory

While the TTM provides a model to understand how change may occur, it does not explain how MI works. Alternative theories such as *self-determination theory (SDT)* do help to conceptualize why MI may work in the way that it does (e.g., Markland et al., 2005). As a generalized theory of motivation, SDT (e.g., Ryan & Deci, 2017) suggests that there are three *basic psychological needs* that influence behavior: *autonomy* (a sense of volition and self-regulation of action/self-control), *competence* (mastery of skills), and *relatedness* (feeling connected to others). As with the TTM, there is significantly more to SDT than is presented here, including *six mini-theories* that describe and predict different aspects of how these basic processes interact within and across individuals, situations, roles, and environments. Despite their conceptual independence, MI and SDT are based on similar assumptions: Humans have an innate desire to engage in personal growth and to become more autonomous. It has been suggested that MI can be used to create the optimal social-environmental conditions to support this innate tendency (Markland et al., 2005) and that SDT may provide the theoretical underpinning to explain MI's effectiveness (Patrick & Williams, 2012).

Concepts consistent with SDT are interwoven in the practice of MI. For example, autonomy is a central concept within the *empowerment* dimension of MI spirit. It is embedded within the discussions of client goals for an encounter. The task of engaging attends to autonomy, as well as requiring practitioners to create safe, comfortable environments within which participants feel connected to the practitioner. Competence underpins ***affirmations*** as a foundational skill and evoking a client's resources for change. Reference to these ideas is integrated throughout the modules in Part II of this workbook.

Another point of value of SDT for MI lies in its conceptualization of what motivation is. It begins with a simple definition of motivation, "what *energizes* and *gives direction* to behavior" (Ryan & Deci, 2017, p. 13). It breaks this down along a *motivational continuum,* with *amotivation* as one endpoint and *intrinsic motivation* at the other. Amotivation occurs when we believe our actions do not meaningfully influence our environment. For example, people who do not vote in elections may fall into this category. Intrinsic motivation describes circumstances when we do things because we find them inherently of interest to us. People with hobbies fall into this area. Sandwiched between these endpoints is *extrinsic motivation* and its four subcategories: *external regulation*, *introjected regulation*, *identified regulation*, and *integrated regulation*. These are the clients we see. As people move through these four subcategories of extrinsic motivation, their reasons for change become more internalized, internally regulated, and coherent with strongly held values. This process may explain why exploring with people what matters to them in an MI-consistent way is much more effective than simply assuming (from a medical or expert opinion) why a person should change or why an external motivator (e.g., jail, a negative health outcome) fails to elicit greater or more sustained efforts to change. These external motivations might start the process, but sustaining and maintaining the changes often require a more internalized form of motivation. Table 2.3 describes these dimensions and subcategories and then provides examples of each.

COM-B Model

There is growing interest in the *COM-B model* (Michie et al., 2011) particularly within the United Kingdom. The model comprises *capability*, *opportunity*, and *motivation* components that are thought to influence *behavior* (hence the acronym COM-B). This model was developed in response to the desire to standardize elements of behavior change interventions such that the *ingredients* that were more effective predictors of change could be better understood and replicated. Yet, COM-B, and the taxonomy that accompanies it, provide a list of *what to do* without guidance on *how to do it.* As such, this model has been criticized because of its lack of attention to the *relational* component, described earlier within the context of MI spirit, which has been consistently demonstrated as predicting favorable client outcomes (see Hilton & Johnston, 2017; Miller & Moyers, 2021). The COM-B model has yet to be associated with a theoretical model that helps to explain observed outcomes of MI. However, some emergent

TABLE 2.3. Forms of Motivation Based on Self-Determination Theory

Type of motivation	Common language definition	Example with smoking cessation	Case example
Amotivation	Person feels unable to meaningfully impact the environment or change the behavior.	I cannot stop smoking. I tried, and it didn't work. Everyone around me smokes.	**Tom** works in the construction industry. He has smoked from the age of 14 years of age. He enjoys smoking and has no intention of trying to reduce his smoking or give it up. His father and grandfather both smoked and lived well into old age. He believes that smoking helps him to relax and reduces his stress levels. He does not believe that stopping smoking would significantly impact his health. His wife is concerned about his smoking, but her comments about his smoking are making him even more determined to smoke. This cycle tends to result in an argument.
Extrinsic motivation			
External regulation	Person's behavior is controlled by external contingencies.	My insurance company will not issue a life insurance policy unless I prove that I have stopped smoking.	**Julie** works in a bank. She has been sent for an occupational health check as part of her annual medical review for her employer's private health insurance scheme. She must undertake a series of physiological tests. These tests revealed damage to her lungs caused by smoking. She has been strongly "advised" by her occupational health department that she needs to attend several sessions with a smoking cessation counselor. She does not want to attend but knows that her boss will bring this up at their next meeting and give her a hard time if she fails to attend. She plans to go to the occupational health check but does not believe this will have an impact on her behavior.
Introjected regulation	Person's behavior is controlled by internal representations of external contingencies or elements.	My children are pressuring me to stop smoking, and I hear their voices in my head whenever I light a cigarette.	**Amari** has worked as a corrections officer for over 20 years. It was when he first started in this job that he also started to smoke. He finds that smoking helps him to relax in what can be a very stressful work environment and generally enjoys a cigarette in social situations with colleagues. Amari now has two teenage children who constantly encourage him to quit. Amari has managed not to smoke a single cigarette for the last week, although if he's honest, he really misses smoking and the only reason he is trying to quit is because of the guilt he feels about his children's feelings toward smoking.
Identified regulation	Person chooses to change because it fits with a goal or identification.	I want to be a father, and I can't do that if I won't be around because of lung cancer.	**Andrew** works as an executive in a life insurance company. He has worked hard to reach a senior position. He is a non-smoker at work. He works hard to hide his smoking behavior at any corporate events. He fully understands why smoking is incongruent with his values and beliefs in terms of risk factors. He is married, and

			his wife is currently pregnant. He wants to completely stop smoking for his own health and because of the potential future impact of his premature death on his family. He is also very concerned about the impact of smoking, like long-term conditions such as COPD. He has attempted to stop smoking on many previous occasions and learned a great deal from his previous quit attempts. He believes that he will be able to stop smoking and has a lot of support from his family. Currently, he only smokes when he has consumed quite a lot of alcohol. This tends to occur when he is *drinking* with one of his single friends from his *college days*. He has spoken to this friend about his smoking and has made it very clear that he is starting to see himself as a non-smoker.
Integrated regulation	Person chooses to change because it fits with core values and sense of self.	To be a good father, I need to model the behavior I want in my children, including addressing tough changes like stopping smoking and making healthy choices.	**Michael** had been a smoker for 20 years. He had managed to stop smoking on several occasions in the past but never for more than a few weeks. Two years ago, he had a *heart attack* and decided to stop smoking *once and for all*. He has managed to stop smoking with the help of nicotine replacement therapy as well as support from a smoking cessation team recommended by his PCP after the heart attack. He is no longer feeling the same urges that he did before and is starting to finally view himself as a "non-smoker." He still has the occasional urge for a cigarette, though. This tends to be at certain times (e.g., after a meal) and when he is with certain people (i.e., his brother still smokes) or in certain situations (e.g., stuck in traffic jams). His wife has been incredibly supportive. She stopped smoking approximately 15 years ago when she became pregnant with their first child. All smoking-related materials have been removed from his home, car, and workplace. His friends and work colleagues have been very supportive. He no longer wants to smoke.
Intrinsic motivation	Person engages in the behavior because of some inherent or intrinsic interest.	The challenge of taking on something hard is interesting to me, and I want to see what I'm capable of doing so I'll stop smoking. [Obviously, this is not a category we typically see with smoking cessation.]	**Kris** was a social smoker when she was a teenager. She is now 42 and works in the fitness industry. She *hates* smoking and believes it is completely incompatible with her life values, but also believes she needs to understand the pull of smoking for people she works with in fitness settings. She reads articles about smoking in trade and professional journals, as well as listens to podcasts and watches videos to understand the dynamics of smoking and smokers, and finds the information fascinating. She has not had a cigarette for 25 years.

literature demonstrates examples of how the COM-B model can be combined productively with MI within intervention studies (e.g., Barrett et al., 2022).

Developing Practice in MI

Beginning in 1993, Miller and Rollnick began training trainers in MI. This process eventually evolved into the Motivational Interviewing Network of Trainers (MINT), which provides annual *train the new trainer (TNT)* events and has sponsored smaller regional networks and trainings. Through this process of workshop training, it became apparent that workshops could enhance practitioner skills in MI (e.g., Baer et al., 2004) and that more would be needed for participants to maintain and enhance their MI skills (Martino et al., 2008; Miller et al., 2004). These findings fit with then emerging evidence in *implementation science* about what was needed to implement evidence-based practices with fidelity (Fixsen et al., 2005), including the importance of continued skill development through supervision, coaching, and feedback (Miller et al., 2004). Knowledge and description of what leads to effective implementation continue to evolve (e.g., Gill et al., 2020; Madson et al., 2019; Schwalbe et al., 2014). What follows is a limited review of three methods—books, artificial intelligence, and coding—that have been used as complements and/or alternatives to ongoing training, coaching and feedback, and supervision over the last 20 years.

Books as a Resource for Learning

Over the last 10 to 15 years, several books/workbooks have been developed to help practitioners learn the how-to of MI skill development and ways to integrate MI skills with specific therapeutic approaches such as CBT. This has grown from texts that have a wide application and can be used as either a stand-alone introduction or an adjunct to introductory training in MI (e.g., Rosengren, 2017) to more targeted workbooks/books designed for specific professions such as those working within mental health (Frey & Hall, 2021), social work practice (Hohman, 2021), health care (Rollnick et al., 2023), and leadership (Marshall & Søgaard Nielsen, 2020). Recently, Manuel and colleagues (Manuel et al., 2022) published a *deliberate practice* workbook for MI. The text's aim is to develop capacity in deploying MI skills. It provides scaffolding for the reader to develop key technical skills and strategies within MI. The exercises build to intermediate and advanced skill development. While an excellent method in developing and automatizing skill proficiency, deliberate practice provides less attention to when and why to deploy skills or the relational aspects of the client and practitioner dynamic; those elements are the focus of this book.

Artificial Intelligence

Another development in deliberate practice is the growth in artificial intelligence (AI) in the teaching and learning of MI. Utilizing AI to support MI skill development has traditionally been limited to the learner being able to recognize MI-consistent and MI-inconsistent responses to given scenarios. Until recently, most AI approaches provided a learner with a client statement and a selection of options for response, some of which are consistent with MI (e.g., open-ended question, complex reflection) and others that are inconsistent with MI (e.g., persuading, warning of consequences of current behavior). This *rote learning* approach (memorization of strategies and repetition) may play a part in helping those newer to MI in recognizing MI-consistent skills and strategies. However, an overreliance on this approach alone may reinforce a formulaic approach with an overemphasis on the technical aspects of MI at the expense of the relational and interpersonal process skills. What may be missing is an appreciation of MI as a *way of being* and a deeper understanding of the nuanced interpersonal processes involved in an MI-consistent conversation (e.g., Hilton et al., 2016).

As technology has grown over the last few years, there is increasing flexibility in learners inputting and receiving feedback about their responses. This science is still in its infancy, but projects are under way currently to evaluate their value in enhancing skillfulness. Until recently, responses had to be preprogrammed and AI's capacity to comprehend the emotional impact of the deployed skills was limited; however, within the last 18 months, there have been tremendous leaps forward in AI's capacity to comprehend human behavior, though its capacity to simulate human behavior continues to lag (Robichaux, 2024). Much as with other forms of deliberate practice, it seems likely there will be value in these methods, and they will serve as a useful adjunct to approaches such as self-practice and self-reflection (SP/SR), helping the learner in developing their own therapeutic intuition via a focus on self-generated responses and self-reflection.

The Use of Coding Tools to Develop Proficiency in MI

Anyone engaged in the process of developing proficiency in MI is likely familiar with commonly used coding tools in MI. There has been growth in the development of such tools since the conception of MI, with Gill and colleagues (2020) reporting 12 available as of 2020. One commonly used instrument is the Motivational Interviewing Treatment Integrity Scale (MITI; Moyers et al., 2016). The initial intention of coding tools was to adequately assess treatment fidelity (i.e., how well a practitioner is adhering to the MI approach) in a clinical trial that incorporated MI into the treatment intervention. However, coding tools are now commonly used for the purpose of supporting people to understand specific areas of strength and opportunities for development in their MI practice. Indeed, the MITI 4.2.1 coding system specifically refers to the utility of the instrument for this purpose. Of course, some coding tools only capture *one side of the partnership* (that of the practitioner) and may be limited to situations when they can be deployed (e.g., coding from a transcript rather than *in vivo*) and by their focus, such as global dimensions (e.g., empathy, cultivating change talk) and behavior counts (specific examples of skills). These tools require careful and skillful communication if interpreted within the context of coaching and supervision. Automation of these processes using AI tools like the *Lyssn* platform (*www.lyssn.io*) provides opportunities to expand their usage and improve practitioner performance, but also carries limitations.

The overuse of an automated coding tool, especially imposed in a non-MI-consistent way, runs the risk of an ***expert trap*** being imposed on the learner. It is something *done to* and *on* the learner, rather than *with* the learner. It raises concern the trainee will neither internalize the learning nor develop MI intuition within their own highly personalized style. This risk is

BOX 2.1. NVivo as a Tool for Self-Reflection

NVivo provides a self-reflective experience using video analysis in combination with synchronized transcripts. NVivo facilitates a thorough review of the encounter with the inclusion of body language and nonverbal communications as part of the detailed observation of the client and practitioner interaction. The inclusion of video invites further exploration of the more nuanced behavioral aspects of an encounter, which are difficult to capture in a written transcript alone (e.g., expressions of emotion; sarcasm; humor or timing issues related to hesitancy, pausing, tone of voice, pitch). This approach also generates opportunities to reflect on the client experience.

—From QSR, NVivo, Version 12, released in March 2020

intensified when the coding instrument provides a pass/fail assessment mark, resulting in trainees learning to perform to the coding instrument rather than developing their internal reflective MI barometer and more nuanced use of MI. A compounding issue is the coding instrument only captures a very small amount of what works in a complex intervention. The easiest-to-measure aspects within any interpersonal dynamic are small in comparison to the unexplained variance in most studies on complex interpersonal processes such as MI. Most variance is explained via the relational aspects that are not easily captured, while the coding focus is only on an aspect of the interaction. The numbers generated from coding instruments can mean very little for the developing practitioner without the context of what the numbers mean for further skill improvement. For these reasons, our prior writing expresses concern about the limitations of some coding tools and how they are being used (Hilton et al., 2016).

Taken as a whole, we draw a few conclusions. First, the problem is not with a coding instrument per se, but in the way it is being applied to help people *learn MI*. The danger lies in overemphasis on the technical aspects at the expense of the experiential interpersonal skills. Second, coding instruments have the most utility when combined with scaffolding, such as ongoing self-practice and self-reflection and in supervision/coaching in MI. Third, coding systems that capture both client and practitioner behaviors and perspectives provide richer opportunities, particularly when they employ a more interactive and self-reflective approach and use video analysis and qualitative data analysis tools. NVivo is an example of such a system (see Box 2.1).

Theoretical Influences in Learning

Let's begin with the obvious: Learning is a brain activity, so to make learning most effective, we should consider how the brain works. Current thinking in neuroscience is critical of an oversimplification of the science of lateralization and presents arguments against a one-dimensional view of brain hemisphericity. Rather, neuroscience now suggests that brain hemispheres work via complex neural networks and subsystems (e.g., Bear et al., 2020) that are not yet fully understood. Reviewing this level of complexity does not help learners scaffold learning transfer. Lucky you!

However, the fact a learner doesn't need to know these things does not negate the need to approach training, and learning, in a manner that considers the ways in which individuals engage in different preferences and approaches to perceiving and processing information across different tasks and contexts. The aim, of course, is to construct learning based on what science indicates is effective. While acknowledging there are debates within neuroscience about best approaches, for pragmatic reasons we build around specific learning theories (e.g., Kolb, 1984) with the aim of helping the reader to use practical questions, learning goals, and tasks to engage and self-reflect on their learning processes. We also recognize individual and context factors, within the complex systems at play from a neuroscience and neurodiversity perspective, that will influence readers (e.g., Armstrong, 2015; Hamilton & Petty, 2023).

Many theories in learning have typically considered the way in which information is both *perceived* and *processed* (e.g., Kolb, 1984; McCarthy & McCarthy, 2005), with the observation that some people, in certain situations, may prefer to start to think through information before experiencing it, whereas others, in another context, may prefer to experience the information first and then think more about it. This has been described as a *thinking–feeling* dimension. A second dimension refers to the way in which learning may be *processed* and suggests that in some situations, certain people will get activity engaged first and then reflect on the experience to help to make sense of it; whereas others may watch and self-reflect first and then get more actively involved by doing. This might be thought of as a *doing–watching* dimension. We do all these things to varying degrees, and the concept of dimensions and cycles of learning is clearly an oversimplification of the multitude of processes that occur in learning and development. While we acknowledge this critique, we consider the use of key questions to be a helpful heuristic to guide learning and skill development. To that end, we use the questions of *Why*, *What*, *How*, and *What If* to guide the learning process.

Why am I doing this?

This question involves our need to understand and engage with *meaning*. This type of learning experience may be encouraged by an interest in people, ideas, and stories; we can often process this type of learning *with* and *through* other people. In each of the modules in Part II of this book, we start each chapter answering an implicit *Why* question. That is, why is a particular concept, technique, or strategy within MI important? Further learning in this way is supported by the *story* element of the traveling companions in this workbook.

What is it that I am learning here?

This aspect of learning is more about facts, data, the evidence base, and it can attract an intellectual format of information exchange—often from theorists and researchers who may be viewed as *experts* in their field. This type of learning context may reflect an organized and structured learning environment whereby the individual is exposed to *academic knowledge* with reference to the evidence base for MI and key conceptual influences; the theoretical influences of MI presented earlier are an example of this process. We highlight some further references to suggested reading within each module in Part II. However, we are conscious that the purpose of this workbook is to deepen the learning and application of MI and is not therefore an academic text filled with many research references. There are already lots of very good texts on MI, and a full list of links to current research on MI can be found on the MINT website: *https://motivationalinterviewing.org*.

How do I use this in my professional practice?

This is the dominant question in a *thinking and doing* dimension. As learners, we want hands-on skills practice and to experience real-world application. At this point, we may prefer to learn with others who have practical, real-world credibility (e.g., clinicians, supervisors, and trainers who work in professional practice). This is the self-practice part of the book, as well as engaging with the self-focused reflective questions, peer or group supervision with others who are engaged in professional practice can be of benefit. For this reason, we recommend working through the modules in Part II of this workbook in a limited-peer practice, in addition to being part of either a small group or under supervision. We have written each module in a way that the material can also be worked through in one-on-one supervision or by individuals who work through the material on their own.

If I do this, what are the results going to be, and then how might I adapt the approach to different situations, contexts, and possibilities?

This is learning set in the *doing* and *feeling* dimensions, often referred to as *dynamic and/or grounded learning*, whereby learners are driven by new possibilities and applications. This is about applying the learning to our personal context or making adaptations to consider new possibilities and applications. This is where we use practitioner-focused self-reflections to cross the reflective bridge and then move these into our work as practitioners. For example, we may want to engage in trying out the implications from self-reflective exercises and perhaps involve colleagues, peer supervisors, and the like in this process. In the modules, there is ample opportunity when reflecting from the *self as practitioner* perspective to think about adaptations to our current professional practice, and we have added self-reflective questions to each module to consistently encourage this type of dynamic and creative learning process.

Figure 2.1 provides an outline of the implicit structure used in each module (e.g., concrete experience, reflective observation, active conceptualization, and active experimentation). The aim is that each module supports the reader to achieve learning transfer via engagement with a learning cycle. To this end, Figure 2.1 draws on Kolb (1984) and McCarthy and McCarthy (4MAT; 2005) to present an integrated learning model.

A final concept in education theory worth a brief mention is ***scaffolding***. Vygotsky's concept of scaffolding refers to providing educational support to help a learner move beyond their current knowledge/skill level into a zone just outside of their reach or knowledge at present, known as the zone of proximal development (ZPD). Practitioners may learn something new by building on their existing foundational knowledge or skill level and, in essence, moving to a new level of understanding. Johnston and Milne (2012) highlighted the central role of Vygotskian scaffolding within clinical supervision, as well as noting the key processes of a Socratic approach to information exchange, the centrality of the supervisory alliance, and the role of self-reflection in how supervisees use supervision within doctoral training in clinical psychology. We refer to the term *scaffolding* at various points within this text and use it to refer to educational support within an individual's ZPD, as Vygotsky intended.

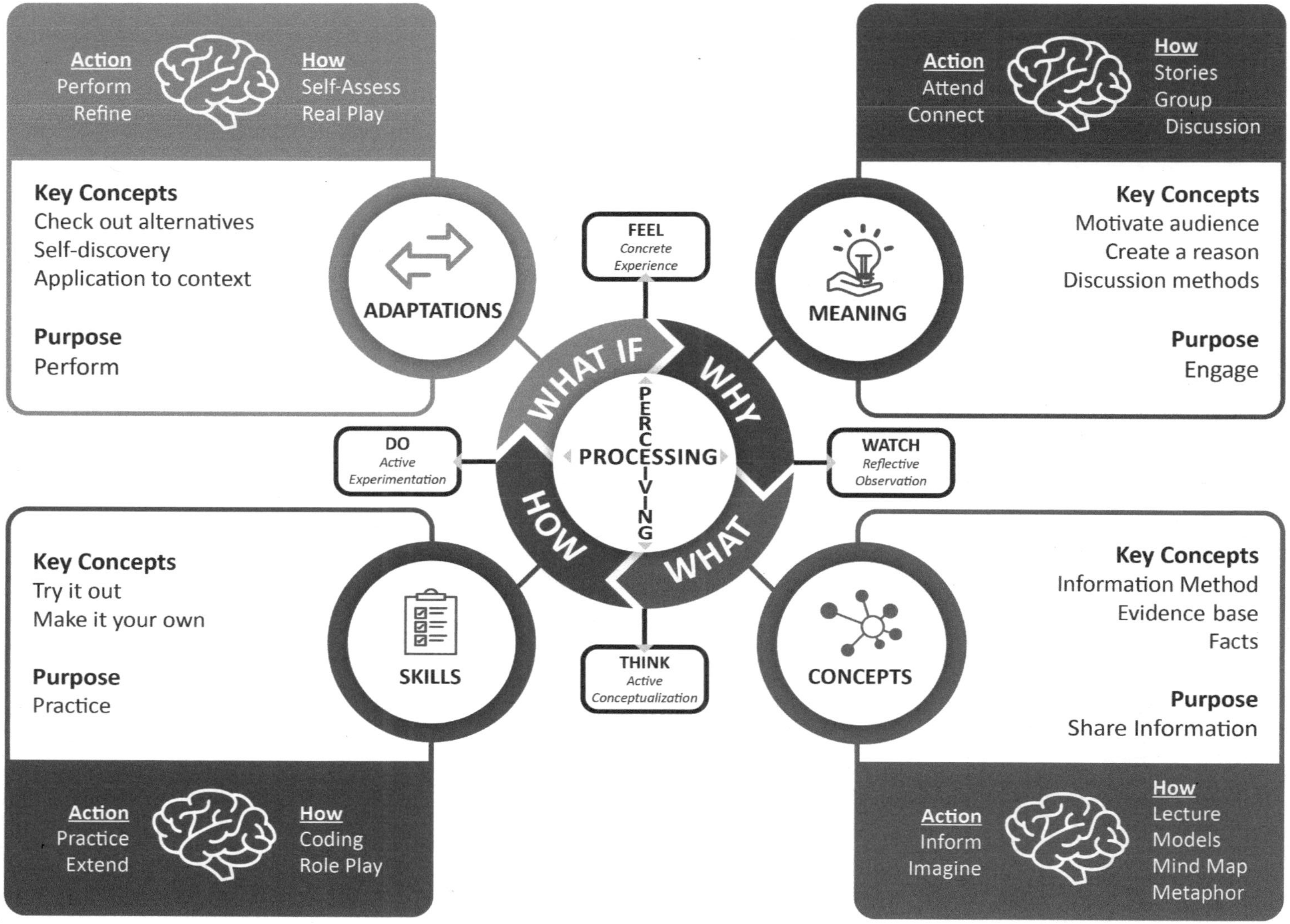

Action
Perform
Refine
How
Self-Assess
Real Play
Key Concepts
Check out alternatives
Self-discovery
Application to context
Purpose
Perform
ADAPTATIONS
Action
Attend
Connect
How
Stories
Group
Discussion
Key Concepts
Motivate audience
Create a reason
Discussion methods
Purpose
Engage
MEANING
FEEL
Concrete Experience
DO
Active Experimentation
WATCH
Reflective Observation
THINK
Active Conceptualization
WHAT IF
WHY
HOW
WHAT
PROCESSING
PERCEIVING
Key Concepts
Try it out
Make it your own
Purpose
Practice
SKILLS
Action
Practice
Extend
How
Coding
Role Play
Key Concepts
Information Method
Evidence base
Facts
Purpose
Share Information
CONCEPTS
Action
Inform
Imagine
How
Lecture
Models
Mind Map
Metaphor

FIGURE 2.1. Integrated learning model (4MAT and Kolb).

Final Thoughts

In sum, as we progress through this text, you will experience a process designed to deepen your understanding of how and why MI works. The learning model provides a way to work through this process, find opportunities for successful engagement, and consolidate the wisdom gleaned. Concepts from the theoretical models will appear throughout the text with the aim of strengthening the fibers of your understanding. The goal is to deepen your proficiency in MI, avoid the limitations noted, and support the development of your highly personal relationship with MI that can be expressed in your own unique practitioner MI style. Chapter 3 describes how the SP/SR process will be used for that process.

CHAPTER 3

MI and SP/SR

Background and Context

As mentioned earlier, we designed this workbook for people who have *some* prior knowledge and training in MI. In this chapter, we provide a rationale for the application of SP/SR for practitioners who want to develop their understanding of MI in terms of deepening their engagement with key concepts, further skill development, and in the application of MI to their own professional context.

Key Questions Discussed in This Chapter

- Why does SP/SR deepen our understanding, and application, of key concepts and practitioner skills within a therapeutic approach?
- What are the key concepts in SP/SR?
- How does SP/SR help MI practitioners to develop their knowledge and skills?
- What if we use SP/SR to enhance skill development in MI?

Self-Practice and Self-Reflection

Why does SP/SR deepen our understanding, and application, of key concepts and practitioner skills within a therapeutic approach?

Picture the scene: Our colleague describes their recent experience of attending an MI training event and we think, *This might be good for my practice, too.* We have been feeling stuck with clients, wondering why they often do not act on our good advice to help them make important changes in their life. From what our colleague says, we think MI could be of value to help us address this issue. We are offered training as part of our ongoing professional development, and there is something about the way that our colleague described MI that feels personally meaningful to us. Our manager arranges for us to attend a 2-day introduction to MI next month and, in the meantime, we decide to gain a better understanding of the approach. We soon learn there are several texts on MI, including a new book from the originators (e.g., Miller & Rollnick, 2023), and a broad range of context-specific applications of MI, including health care, diabetes, fitness, sport coaching, and so forth (see *www.guilford.com/browse/psychology-psychiatry-social-work/applications-motivational-interviewing-series*). We also identify several examples of positive clinical trials that have utilized MI (see *https://pubmed.ncbi.nlm.nih.gov/?term=%22motivational+interviewing%22*) and a community of those who are proficient in the method on the Motivational Interviewing Network of Trainers (MINT) website (see *https://motivationalinterviewing.org*). We discover videos of MINT members demonstrating various skills, and these sources of information increase our interest in MI and our confidence that these are skills worth learning.

Following the 2 days of training, we leave enthused about the prospect of using MI within our practice. To improve, we watch several video demonstrations of practitioners who are proficient in MI using a range of skills. However, we are left feeling this method is more difficult than we originally thought, and it is going to take some practice to master. We also wonder, *How do I know when to do what? And why am I doing it?* Three months have passed by, and we have made several attempts to use MI, with some success. Yet, it remains a challenge to use it consistently and well. We have yet to actively transfer the new knowledge into our professional practice, via the implementation and refinement of the MI skills that we initiated in the introductory training course.

Why might these events have happened?

For early career and or novice MI practitioners, it might be that some of the foundational skills in MI (e.g., complex reflections) feel unusual, unfamiliar, and were not well learned. If we are in this category, we may need more self-practice with the additional aid of a workbook, video or audio recording, or an AI trainer to *scaffold* or prompt for our self-reflection. For example, we might use prompts to help us *self-reflect on action* (after the event) to enable us to become conscious of our current skill level. Prior research in clinical supervision shows that in their earlier developmental stages of learning, trainees find it easier to self-reflect on action (after the event) rather than *self-reflect in action* (in the moment). This suggests that self-reflecting in the moment may be a skill that advances alongside the development of practitioner expertise (e.g., Johnston & Milne, 2012).

Those of us with slightly more experience may struggle to understand what strategies are useful within a particular context or situation. For example, when to use an ***amplified reflection*** or a ***complex affirmation***. If we are proficient in other therapeutic approaches (e.g., CBT), it may be difficult to integrate the use of MI with aspects of our particular model, for instance, integrating the elicitation of ***change talk*** in discussions around the role of ***behavioral activation***. It may be hard to move away from our existing prelearned habits and models, to try something new that feels clunky and less automatic than our existing skill set, like ***recognizing***, ***eliciting***, and ***strengthening change talk***, as well as eliciting key cognitions and emotions. This is much like the experienced sportsperson who makes alternations to their technique only to find it is highly uncomfortable and that it might negatively impact their performance in the short term; yet with sustained practice, the new technique becomes integrated, natural, and automatic and performance subsequently improves in the longer term.

What do we already know about learning MI?

William Miller is often asked how long it takes to become highly proficient in MI. While this is an almost impossible question to answer, due to individual, contextual, and situational factors, he estimates that it can take several years (personal communication, TNT Training Event, 2022). Miller and Moyers (2006, p. 3) postulated a series of eight stages, now referred to as tasks, in learning MI, as shown in Box 3.1. This is based on many years of *practice-based training evidence* rather than longitudinal training studies per se. However, there is a consensus within the MI community of trainers that although MI may appear simple, it can take several years to develop proficiency in the consistent skilled use of MI, and time alone is insufficient. To use a further sports analogy, this situation is akin to that of the experienced golfer who has played golf for 30 years but continues to practice with the same technique they have had for the last 29½ years; without good feedback, reflection, and refinement, their performance does not improve.

So, what counts as experience, and how do we shine a light on the areas of knowledge and skill that we are still unaware of? To improve performance in MI, skills, knowledge, and understanding are deepened in an iterative manner, which might be accomplished through a variety of methods. As Will Durant quipped, "Education is the progressive discovery of our own ignorance." The more we understand, the more we discover the layers of complexity. Perhaps only when we understand the complexity can we aim for simplicity. This is why after 40 years of writing about MI, Miller and Rollnick (2023) now emphasize simplicity and a broadening of application of MI in their latest text.

BOX 3.1. Eight Tasks in Learning MI

1. Openness to collaboration with clients' own expertise.
2. Proficiency in client-centered counseling, including accurate empathy.
3. Recognition of key aspects of client speech that guide the practice of MI.
4. Eliciting and strengthening client change talk.
5. Softening sustain talk and discord.[1]
6. Negotiating change plans.
7. Consolidating client commitment.
8. Switching flexibly between MI and other intervention styles.

[1]*Rolling with resistance* was a term used in the original Miller and Moyers (2006), but has been replaced by this term.

Declarative and Procedural Knowledge

Knowing what MI is, why it is useful, and its key ingredients are insufficient to enable a practitioner to conduct MI-consistent conversations with proficiency and fidelity. Knowing about a therapeutic approach demonstrates *declarative* (factual) knowledge. This may enable the practitioner to describe and explain information about an approach, its component parts, and the associated evidence base. This practitioner may also be able to describe, differentiate, and assess practice with the aid of coding systems, like the behavioral counts in the MITI. However, this type of declarative knowledge of the *Why* and the *What* of MI provides little guarantee that the person can execute the skills required to embody and deliver MI in a consistently skillful and therapeutically effective way (i.e., the *How*, as described in Chapter 2). Being skillful requires *procedural knowledge* (Bennett-Levy, 2006). This refers to our ability to perform skills in action, by implementing the skill proficiently whether this be in sports, therapy, or any other skill-based practice, such as cooking or playing music. Any learner requires practice, feedback, and repeated continual refinement. Learning MI takes time, and there are many suggested ways in which to do this. Further information on some existing approaches to learning MI can be found at the MINT website (see *https://motivationalinterviewing.org/learning-motivational-interviewing*).

As mentioned in Chapter 2, one solution to helping learners actively shift from knowing about MI (declarative knowledge) to doing MI (procedural knowledge) has been through deliberate practice (see Manuel et al., 2022). This approach offers learners the opportunity to practice MI skills via set methods that help the learner develop confidence in using MI-consistent skills across a range of scenarios. This is the tennis player practicing forehands, backhands, overhands, and lobs until they can do them with precision and without thought. Although this method is helpful for learners moving from novice to more intermediate skill levels, it has not necessarily aided the player to understand when to execute a specific shot, in what type of game, on what type of surface, and with what type of player. Self-reflection and refinement in this deliberate practice process are about building technical virtuosity and not deeper understanding of self, the therapeutic intervention, and the interaction of the two; this requires something more.

What if I learn more about SP/SR to further develop my knowledge, skills, and experience of using MI?

Figure 3.1 offers a summary of how learning may take place for many, early in acquiring knowledge about MI. Indeed, this may reflect the learning stage of the hypothetical post-workshop learner described above. The current workbook is targeted toward learners who may now be thinking more about the *What If* of MI in application and integration within their work/practice context. In picking up this workbook, the question that may have led you to this point could be: *How can I further deepen/develop my skills as an MI practitioner using SP/SR?* It is the application of a therapeutic approach to a personal or professional issue that is crucial to SP/SR. In practical terms, this is reflected in the difference between the use of *role-play*—playing a client whom we might or might not have direct experience working with or a change issue that we have not experienced personally—versus *real-play*—engaging with a change issue we are experiencing personally. This has relevance in training, supervision, mentoring, and ongoing development, but from the perspective of being in the *client's chair* rather than the *therapist's chair*. It is the change in perspective that is vital.

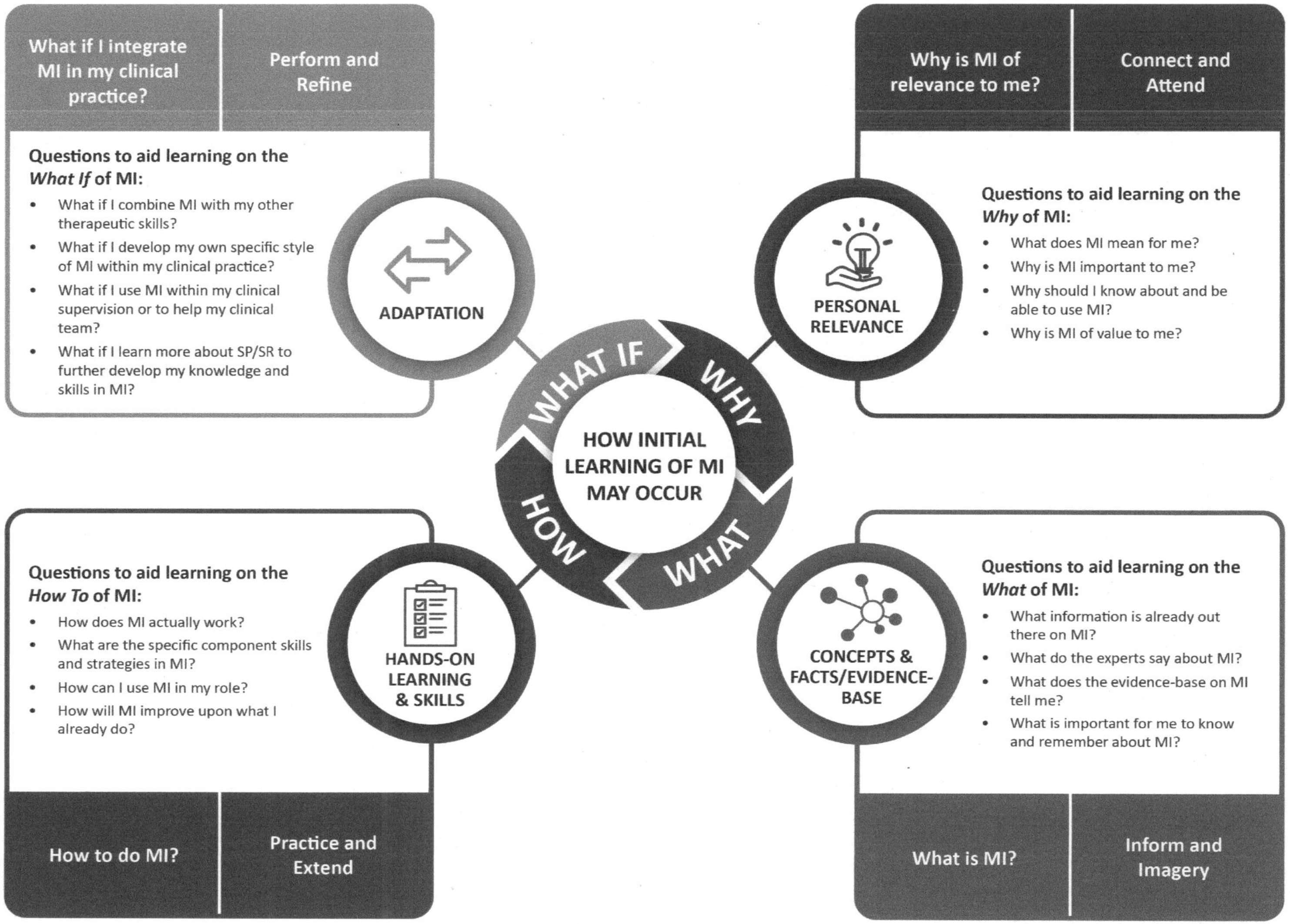
What if I integrate MI in my clinical practice?
Perform and Refine
Questions to aid learning on the What If of MI:
What if I combine MI with my other therapeutic skills?
What if I develop my own specific style of MI within my clinical practice?
What if I use MI within my clinical supervision or to help my clinical team?
What if I learn more about SP/SR to further develop my knowledge and skills in MI?
ADAPTATION
Why is MI of relevance to me?
Connect and Attend
Questions to aid learning on the Why of MI:
What does MI mean for me?
Why is MI important to me?
Why should I know about and be able to use MI?
Why is MI of value to me?
PERSONAL RELEVANCE
WHAT IF
WHY
HOW
WHAT
HOW INITIAL LEARNING OF MI MAY OCCUR
Questions to aid learning on the How To of MI:
How does MI actually work?
What are the specific component skills and strategies in MI?
How can I use MI in my role?
How will MI improve upon what I already do?
HANDS-ON LEARNING & SKILLS
How to do MI?
Practice and Extend
CONCEPTS & FACTS/EVIDENCE-BASE
Questions to aid learning on the What of MI:
What information is already out there on MI?
What do the experts say about MI?
What does the evidence-base on MI tell me?
What is important for me to know and remember about MI?
What is MI?
Inform and Imagery

FIGURE 3.1. How initial learning of MI may occur.

Where Did SP/SR Come from and Who Developed It?

SP/SR emerged from the real-life learning transfer and development of clinical skills for James Bennett-Levy. It began where he applied CBT, in peer supervision, to help him to experience the receipt of a CBT intervention with a co-trainee. The rationale for SP/SR is to support the enhancement of practitioner skills and practitioner self-care *from the inside out*. It has been defined as a "structured self-experiential program in which therapists practice therapy techniques on themselves and reflect in writing on the implications of their self-practice" (Bennett-Levy & Finlay-Jones, 2018, p. 188). Bennett-Levy developed the *declarative–procedural–reflective (DPR) model* of therapist skills development in 2006. A central aspect in this model is the *reflective system* to aid therapist self-development as the "engine of lifelong learning . . . [in helping therapists to] navigate the 'low swampy ground' to determine which problem to address with which person, in which situation at which time in therapy, drawing on which kind of conceptualization for selecting which therapeutic skill" (Bennett-Levy & Haarhoff, 2019, p. 383). In essence, the reflective system in the DPR model is the engine that drives the learning process for both declarative (i.e., theory, facts, information about an approach such as CBT or MI) and procedural (i.e., skills in action or the "how-to" of CBT or MI) knowledge systems; this is thought to be particularly true when basic therapy skills have been learned.

Bennett-Levy et al. (2015) emphasize the importance of various authors in CBT (e.g., Judith Beck; Christine Padesky; Jeremy Safran and Zindel Segal) in influencing a *paradigm shift*, in the 1990s, toward greater attention to both interpersonal processes (procedural) in CBT as well as a greater focus on how *self-practice*, as a more general approach, can enhance skill acquisition, development, and refinement. Interestingly, a similar paradigm shift has started to emerge within MI over the last 10 years (e.g., Hilton et al., 2016; Miller & Moyers, 2021; Moyers & Miller, 2013). Prior to this, the MI training literature had a relative focus on technical skill development, coding, and fidelity testing (e.g., Fixsen et al., 2005) to support large-scale randomized controlled trial (RCT) research incorporating best-practice recommendations on treatment fidelity (e.g., Bellg et al., 2004).

Using SP/SR to Develop a Deeper Level of Learning in MI

SP/SR can facilitate a more effective learning transfer by helping learners to engage their reflective system in a way that aids their understanding of concepts (declarative) and skills (procedural) at a deeper, more personally meaningful level. To date, most published studies using the SP/SR approach have been conducted within the context of CBT. Research findings offer support for positive outcomes on therapist skill development (conceptual/technical), especially interpersonal skills and increased levels of therapist self-awareness (Bennett-Levy & Finlay-Jones, 2018). Experiencing MI from the *inside out* (i.e., as a *real-play* from the position of the client) offers the potential to reach a deeper level of learning because it is *experiential* and produces a personal connection compared to other approaches to learning MI that keep personal application at a distance.

Most existing MI texts and associated learning support materials are written and narrated from the perspective of an MI practitioner. Role-play examples in workshop training, and the coding tools that have been developed to assess fidelity in MI (e.g., MITI), also typically approach the learning experience from the position of the developing practitioner perspective. Learning in this way results in the client perspective (inside out) being omitted. The current workbook, through a series of exercises, will demonstrate that learning from the client's perspective is a crucial process in learning and developing proficiency in MI. SP/SR is different because it is personal. It positions the learner in the *client's chair.*

The Personal Practice Model

In recent years, the personal practice (PP) model (Bennett-Levy, 2019; Bennett-Levy & Finlay-Jones, 2018) has evolved from the DPR model to highlight the increased recognition of the role of personal practice (including SP/SR) on the development of therapist skills. The PP model highlights *four motivations to engage in PP,* including *personal problems, personal growth, self-care,* and *therapist skill development.* It identifies *two selves* as structural elements: *personal and therapist,* which we refer to as *practitioner-self. Self-reflection* is a key process. There are *five core outcomes* of the PP model: *personal development and well-being, self-awareness, interpersonal beliefs/attitudes/skills, self-reflective skills,* and *conceptual/technical skills.* The primary motivation to engage in SP/SR has tended to focus on practitioner self-development. The two *selves,* personal and practitioner, are viewed as both distinct and overlapping with common elements in the overlapping area, including self-awareness, interpersonal beliefs/attitudes/skills, reflective skills. The other elements are situated only in either the personal-self, like personal development and well-being, personal self-reflection, or the practitioner-self, like conceptual/technical skills and therapist self-reflection. The PP model suggests that both selves impact reciprocally on each other via the engagement of the reflective system. As such, it is hypothesized that they have independent and overlapping impact on practitioner skills development. The reflective system views reflection as a process, which acts as a bridge between the personal-self and the practitioner-self. An important distinction is made between reflection as a process (i.e., the reflective system) and self-reflection as a practitioner skill; the latter being viewed as one of the five core outcomes in the PP model. Thus, the PP model highlights the distinction and the interaction between the personal- and practitioner-self, noting that both components contribute to how a practitioner works with clients.

Integrating MI into the PP Model

This application of SP/SR to MI is novel, although highly transferable, particularly if we view the PP model through an MI-specific lens. Therefore, for ease of understanding, Figure 3.2 presents a proposed PP model for MI that we have formulated for the purposes of this text.

There are specific examples of what might comprise interpersonal beliefs, attitudes, and skills (e.g., partnership, acceptance, compassion, empowerment) included in the PP model for MI. The rationale being that if we consider these elements as interpersonal alliance factors that are *process-related,* this presents a good fit in terms of internal consistency for MI. We explored the possibility of including the term *values* because it is so central to MI researchers, trainers, and practitioners. However, there is scant empirical research for it as a separate concept in this PP context, and therefore, we offer this as a suggestion for future scholarship. We have also offered further specificity regarding personal and practitioner self-reflective skills to avoid confusion with reflective listening skills in MI. What is meant here is the purposeful and iterative

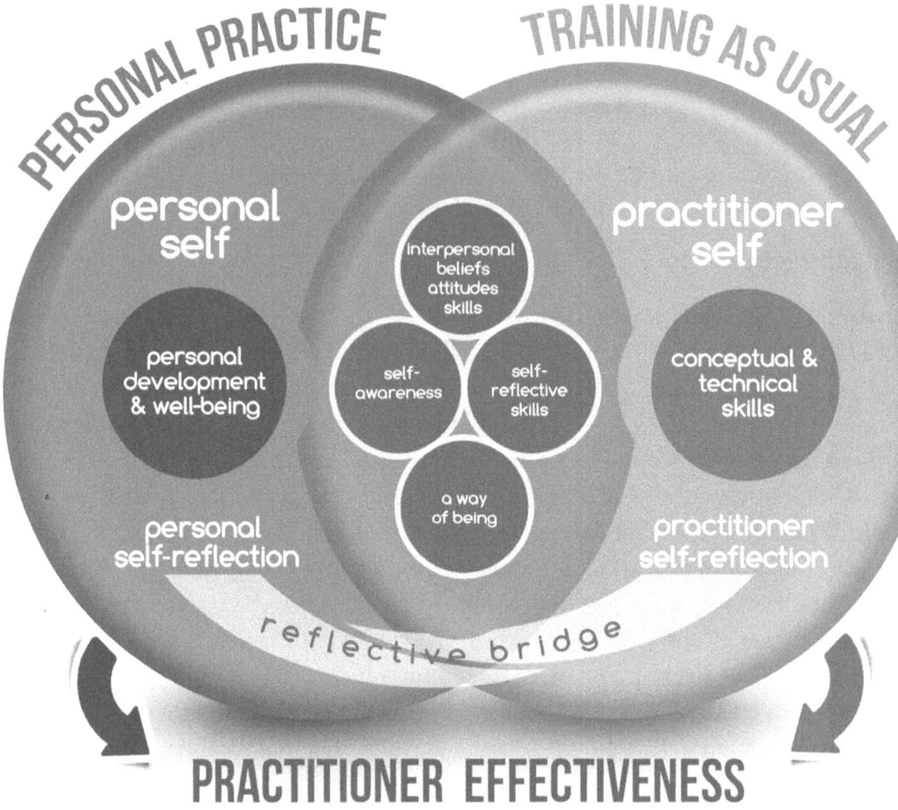

FIGURE 3.2. Proposed personal practice model for MI.

process of self-questioning and logical analysis to either confirm or refute certain ideas, beliefs, feelings, behaviors, and skills. Our intention is that the specificity of the application of the PP model to MI is enhanced by the inclusion of technical skills such as (***OARS+I***), although this may also include conceptual skills such as the integration of the ***four tasks*** in MI in addition to other key components of MI such as, for example, avoiding the ***fixing reflex***, eliciting and strengthening change talk, and ***softening sustain talk***.

A key MI component relevant to both the technical and conceptual aspects in this model is ***ambivalence*** (uncertainty about change) as a normal part of the change process. MI actively explores ambivalence and directionally responds to it by eliciting and strengthening change talk and softening sustain talk. This differs from other person-centered approaches, such as solution-focused therapy whereby the benefits of not changing are not actively explored. Finally, there is ***a way of being*** shared by the personal-self and practitioner-self.

Motivational interviewing as a way of being is perhaps best thought of in two main ways: One reflects how we are rather than what we do in our professional-self. We consider a way of being as consistent with MI spirit. MI trainers encourage practitioners to view MI as a way of being with clients and not simply a set of techniques or concepts. A second perspective is a way of being as who we are at the core of our personal-self. Indeed, it is learning this way of being that is often thought to change how people relate more broadly in the world, which also makes it appropriate for the personal-self, too. It becomes a way of being in the world. This is akin to the inclusion of compassion as a way of life in the PP model for compassion-focused therapy (Kolts et al., 2018). It is not uncommon after an introductory workshop in MI training for some participants to report that MI is a helpful way of interacting with people, not simply those they are supporting professionally. Consistent with these ideas, Bennett-Levy and Haarhoff (2019) suggested "the aim of SP/SR should be for therapists to create new ways of being that enhance their personal and professional wisdom and skills" (p. 392). Indeed, a way of being for some reflects *not what I do, but who I am.*

How Does SP/SR Work within the PP Model?

It is the *process* of transitioning between experiential learning, via personally relevant and grounded self-reflections from the perspective of the client, that enhances, widens, and deepens the self-reflective lens of the practitioner. For example, a practitioner engaging in SP/SR experiences receipt of a specific MI interaction from the position of client on a meaningful personal or professional issue. Then we self-reflect on this experience via the perspective of our personal-self (as client). Once this is fully in mind, we *cross the reflective bridge* by reflecting on our client learning experience (personal-self) via the lens of ourselves as practitioner (i.e., practitioner-self). In addition to enhancing practitioner skillfulness, it is also proposed the PP model may support personal development, well-being, enhanced self-awareness (interpersonal beliefs, attitudes, skills), self-reflective skills, as well as conceptual and technical skills.

There is growing support for SP/SR as a method for therapist skill development including research evidence (e.g., see Bennett Levy & Finlay-Jones, 2018) and learning materials via the Inside Out workbooks for CBT (Bennett-Levy et al., 2015); CFT (Kolts et al., 2018); schema therapy (Farrell & Shaw, 2018); and ACT (Tirch et al., 2019). However, the current text is the first of its kind to apply the SP/SR approach specifically to MI.

While SP/SR may resonate with some aspects of personal therapy, its primary purpose is to receive an intervention in service of creating greater practitioner skillfulness. It is not unusual that therapists working within certain traditions (e.g., psychodynamic psychotherapy, cognitive analytic therapy) undertake personal therapy as part of their training, personal growth, self-reflection, and self-care. However, the developers of SP/SR suggest that it differs from personal therapy in that, via self-reflective bridging questions, SP/SR encourages an active process of utilizing the reflective bridge to transfer experiential learning from the personal-self to the practitioner-self, whereas personal therapy tends to remain within the personal-self.

In the modules to follow, we designed reflective bridging questions to help you transition from self-experience to defining its relevance as MI practitioners (practitioner experience). We introduce traveling companions, practitioners with differing levels of practitioner and MI experience, and their personal circumstances to help exemplify the SP/SR approach within each of the modules. However, the traveling companions are no substitute for our personal, active, and felt experience of the SP/SR process—it is this experiential engagement with the examples in this workbook that allows us to travel across the reflective bridge and thereby develop proficiency in MI.

CHAPTER 4

Guidance for Participants

Background and Context

In the previous chapters, we have outlined the rationale for integrating SP/SR into a program of MI skill development. We have also included established adult learning theory to help guide the process of understanding common approaches to knowledge and skill acquisition. What follows in this chapter is an overview of known principles with regard to how SP/SR should be designed, adapted, and implemented and a suite of SP/SR options to consider. Adult learning theory and professional practice literature inform the principles and options. We review *how* and *why* the SP/SR options may be used either in isolation or in combination, and we discuss important considerations for participants.

Key Questions Discussed in This Chapter

- Why is the learning process set up in the manner it is?
- What are the guiding principles for SP/SR?
- What are the reflective system and self-reflection, and how do I do them?
- Why is writing important in this process?
- What are the options for doing SP/SR, and how might I engage in this process?
- Why might this process be different for me than others in training, and what do I need to know to take care of myself in this process?

The Guiding Principles of SP/SR

Let's start with some useful clarification of terms. Bennett-Levy and colleagues (2009) identified that the interchangeable use of the terms *reflective* and *reflection* have been problematic without adequate clarification of meaning and context. This presents a particular challenge for MI given the specific reference to reflection or ***reflective listening*** as a purposeful (micro) skill.

In Chapter 1, we describe our rationale for the deliberate use of the term *self-reflection* within an SP/SR context to avoid confusion. However, as we now shift into focusing on the specifics of what it means to self-reflect, it is helpful to elaborate on some key terminology identified by Bennett-Levy et al. (2009).

Reflective practice is typically used to refer to the process of reflecting on clinical experience. This may include *aspects of self*, such as how our attitudes/beliefs may have influenced the experience, and encompasses activities undertaken either alone or with supervision (e.g., writing journals, blogging, or reviewing audio/audio-visual resources). *Reflective skill* refers to our ability to reflect on ourselves and our practice. This comprises our *general reflective skills* and *self-reflective skills*. General reflective skills describe our ability to reconstruct and explore events (e.g., a specific MI encounter) and make sense of the information. Self-reflective skills include this, but also our ability to identify and explore our feelings and thoughts.

The *reflective system* comprises interpersonal perceptual skills, our attitudes/beliefs, interpersonal and relational skills, declarative knowledge, and procedural skills. We address this system in Chapter 3 and in the exploration of the *personal practice (PP) model for MI* there (Figure 3.3). It is via the reflective system that we can refine our declarative knowledge and procedural skills. Self-reflection on MI encounters develops our proficiency to understand what skills are most helpful for a particular client problem, within a particular context in an MI conversation.

Finally, considering reflection as a process helps to reduce some of the confusion caused by interchangeable terminology. For example, Bennett-Levy et al. (2009) suggest that rather than considering terms in isolation, we think of the reflective process as three phases: (1) focus attention, (2) reconstruct and observe, and (3) conceptualize and synthesize. It is this complete process that accurately describes self-reflection and should be linked to action. The learning modules within the current text are designed to guide you through this process.

What we know about successful approaches to SP/SR has been derived from iterative phases of testing and implementation, largely within the context of psychology and therapy training programs in academic settings. Bennett-Levy and Lee (2014) suggest various expectations of and benefits from SP/SR, including engagement with the process, course structure and requirements, feeling of safety within the process, group process, and available personal resources. We draw on this, and the expertise and recommendations of Freeston et al. (2019), to outline guiding principles of SP/SR suitable for learning MI, as well as to target the practice context in which we anticipate most people will be engaging in the process. Further details regarding the different options and approaches to SP/SR follow.

Process, Content, and Structure

Effective learning occurs when the type of task or learning activity is matched to the practitioner's stage of development. Often referred to as the zone of proximal development (ZPD), Vygotsky (1978) (see Chapter 2) held that with appropriate scaffolding, we can learn tasks that are outside of our current knowledge or skills. For example, Takeshi (whom we meet in Chapter 6) feels confident in his clinical work generally, but feels less knowledgeable and confident in his work with older men. With appropriate scaffolding, we can support him to improve in this area. We designed the exercises presented within the modules of this current text to provide such scaffolding. As part of the learning process, each module encourages us to choose an aspect of change that is personally relevant. The level of difficulty we choose is important not only to reduce the possibility of distress, but also to enable access to our personal ZPD and to continually enhance our knowledge and skills. It is likely that this will shift and move across the modules, and therefore, it is helpful for us to adjust the level of difficulty and assess how well this reflects our ZPD as we progress.

That said, it is important to acknowledge that the learning progress is not linear, and it is typical to experience dips or delays to learning that may be accompanied with feelings of lowered confidence and competence. For example, a golfer changing their swing may experience a process of de-skilling as the learning progresses. That is, the golfer might experience a period of feeling that their swing has worsened before recognizing the enhancement beyond the starting skill level. Such an analogy also has relevance here. As we improve in our self-reflective skills, we may notice that more areas are challenging, or aren't going as smoothly as we previously perceived, and so may feel a bit de-skilled. It will come as no surprise that the ability to self-reflect is a critical component of the SP/SR process, and it comes with challenges. Indeed, the primary aim of SP/SR is to develop self-reflective knowledge and skills (Freeston et al., 2019). We will discuss this in more detail in the next section.

We mentioned earlier that the current text is aimed at readers who have some familiarity with MI. This is no accident because the adult learning theory underpinning SP/SR for MI is rooted in the requirement of having familiarity with the method. Thus, the module exercises are grounded in a level of familiarity with MI. It is usually helpful to have access to someone who is proficient in MI, to check that our understanding is accurate or that a demonstration of a particular skill is consistent with recommended practice. It may also be helpful to have access to materials and resources that refresh or confirm our understanding (e.g., MI texts, trusted video demonstrations). Finally, SP/SR is most effective when it is tailored to the specific context in which we work. Thus, as you work through the modules, we encourage you to apply your self-reflections not simply to work in general, but rather to your specific work setting, which might include tasks such as supervising others.

The module exercises within the current text are repeated in a familiar way and are designed to engage the reflective system from the perspective of you as the client (personal-self) to you as the practitioner (therapist-self) across the reflective bridge as outlined in Figure 3.3. The self-reflective questions contained within the modules have been carefully formulated to scaffold the process of reflection from personal-self to practitioner-self and to extend the ZPD. L. H. J. prefers to call this personal-self the *client-self*, which reflects the role that we step into as the learner. That is, we are the recipient of the MI intervention and therefore are the *client*. However, we are not role-playing as a client. For example, in Module 2, Takeshi self-reflects on his experience of engaging in real-play (as a client) with his limited-practice partner and then crosses the reflective bridge using further self-reflection to integrate this information into his practitioner-self and specifically into his practice skills. Recall that in Chapter 1, we explain why real-play (rather than role-play) enhances the felt component of the client experience and thereby deepens learning.

There is repetition through the modules to allow this process of experience and self-reflection to become internalized. Similarly, we designed the modules to link across one another (across session). The *golden thread* that runs across the modules is the progressive development of MI skills via the ability to engage the reflective system from personal-self to practitioner-self. For a comprehensive exploration of the application of these guiding principles, see Freeston et al. (2019).

How Do We Self-Reflect?

Perhaps since the publication of Donald Schön's seminal book *The Reflective Practitioner* (2017), considerable literature has been generated that has sought to explore what self-reflection is, how to do it, what the benefits are, and even how to measure it (e.g., Bennett-Levy et al., 2009, 2015; So et al., 2018). We also know that in much the same way that initial empathy levels differ (e.g., Zaki, 2020), people have differing initial abilities to self-reflect (Bennett-Levy et al., 2015) and learning can enhance these capacities (e.g., Duke et al., 2015). Combining theoretical knowledge with practical experience requires that we self-reflect in the moment, as we are doing it (*in action*) and after the event (*on action*) (Haarhoff & Thwaites, 2016). In addition to recognizing differing abilities to self-reflect, it is also important to acknowledge that our desire to self-reflect may differ depending on circumstance. For example, reflection in action during difficult encounters with clients (perhaps those who present with complex needs or those we identify with more personally) may mean that we wish to protect ourselves from the sensory and emotional experience of self-reflection (e.g., Ferguson, 2018).

Remember that self-reflection is best considered as a process, and this is the reflective system referred to earlier. Three distinct phases comprise this system: focused attention on the problem (stimulated by curiosity, goals, or mismatch with expectations); reconstruction and observation (e.g., via self-questioning, role-play or real-play, video review); and conceptualization and synthetization (e.g., self-questioning, elaboration, problem solving imagining alternatives). Self-reflection is a representation of all three phases—the complete process.

Bennett-Levy et al. (2009) suggest the following structure as a useful guide to the self-reflective process. This structure is evident in the exercise modules in the current text:

- Observe the experience (e.g., How did I feel? What did I notice?).
- Clarify the experience (e.g., How helpful was it? What did not change?).
- Implications of the experience for practice.
- Implications of how I see myself as *person* or *self as the practitioner.*
- Implications of this experience for my understanding of MI theory and practice. This may also include *MI as a way of being.*

Within the context of CBT, Bennett-Levy et al. (2015) provide some useful practical "how-to" guidance for self-reflection (see Box 4.1).

A fundamental component of self-reflection is that it allows us to critique and explore the utility of our interpersonal skills. In the PP model for MI (Figure 3.2, p. 32), we see that interpersonal beliefs, attitudes, and skills feature as key components alongside self-awareness, self-reflective skills, and a way of being. The intentional use of our personal characteristics can be thought of as the practitioner's therapeutic use of self and, in Rogerian terms, is strongly linked to genuineness. Within the context of the DPR model (which preceded the PP model; see Chapter 3), interpersonal skills are conceptualized into four elements: perceptual skills, practitioner attitudes, relational skills, and interpersonal knowledge (Bennett-Levy & Thwaites, 2007). Perceptual skills, the ability to pay attention to both the client's and practitioner's internal state, are linked to therapeutic proficiency, and SP/SR helps to develop such proficiency. However, paying attention to this alongside additional technical and relational skills can be difficult for those who have yet to develop automated procedural skills (e.g., Johnston & Milne, 2012).

BOX 4.1. Guidance for SP/SR

- Find a time and place where interruptions or distractions are unlikely.
- Transition from the self-practice exercise to the task of self-reflecting. Some people find focused breathing and/or mindfulness exercises helpful.
- Use whatever works best to assist in the recall of situations/events and awareness of our thoughts and feelings.
- Stay with our thoughts and feelings.
- Notice the unexpected.
- Notice if we are self-reflecting or ruminating. The latter may occur if our thinking drifts and lacks purpose/direction.
- Remain compassionate toward ourselves.
- Use SP/SR to address critical thoughts.
- Remember that self-reflection can occur in stages and when least expected.
- Pose questions to ourselves as we self-reflect on our experiences.
- Aim to link the personal and the professional.

Our practitioner attitudes influence how we understand what the client tells us, which might be why skillful use of reflective listening is so important. Among other factors, it provides a check on our attitudinal lens by inviting the client to clarify our understanding via the reflective listening statements offered (that will be filtered through our attitudes). Our relational skills also directly influence the demonstration of ***MI spirit***. Finally, there is our interpersonal knowledge. Specifically, our understanding of the dynamics of how people in general interact, as well as how particular individuals situated in their life circumstances interact. This knowledge can support us in understanding why things might work the way they do. For example, why seeking permission before sharing information is always encouraged and why it might be handled differently across situations, with particular clients, at a specific moment in time. It is noteworthy that reflecting on our lack of technical skill may feel easier than becoming aware of limitations in our interpersonal skills because they are so closely aligned with who we consider ourselves to be as people. Consequently, as we engage in a process of SP/SR, it may be useful to raise our awareness of this potential challenge or discomfort, understand its normality, and engage in self-compassion if it arises.

Self-Reflective Writing

Writing is central to the SP/SR process (e.g., Chigwedere, 2019; Gale & Schröder, 2014). Arguably, writing *is* thinking and reflection, and through the writing process, participants often identify new perspectives and a broader, deeper understanding of an experience. Practically, it is useful to write in the first person (e.g., "I felt," "I noticed"). Doing so helps us to connect on a deeper, personal level with the experience. The more honest and authentic we can be, the more meaningful and effective this work is (Bennett-Levy et al., 2009).

Writing also allows for a far greater appreciation of, and difficulty in avoiding, the emotional experiences associated with the process because of the attention to detail the writing process requires (Fraser & Wilson, 2011). Documented reflection enables the opportunity for learners to review their journey of increased competence and skill enhancement over time (Farrand et al., 2010). Sharing anonymous written reflections within group settings can further enhance reflective learning (McGillivray et al., 2015). In general terms, the reflective practice literature contends that reflective writing can develop critical writing, thinking, and analytical abilities; contribute to cognitive development; enhance creativity; and enable unique connections to be made between seemingly separate things such that new perspectives develop (Jasper, 2005).

Options for Engaging in the Process of SP/SR

It is a participant's mode and level of engagement that determine the benefit of SP/SR (e.g., Bennett-Levy & Lee, 2014), and how a person engages in SP/SR can take many forms. For example, individually (self-directed), with a friend or colleague in a limited peer practice, in groups, or with a coach or supervisor are all forms of SP/SR. It is likely that feasibility and practicality will guide the process of selecting the most appropriate approach for us in practice. In our experience, those who attend a sole introductory-level workshop training in MI may find it difficult to further develop their MI skills due to a lack of posttraining supervision, coaching, and mentoring. Lack of dedicated time to practice and reflect on developing skills also hinders progress. As described earlier, ongoing deliberate self-practice (with feedback) is necessary to help people move from a position of *knowing about MI* to becoming a more competent and skilled practitioner in the implementation of MI skills. Further engagement in SP/SR will support developing practitioners to enhance the shift from knowing to doing. However, in our experience, this crucial aspect of training has been neglected in professional development training. We anticipate therefore that some readers will undertake SP/SR individually as self-directed study and guided by this text.

Those familiar with qualitative research methods may be aware of the process of repeatedly listening to audio recordings to gain familiarity and a deeper understanding of data. Thus, there may be some benefit in the use of audio as a method of recording (perhaps alongside written) self-reflection. Such recordings could be integrated into the SP/SR process as a method of documenting self-reflection and as a tool to generate discussion in paired or group settings. However, we make this suggestion based on good-practice qualitative methodology and our experience of handling qualitative data as a transferable opportunity to consider. To our knowledge, this has not been formally integrated into taught SP/SR programs yet. For a detailed and practical exploration of self-reflective practice including common approaches, see Bhola et al. (2022). Most importantly, through SP/SR, learners experience the power of an approach through its receipt, the careful consideration of its effect on them, and the transfer of this experience across the reflective bridge to their professional practice setting. The careful, thoughtful consideration of these questions, and the written responses, are the mechanism by which the learner crosses the bridge into enhancing their understanding of MI and thereby becoming a more discerning MI practitioner.

Toward this end of a greater understanding of the Why, What, and How of MI, this text provides a range of reflective questions at the end of each exercise module, which act as a support structure (i.e., Vygotskian scaffold; Vygotsky, 1978) to help guide us, as learners, to explore and deepen our reflective experience. The self-reflective questions are written to enable us to engage the reflective system and to move beyond our current levels of learning, akin to the scaffolding role of clinical supervision, or coach, or mentor (refer to Johnston & Milne, 2012). The completed exercises also become a written diary of personal learning experiences.

The traveling companions (Chapter 6) assist us, as learners, in moving through the SP/SR process. They reflect individuals with differing levels of expertise. Our aim is that we all find ourselves reflected in at least one of these companions and where they are in either their career or their learning process. These companions may also provide insights for supervisors working with practitioners at different stages in their career.

As with MI, we respect people's ability to select what is best for them in utilizing this workbook and in engaging with their own *inside out* journey. We know ourselves and how we tend to learn best. Yet, the purpose of the ZPD is that we need to move slightly beyond our comfort zones to grow. Therefore, it might also be useful to consider if there are ways in which we need to stretch as we review the options below.

Individual (Self-Directed) SP/SR

Opting to undertake self-directed SP/SR with the aid of a workbook has several advantages. For example, time and place do not constrain when to practice or work deliberately through self-reflective prompts. Moreover, we select the modules that feel most beneficial to us and take greater ownership of building personal and professional skills over a time of our choosing. Our SP/SR timeline can expand or contract based on other demands in our lives. Some people may prefer the safety of thinking things through themselves first before doing so with others. A self-study approach clearly provides more autonomy, requires greater self-discipline, and may permit greater ownership over learning and development.

There are also limitations to self-directed SP/SR work. Although there may be opportunities during the process, no immediate opportunity exists to share experiences with peers/colleagues/supervisors. Sharing self-reflections with others deepens our experience. This creates opportunities for alternative perspectives that enrich our insight and enhance our self-reflections. The absence of this immediate opportunity to share may also permit blindspots to remain in what we don't know about unknown strengths or weaknesses—we don't know what we don't know. For some people, not having the encouragement (or accountability) of others may result in a lower level of commitment or quitting the process altogether. Yet, the biggest limitation is that MI involves an interpersonal process—a way of being with people. Without a practice activity involving another, we may not experience the full power of MI and therefore the SP/SR process. That said, even with these limitations, self-directed study is a feasible and beneficial option for some learners.

SP/SR in Pairs (Limited-Practice Partner)

With SP/SR in pairs, there is an opportunity to experience MI from the *inside out*, to share our experiences of SP/SR in a safe place with someone we trust and deepen our learning experience. Practically, working in limited-practice pairs within a real-play context allows for each person to undertake the role of practitioner and client (Bennett-Levy et al., 2003). This practice process allows us to experience what the application of MI concepts and skills feels like as a recipient and how this, in turn, influences our thoughts, feelings, and bodily reactions, as well as to practice our application of these same tools. Additionally, this can help us to stay committed and enthused about the process and normalize any discomfort experienced. It is beneficial to pair with someone who has a similar level of skill as yourself. It is likely that less experienced MI practitioners will want to focus on conceptual and skill development practices, whereas those who are more experienced may seek to develop a deeper level of self-awareness around their advanced skills in action (Johnston & Milne, 2012).

In practical terms, it is possible to undertake SP/SR sessions either virtually or in person. The confidentiality and anonymity of any clinical case materials shared remain paramount, regardless of the meeting venue, and should be maintained throughout this paired relationship. Matching of skill level can assist in exploration of similar issues. Regardless, each member encourages equitable contributions within the reflective meetings. Perhaps the most obvious practical limitation of conducting SP/SR in pairs is access to a suitable partner who has a comparable skill level.

SP/SR in Groups

An established SP/SR group can create opportunities for a supportive learning community and reduce the risks associated with solo work or when practitioners work in silos within larger organizations and teams. The practical considerations and benefits of a deeper reflective learning experience described in working in pairs also apply to learning groups. The breadth of, and differences in, perspectives in a learning group can provide an additional element to the learning process. Moreover, learners benefit from deeper insight and more advanced skills of some group members. However, this approach requires careful consideration and management of group processes.

There are well-documented costs and benefits to any learning group. As with any group, close attention to group dynamics and process factors (e.g., composition, readiness, expectations, challenges cohesion, ruptures) is critical to success, and we cover this in more detail in Chapter 5. A group may take longer to develop trust and to establish helpful patterns of meaningful engagement than does a limited-practice partnership. SP/SR work requires sharing self-reflections, which increases a sense of vulnerability. Sharing vulnerabilities in a group, especially in the context of peers and coworkers, takes time. This can impact the depth and quality of the reflective process if not well addressed by the SP/SR facilitators.

Chapter 5 will discuss the sharing of public self-reflections (process) and their difference from private self-reflections (content), as well as considerations for facilitators in leading an SP/SR group. While online platforms are not immune to these limitations, the use of online blogs whereby other SP/SR participants can read the written reflective commentaries of others can generate peer support, encourage participation, and normalize the experience (Farrand et al., 2010). It is noteworthy that with the rise in interest in utilizing online approaches to teaching and learning, the online experience of SP/SR has been reported as comparable to an in-person experience. However, some trainees may find it more difficult to show vulnerability online and some supervisors may be less likely to encourage trainees to experience and express difficult thoughts and emotions (Jona et al., 2022b). Supervisor comfort and capacity with online service provision seem to be important considerations in this process. Certainly, there is a growing sensitivity to, and awareness of, how individual differences (i.e., gender, age, race) impact the group dynamic. An SP/SR facilitator will need to be attuned to these factors and their potential impact on the group dynamic, in addition to finding an appropriate balance of vulnerability for the deep, self-reflective learning to occur. A blended approach to group sessions (either virtually or in person) with online supporting materials/blogs may offer a level of compromise with a rich experience for SP/SR and with skillful facilitation, an opportunity for greater participation by less dominant members of a group (Farrand et al., 2010).

When possible, if a learning community is created via attendance at an initial MI training, we encourage this group (with limited pair practice) to be maintained thereafter for ongoing coaching and supervision. The reasoning is twofold. First, doing so means that (if the confidentiality, anonymity, and facilitator skillfulness considerations mentioned earlier can be met) trainees benefit from continued growth and development within a learning group that has some level of familiarity with, and some early development of group dynamics. Second, developing an MI learning culture that routinely encourages continuous learning, post initial training, supports a shift away from MI training as a single event to something that requires an ongoing commitment such as the SP/SR approach offers. Learning is an iterative and reflective journey rather than a single event.

SP/SR with a Coach or Supervisor

The degree to which trainees have ready access to continued coaching and/or supervision following initial training in MI varies considerably. In our experience, this is typically influenced by the commissioner's/organization's understanding of the evidence base for ongoing coaching and supervision, training budgets, cultural differences, whether this is offered by the training provider, and the motivations of trainees to develop their skills to proficiency in a method. The danger of not having access to an experienced supervisor is that the trainee remains unconsciously incompetent (i.e., we remain unaware of the skills that we do not (yet) know or are practicing without competence) and that skills will erode (Schwalbe et al., 2014). Alternatively, the trainee may also remain consciously incompetent (i.e., aware of skill limitations but unable to access or prioritize development via supervision).

Often, supervisory discussions between experienced supervisors and novice practitioners can be "typified as attempts made by the consciously incompetent to learn from the unconsciously competent" (Green, 2003, p. 103). This reflective process of working through a detailed discussion of experiential tasks offers as much educational potential for the supervisor as the supervisee. This is the original process that Bill Miller describes in the *discovery* of MI via his supervision sessions with highly inquisitive postgraduate students and psychologists during a sabbatical in Norway. Essentially, Miller derived inductively, through an iterative process of observation, questions, and reflection on the processes involved in clinical encounters, the conceptualization of a helpful therapeutic process that came to be known as MI (Miller, 1983, 2023). Chapter 5 addresses the process and skills associated with the supervision/coaching of SP/SR in more detail.

Taking Care of Yourself

Prioritizing our needs is an important part of SP/SR. As we start to engage in the exercise modules, it might be that we feel emotionally or practically unable to start a particular exercise, and if this should occur, we suggest taking time for self-care. Similarly, and perhaps most importantly, remember that SP/SR often includes periods of de-skilling and in increased awareness of deficiencies that we might have previously been unaware of. This can evoke feelings of incompetence and self-doubt, so it is important for us to trust that perfection is unattainable and that the process of SP/SR typically becomes easier as we progress (Bennett-Levy et al., 2009).

As noted earlier, some clients or topics might have emotional relevance for us, which might make self-reflection, either in action (during) or on action (afterward), more challenging for us. While understanding and working through these areas may be of critical importance in working effectively with clients over the long term, it does not mean this is the correct choice for this process at this time. Choice of topic for this workbook is important. We encourage you to choose something that doesn't cause too much discomfort (see Module 1).

Even when thoughtful about our topic selection, learners need to be mindful of exploring material or situations that can trigger unexpected and strong emotional responses that, without support, may be difficult to manage. In general terms, SP/SR requires self-disclosure that, while beneficial in empathizing with the client perspective, can also be challenging (Jona et al., 2022a). The process can also give rise to distressing experiences, and there should thus be access to support and the option of pausing or ending the process (Bennett-Levy et al., 2001). We encourage you to consider making someone you trust, and are comfortable being vulnerable with, aware that you are undertaking the SP/SR process. We recommend this plan for all SP/SR learners and especially for those working independently; of course, you will be the one that makes this decision.

Final Thoughts

The reflective bridge is an essential element in this learning process. The self-practice element gives practitioners a powerful but limited experience for the personal-self. However, we must actively transfer this experience across the reflective bridge. This happens through the self-reflective component. That is, answering the questions at the end of each module. We designed these questions to explore practitioners' thoughts, feelings, and bodily experiences as they go through this process. The modules are also designed to follow the four steps in learning described earlier: What, How, Why, and What If. The aim is to help the learning process move implicitly and intentionally through these dimensions.

As you might expect, there are advantages with, and limitations to, whatever approach you decide is right for you. There is more than one right way. Practitioners using SP/SR report it can be difficult and life-changing. Similarly, MI trainees sometimes describe MI as appearing deceptively easy, and unexpectedly eliciting powerful thoughts and feelings that can be difficult and life changing.

CHAPTER 5

Guidance for Facilitators

Background and Context

In Chapter 4, we outlined several approaches to undertaking SP/SR. Some of these approaches (i.e., within groups or as part of an educational program) require skillful facilitation to guide participants through the process. What follows are some key considerations for the facilitation of SP/SR. Some of these considerations are shared with those for any group learning experience and some are unique to SP/SR. It is intended that the guidance presented here will have most relevance for those who plan to facilitate SP/SR, although it is likely that anyone with an interest in SP/SR will benefit from incorporating this guidance into the learning process.

Key Questions Discussed in This Chapter

- Why does modeling the method matter for SP/SR group facilitation?
- What is the role of a group facilitator in SP/SR?
- What are important practical and interpersonal considerations?
- How might facilitators need to prepare for, and look after, participants in an SP/SR process?
- What additional resources might be helpful to undertake this work?

Modeling the Method

It is generally accepted that the key to developing and sustaining MI skills is a process of post-training coaching and supervision (e.g., Miller, 2023; Schwalbe et al., 2014) and that real-world integration of the skills into routine practice enhances fidelity (DeShaw et al., 2024). However, it is *how* this process is undertaken that is important. Ask any proficient MI trainer what one of the most important aspects of facilitating training is, and their answer is typically *modeling the method* (i.e., actively demonstrating ***MI spirit*** and skills as part of the learning process). Doing so offers a parallel learning process for trainees such that they can experience an MI-consistent conversation as they learn what it is and, crucially, *how* to do it. This consideration has both a general and specific relevance to SP/SR. In general terms, it is the experiential aspect of learning that is demonstrative of SP/SR and is linked to the process of self-reflective learning as presented in the PP model in Chapter 3 (see Figure 3.2). Specifically, modeling the method relates directly to the guidance offered in this chapter. It represents the practical and interpersonal aspects of group facilitation and is the *golden thread* of *how* to facilitate SP/SR.

The Role of the MI SP/SR Facilitator

The role of the MI SP/SR facilitator may be both practical (arranging times and venues) and interpersonal (facilitation skills). We will explore this more in the next section. However, an important early consideration is that because of the level of vulnerability and some of the personal and professional challenges that can be experienced during SP/SR (described in Chapter 4), SP/SR facilitation requires a greater level of sensitivity to individual needs than a more general training situation. Within the context of CBT, Bennett-Levy and colleagues (2015) have previously emphasized the importance of the *collaborative relationship* as central to the facilitator role. The facilitators' creation of *psychological safety* is also an essential component of the group dynamic and depth of experience (e.g., Cave et al., 2016).

The principles, processes, and skills of MI have direct relevance to supporting the safe engagement of trainees into a group SP/SR program. For example, being persuaded or coerced into participation negatively impacts on ***engagement*** and the experience of SP/SR. Facilitators should focus on enhancing participant ***autonomy*** whenever possible, but especially within a mandatory learning program. The facilitator's modeling of MI methods is also important for observational purposes, experiential aspects of SP/SR, and supporting trainees in this process. Not surprisingly, the ***four tasks, MI spirit, and OARS+I*** are all valuable, particularly in the context of early engagement for SP/SR and if people are ambivalent.

Practical and Interpersonal Considerations

Preparation for SP/SR

SP/SR program participants benefit from prior written communication to clearly explain the rationale for SP/SR, what to expect, the personal and self-reflective nature of the program, that SP/SR may include group and/or online disclosure, and issues around courage, safety, and confidentiality. Encouraging trainees to access preparatory written guidance prior to commencement may help alleviate concerns and enhance engagement. A preprogram meeting that addresses the rationale for SP/SR and program requirements and promotes feelings of safety and courage may also be beneficial (Bennett-Levy et al., 2015).

Providing a Strong Rationale for SP/SR

There isn't a standardized training pathway in MI, and for those who may have attended introductory training, posttraining opportunities to continue skill development are not always offered. It is important that we have access to information that helps us understand why we might want to engage in SP/SR rather than, or possibly in combination with, another approach such as deliberate practice (Manuel et al., 2022) or practice-based supervision. It may also be helpful to consider those who would benefit from additional information about the primary literature (e.g., Bennett-Levy et al., 2009; Bhola et al., 2022) from those who have experienced SP/SR (e.g., Farrell & Shaw, 2018).

Pre-program meetings offer an opportunity for facilitators and co-learners to share examples of SP/SR experiences and critically reflect on research demonstrating the rationale for SP/SR (e.g., Gale & Schröder, 2014; Haarhoff & Farrand, 2012; Thwaites et al., 2014). Box 5.1 contains an example that C. E. H. often includes in her MI training that illustrates the power of a particular technique—a ***complex reflection***—in shifting understanding within her life. While not specifically designed as a full SP/SR activity, it contains the essential elements and illustrates how *inside out* work happens. C. E. H. engaged in a real discussion about a then current and important challenge in her personal life about which she was struggling to make a decision. The receipt of a complex reflection had a powerful impact on her decision making. Self-reflection on this impact allowed her to more deeply understand the value of accurate empathy in connecting to her identity and values. She considered how to bring this new comprehension into her work and training. She then implemented and refined how she used this approach through further self-reflection in action (when working with clients and trainees) and after action in how she designed her training and does her work.

Of course, our aim is not to persuade participants because this would challenge modeling the method of MI as part of the facilitation process. Rather, consider the provision of evidence-based materials and the experiential examples—our own and others—as ***empowering*** participants to make an informed choice about whether engagement in SP/SR is right for them.

Aligning SP/SR to the Participants' Competencies and Needs

Aligning SP/SR to participant competencies and needs is more challenging within groups. Working with individuals allows for a focused, ongoing assessment of key considerations such as ability and comfort level in the self-reflective process (i.e., engaging the reflective system; see Chapter 4), MI skill proficiency, and the context in which the person is undertaking SP/SR. Facilitating within a group context requires attention to each of the participants' individual competencies and needs, while maintaining a larger focus on the group's progression. Wherever possible, it is useful to create a group that comprises learners working within similar contexts who have comparable levels of experience of reflection and MI skill; however, this may not always be possible. For this reason, it is likely that preparatory materials, time, and discussion will be more important for less experienced participants, or for those who may not have joined the program voluntarily (Bennett-Levy & Lee, 2014).

SP/SR programs are best considered as flexible and facilitated in a manner that responds to differing contexts, competencies, and needs. One relatively easy and practical adjustment might be to amend the self-reflective questions, so they target the context and relevance for learners

BOX 5.1. Buying a House

C. E. H.: I often share my experience of being ambivalent around a house purchase and how being offered a complex reflection during a real-play practice affected me from both a personal and professional perspective. The reflection invited deep thinking around identity and core values, which hadn't been considered before. Consequently, two things occurred. First, I resolved my ambivalence and purchased the house. Second, a process of SP/SR led me to a renewed appreciation of the value of complex reflections—particularly those that help the unseen or yet to be considered, become visible.

The context of the experience is that during a real-play training activity, I was talking through my ambivalence around buying my first house. I was fortunate enough to have saved a deposit and despite living in several places across the UK, I had settled on my location. Practically everything pointed toward now being the right time to buy. However, something was holding me back and I really couldn't figure out what. A MI practitioner offered a reflection that captured aspects of my ambivalence around identity and values that I hadn't fully recognized at that time. The reflection sounded something like this: *It sounds like buying a house is inviting you to consider what that would mean about who you are. It's almost like you're asking yourself, can I be a homeowner and still identify as a free spirit who can live and work wherever they would like?*

Observation of the experience: The reflection opened a new way of thinking about my uncertainty. In my body, it was like something was released. I became *unstuck* in that very moment because I was able to feel and see the source of my ambivalence. While I had considered that buying a home would mean I would settle in a particular area for some time, I hadn't fully recognized how this was so deeply linked to the value I had placed on my identity as someone who was *free-spirited*. I remember experiencing very strong feelings of being truly seen, heard, and understood, yet also feeling vulnerable and somewhat exposed; I recall being aware of this at the time in my body, feelings, and thoughts. I noticed that it took some time to respond because of the deep cognitive and emotional process I experienced.

Clarification of the experience: I found that purposefully and consciously undertaking a full self-reflective process at the time of the real-play (in action) and following (on action) particularly helpful. This experience shaped both my MI practice and training in terms of reaffirming the value and transformational power of hearing complex reflections from a client perspective and how I might help trainees experience this for themselves.

Implications for MI practice: This experience reaffirmed what thoughts and feelings clients may experience when in receipt of a skillful complex reflection that captures something at a deeper level and that they may not have considered before. Although I knew this at the time, the *felt* experience and purposeful self-reflective process deepened the value I attributed to this skill. I also benefited from a much deeper appreciation of "trusting the process"—that people may need time to respond to complex reflections because of the level of cognitive and emotional processing they evoke. This has also helped me to trust the silence that I offer during these times to allow that to happen. This is reflected in my work and MI training to this day.

(continued)

BOX 5.1. *(continued)*

Implications for how I see my practitioner-self: I am generally comfortable with low levels of detail and structure. This is often evident in my MI training whereby I am comfortable with responding to the needs of trainees, rather than having a highly structured, predetermined content plan. This experience invited me to recognize that although I consider myself a person who enjoys unstructured exploratory and curious self-reflection, the structure that was offered by this process allowed me to benefit more fully. It invited me to self-reflect in a more systematic way. I learned that while I am still comfortable with flexibility and less structured approaches to learning, SP/SR offers me a process that I enjoy following and that benefits my work. I now routinely apply this approach to other areas of my professional practice and training.

Implications for understanding MI theory and practice as a way of being: This process supported a deeper appreciation of translating the "what to do" of MI into the "how to do it" (reflective listening skill). I actively encourage trainees to experience MI skills through real-play and to make sense of their experience by engaging the reflective system as I did. I also have a heightened awareness of the thoughts, feelings, and bodily responses that clients may process as part of an MI-consistent conversation and the safe space and time that are needed to do this. It was the spirit of MI that, when coupled with the reflection I heard, contributed to the experience I had. I felt safe enough to be given the time to process this experience in the moment. There was compassion in the curious nature of the reflection offered and an acceptance of the felt experience I had in response. I consider the spirit of MI—a way of being—to be critical to both my personal and professional life.

(Freeston et al., 2019; Thwaites et al., 2014). For example, learners looking to improve their approach to supervision might be asked self-reflective bridging questions that have relevance for facilitating supervision. Alternatively, learners working in areas of behavior change (e.g., addiction, diabetes, probation) could be invited to reflect on the implications of the personal learning experience for their practice with those clients.

Generally, Bennett-Levy et al. (2015) suggest that early career practitioners (e.g., traveling companion Takeshi, whom you'll meet in the next chapter) may benefit more from transferring declarative knowledge into procedural skills, with an emphasis on therapist-self. More experienced practitioners (e.g., traveling companion Sam) may benefit more from a greater focus on personal-self to enhance self-awareness, interpersonal skills, and self-reflective capacity (Davis et al., 2015). Doing so is also likely to support practitioners who work with individuals presenting with particularly complex needs and/or who may be unexpectedly triggered (i.e., experience a strong emotional reaction) (Safran & Muran, 2000) by increasing awareness of how they're impacting clients, how clients are affecting them, and how their physical, emotional, and cognitive states, for example, influence their responses to clients.

Finally, given the critical role of engaging the reflective system and that we differ in our ability to do this initially (see Chapter 4), it is important that facilitators explain the importance of developing these skills. Anonymous practical examples from previous learners, those shared by fellow learners, and signposting to methods of enhancing self-reflective skills—all contribute to building reflective capacity (Bennett-Levy et al., 2015).

Communicating Clear and Agreed-Upon SP/SR Requirements

The context and requirements of an SP/SR program influence what and how we communicate. For example, if SP/SR comprises part of a required and assessed program of study (e.g., doctoral degree program), there will be practical considerations regarding when to introduce SP/SR, how much time should be dedicated to this component of the program, and what appropriate competency criteria and assessment should be. SP/SR programs facilitated outside of the academic context might have similar considerations, though they may be potentially less complex and/or limiting. Allocation of adequate time is essential to the process of SP/SR as it allows the depth of reflection and application of learning to the practitioner context. One useful approach to reducing barriers and enhancing learners' exposure to SP/SR is to include a self-reflection exercise as part of introducing a skill or strategy. For example, participants attending a 2-day MI introduction training could be invited to experience what it feels like to be in receipt of an ***affirmation*** and to consider how this might influence their own MI practice.

It is a challenge when SP/SR assessment is required. For example, evaluating the quality of participant self-reflection is of questionable value in a required training context (Bennett-Levy et al., 2015). It runs the risk of unintentionally creating demand characteristics regarding self-reflective content and potentially increasing the anxiety of participants by focusing on depicting competency, instead of demonstrating the vulnerability necessary for growth. Learners may disengage or censor what they share, which will cause their self-reflections to be more surface-level or self-protective. It may be more helpful to consider process-related indicators, such as the level of engagement in group or online discussions, or completion of activities. Regardless of context, we recommend clear communication of program requirements, including time commitment and assessment requirements, within the preparatory materials and during any pre-program meetings.

Creating Safety and Conditions for Supportive and Enriching Group Interaction

Facilitating feelings of safety should start early in the SP/SR process. At a practical level, it begins with making clear what participants will share in the group setting. The focus will be on sharing reflections about the process (e.g., *What did it feel like to think or talk about a mistake?*) and not about the content (e.g., *What is a mistake you made, and what made it memorable for you?*). Facilitators make clear this is not a group therapy program, although at times participants may experience the power of connection and universality that comes from being part of a shared experience, and people may also experience a sense of vulnerability and anxiety as part of this process. As facilitators, we explain and normalize feelings of vulnerability and anxiety within the preparatory materials and meetings, as well as the importance of mutual care and support among members.

The creation of safety alongside a supportive, enriching, and brave interaction space is an ongoing consideration for facilitators; indeed, this facilitator behavior is perhaps the most demonstrative of facilitator interpersonal skill. SP/SR groups typically meet either in person, online, or both and can often be the most enriching aspect of the program (Bennett-Levy & Lee, 2014; Haarhoff & Farrand, 2012; Farrand et al., 2010). As we described in Chapter 4, there are both benefits and limitations to experiencing SP/SR in a group and individually. From the facilitator perspective, a group requires careful management of participants such that contributions are equitable and that any group-formulated agreements are upheld. Such agreements may include the role of participants and the facilitator; confidentiality; anonymity; safeguarding; and, if context allows, how the group should meet (i.e., in person, online, or both). Practical online facilitation considerations include committing to regular prompts for participants to engage with online material, referencing and integrating reflective posts shared by others, and timely responses to comments and questions (e.g., Thomas & Thorpe, 2019).

With respect to in-person facilitation, Bennett-Levy et al. (2015) recognize that group facilitation represents a sophisticated skill set and recommend that facilitators seek appropriate training. There is a wealth of literature on group facilitation skills (e.g., Cave et al., 2016; McDermott, 2020; Ritchie et al., 2020), transferring group therapy facilitation skills to a learning group (e.g., *www.apa.org/monitor/2019/04/group-therapy*), and MI group facilitation skills in general (Wagner & Ingersoll, 2012) and in leadership contexts (Marshall & Nielsen, 2020). Again, modeling MI in groups may enhance group safety and support, encourage interaction, and reinforce the structure and content of SP/SR groups, including trainees experiencing the *skills in action*. Figure 5.1 provides a visual representation of how MI tasks and skills might be integrated into an SP/SR group facilitation context. Given the importance of these skills, facilitators may find value in ongoing coaching and supervision in group facilitation skills, including deepening their knowledge and recognition of group processes, enhancing skill use and application of techniques, and handling challenging situations (Wagner & Ingersoll, 2012, 2025).

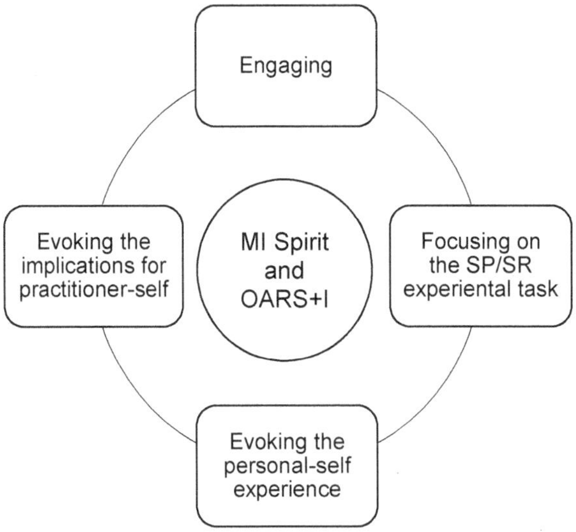

FIGURE 5.1. Tasks and skills of MI within a SP/SR facilitation context.

Looking After Participants

While SP/SR can be extremely beneficial to skill development, the process places more emotional demand on trainees than conventional training (e.g., Fraser & Wilson, 2011). As such, it may be helpful to agree about procedures to contact participants who appear to be struggling during the early preparation meetings. Similar agreements may identify when and how the facilitator can be contacted as part of personal safeguarding strategies for learners. Supportive discussions providing options for participants to delay or to reduce the intensity of the SP/SR can also be helpful and reflect a further opportunity for modeling the MI method by enhancing participant autonomy and choice. Finally, giving forethought to appropriate referral mechanisms and processes is also prudent.

Final Thoughts

Skillful group facilitation is an area of expertise that requires mastery. However, the transferability of MI processes and skills has a lot to offer in this regard. The facilitation of SP/SR is perhaps best considered as a combination of both practical and interpersonal skills and Box 5.2 below presents a useful summary of the key components.

BOX 5.2. Summary of Considerations for SP/SR Facilitation

Preparation for SP/SR

May include preparatory written materials and preprogram meetings with participants.

Providing a Strong Rationale for SP/SR

Support participants to understand how and why SP/SR can enhance skill development. Communicate using written materials and preprogram meetings with participants. Use storytelling and experiential examples of impact.

Aligning SP/SR to the Participants' Competencies and Needs

Create a homogenous group wherever possible. Respond to individual needs and adopt a flexible approach to SP/SR delivery. Amend self-reflective questions to suit individual context. Assess and respond to participant reflective capacity.

(continued)

BOX 5.2. *(continued)*

Communicating Clear and Agreed-Upon SP/SR Requirements

Utilize preparatory materials and meetings. Wherever possible, introduce SP/SR exercise early in the learning process and in parallel to the introduction of skills (e.g., a SP/SR exercise for reflective listening). If assessment is required, consider levels of engagement as more useful than ability to self-reflect per se.

Creating Safety and Conditions for Supportive, Enriching, and Brave Group Interaction

Practical considerations include facilitating the co-production of agreements within the group. Explain and normalize any discomfort within the preparatory materials and meetings. Consider how MI processes and skills can be utilized within group facilitation to model the method and enhance safety, support, and enriching group discussion.

Looking After Participants

A facilitator should uphold a duty of care. Agree to methods of contact between facilitator and participant should there be any welfare concern. Support participants' autonomy by offering choice in how and when SP/SR is undertaken.

CHAPTER 6

MI Companions for SP/SR Travel

Background and Context

To learn MI from the *inside out*, it is helpful to have *traveling companions* in the process. While having a limited-practice partner deepens our understanding from the *personal-self* perspective, it is also helpful to have models assist us in the learning by moving through the process as we do. These personas reflect learners at various developmental states of their career and in learning MI. We introduce these companions here.

Key Questions to Consider in this Chapter

- Why are traveling companions helpful in the SP/SR process?
- Which of the companions fits best with where I am in either the learning process or my career progress?
- What characteristics can I relate to?
- How might I use these companions to help me as I move through this book?

Common Ground

Our traveling companions are people working in the helping professions like us. They are compendiums of ourselves, as well as trainees, supervisees, and colleagues we have known. They will model some of the struggles we encounter in our lives, in our clinical work, and in supervision and training. The companions' circumstances are adapted to fit our work. We will begin by providing background to give you a sense of their lives and work, but by necessity this will be incomplete. We want the space for imagination and the opportunity to insert ourselves into these characters, which will assist us in experiencing the personal relevance, power, and effects of these interactions.

Takeshi

Takeshi is a 24-year-old, cisgender, straight man and graduate student working on his doctorate in clinical psychology. A fourth-generation Japanese American, his father is a dentist and his mother, with a degree in business, is an office manager. Both were warm and encouraging, but also set certain expectations for Takeshi: that he would do his best and work hard in his endeavors. In addition to his studies, he played violin in the orchestra and spent time daily practicing his instrument, as well as participating in clubs and sports. The stress associated with these activities caused him to seek out his school counselor intermittently. While he found these sessions helpful, he never settled into a regular routine. There are, and have been, a core group of friends throughout his life, though the size and membership of this group have changed. With strangers he can be reserved, but among his friends he is outgoing and joins the conversation easily. Still, he finds that his willingness to share extends only so far. Like many young men, he finds it difficult to reveal himself deeply.

Takeshi worked hard academically, attended a highly competitive university for his undergraduate degree, and chose to attend graduate school as the logical next step. Originally intent on being a researcher of anxiety disorders, he nonetheless retained a curiosity about clinical work given his positive experience with the school counselor. His graduate program has a primary focus on CBT, and he has been seeing clients through the campus clinic. He finds himself quite adept at identifying issues and appropriate interventions but is feeling frustrated by his clients' nonadherence to the plans he's created for them. At his supervisor's suggestion, he enrolled in the MI seminar his program offered. He found himself intrigued and spent time talking with fellow graduate students about MI, sought out some journal articles on it, watched some related videos online, and decided this might be worthwhile. As part of his training, he sees clients and finds himself feeling anxious about his proficiency in MI because the roadmap seems much less clear than with CBT. He feels as if his listening stays on the surface and is unsure when he should be doing things.

In summary, Takeshi is a 24-year-old cisgender, straight man of Japanese descent in graduate school, working on his doctorate in clinical psychology. He maintains high expectations for himself, and at times this causes him stress. He is a strong student and shows promise as a counselor. He feels some frustration about his clients' lack of change at times. He sought out MI training at the suggestion of his supervisor and sees the value in it, though he doesn't feel as confident in this approach as he does in CBT.

Quincy

Quincy is a 38-year-old, cisgender, straight woman of African descent who grew up in a community where issues of racism and economic challenge stood shoulder to shoulder with strong activism, spiritual leadership from local church congregations, and a vibrant cultural community. Quincy's father is a successful business owner and her mother a nurse. They worked long hours, but alternated shifts so that someone was always there when Q (as she's known in the family) and her two younger sisters were home. Church was a part of Q's life growing up, as were clear and strong moral values, the necessity of school to achieve success in life, and the importance of being part of and giving back to the community.

Early on, Q saw the devastation wrought by alcohol and other substance use among people and decided to become an addiction professional. She's been working in the field for 15 years now and has begun to feel burned out. The constant relapsing and recycling of people through her program have left her feeling dispirited. She's begun to believe that her clients are lying to her consistently, and this makes her discouraged and more irritable than is her nature. She's noted her increasingly confrontational tone at work, which she doesn't like but feels is needed to get through all the denial and deceit. While addiction has never been an issue for her, she's found her occasional drink has now become a nightly routine. While she doesn't think it's an issue, it concerns her and she's thus decided to seek some help to manage her stress.

Because of the work she does, Q decided it would be best to find a counselor in a nearby community who has a good reputation and whom she does not know. She took a 90-minute "Taste of MI" course over Zoom, which led her to recently attend a 2-day, introductory MI training workshop. She was interested, but remained skeptical about whether it would work with her clients and never really implemented it with them. She decided to seek out someone who knew MI to be her counselor so she could see firsthand whether it had merit.

In summary, Quincy is a 38-year-old, cisgender straight woman of African descent who works as an alcohol and drug (AOD) counselor. Growing up in a vibrant community, she has strong family ties and a foundation of giving to others. She was feeling some burnout with substance use clients and has taken an MI workshop, but the approach hasn't yet found its way into her work. Because of her feelings of stress and burnout, she sought personal support and decided to find a therapist skilled in MI to learn more about the process.

Sam

Samantha, or Sam as she is known by virtually everyone outside her family, is a retirement-age, cisgender, gay White woman who has been a successful counselor for many years. Sam worked in the family business for many years after high school. She found that others turned to her for counsel and advice, and perhaps she had a natural talent for this kind of work. Besides, she enjoyed being of service to others. These considerations, in combination with her restlessness in the family business, spurred her to go back to school to obtain a degree in counseling. After graduation, she worked for mental health agencies in the area, but eventually continued restlessness led her to decide to open a private practice. The aim was to pursue her other life interests, while focusing on the work she does 3 days a week.

Sam has always been interested and taken part in active life pursuits during her leisure time. About 15 years ago, Sam suffered a fall on an adventure trip and injured her back. The recovery was slow and arduous, and included a prescription for opiates for a period of time. With concern rising about opiate misuse in the media, Sam decided to pursue information about other forms of pain relief. This led her specifically to mindfulness and meditation, but more generally to how people manage pain. Over the last 10 years, her practice focus has migrated into health practices and right now this is its almost exclusive focus.

As part of this health focus, Sam completed introductory MI training. She immediately felt as if this process was a fit for how she worked and began looking for other opportunities to learn. She purchased several MI books, including a workbook, as part of intermediate MI training; she regards her skills as improving. She occasionally acts as a consultant to younger colleagues and has found MI quite helpful in this work as well. Lately, she has begun wondering how one becomes proficient in MI.

At the same time, Sam is currently of retirement age. Her wife Debra retired this year from a job she disliked and would like Sam to do the same. There was a health scare last year when squamous cells were discovered on Sam's arm and stomach, but they were removed successfully and now Sam is checked regularly for their return. Debra saw this as evidence that the couple needs to take advantage of the time left and retire, but Sam still loves the work she does and feels the value it has for the people she interacts with. Sam and Debra talked with their accountant, and they could afford—with sacrifices—for Sam to retire now. However, these sacrifices would be unnecessary if Sam worked a few years longer.

Sam is ambivalent about retiring. She sees the value of it, as well as the worth of working for a few more years. She believes that Debra's experience with less fulfilling work makes her unable to understand why Sam sees things differently. Debra has been putting pressure on her, and Sam's response has been to dig in her heels. Attempts to discuss this led to point–counterpoint arguments, with both sides feeling resentful. Debra is now pressing Sam to see someone professionally so she can "make a decision." Sam has agreed but is dubious about the value of it. She feels stuck.

In summary, Sam is a retirement-age, cisgender, gay White woman of European descent who has been a successful counselor for many years. Fifteen years ago, she injured her back and because of that experience has shifted her private practice to health-focused care. She became interested in MI as part of the learning she did post injury, engaged in a variety of training and learning, and has recently been considering ways to advance her expertise. She had experienced a cancer scare last year, and her wife is encouraging her to retire. Sam is ambivalent about making such a change, and this has become a point of contention for them.

Final Thoughts

We intentionally made our traveling companions a diverse set of characters. Our aim was to move beyond our limited boundaries of White, European-descent, cisgender, straight and gay people to better reflect the breadth and experience of all the MI practitioners in the United States and around the world. In so doing, we acknowledge that our backgrounds shaped the identities we created, that all people have many identities, and we have described just a few. We have reflected neither every group nor every important identity. It is possible we have unintentionally given offense, despite our best efforts to be thoughtful and self-reflective in this process. If that is the case for you, please accept our apologies and let us know so that we can do better.

PART II

MI from the Inside Out

MODULE 1

Identifying and Formulating an Area for Growth

The Evolving Focus within MI

Module Purpose

This module invites you to identify an area of either personal or professional growth. Doing so provides a highly relevant and personalized focus for us to experience the ***self-practice/ self-reflective process (SP/SR)*** as we work through the remaining modules. By the end of this module, it is our hope that you will have experienced what it might be like for clients to undertake the process of identifying areas of growth and their ***readiness to engage*** in the process of change. Formulating a specific, personal/professional area for growth and change also supports your *experience* of the SP/SR process.

The *Why*: How MI Begins

Often in our helping encounters, we begin with the assumption that people arrive ready to start. Yet, a moment's thought tells us this is not the case. People arrive in varying states of readiness to change because change is often complex. Moreover, they may be at various states of readiness within a particular domain of change, and initially there may be a lack of awareness regarding what the specific focus for change is or what the causal factors might be. As a result, we regard readiness to change as a fluid concept and the targets of change as evolving over time as our collaborative understanding of the presenting difficulties unfolds (Rosengren, 2017). Thus, initial assessment can be simple, complex, and everything in between depending on a range of factors within the broad target area. Whatever the focus, MI always begins with where the client is. For example, if we are working with a client who does not see the benefit in doing so, we might begin our conversation with a very simple statement and question: "I know you're unhappy about coming to see me. What do you have to do to not see me any more?" Doing so specifically acknowledges and accepts the client's current situation/feeling state. By expecting and demonstrating understanding, and then from the beginning, aligning with the client's goal—*not coming to see me any longer*—this begins the ***task of engaging***.

The *What*: Assessment within an MI Frame of Reference

There is no battery of instruments associated with MI. However, there are some commonalities for assessment within an MI working framework. First, we are much more concerned with the person and engaging them in whatever process we are undertaking (discussed more in Modules 2, 7–10). Second, MI is not the only thing we do as practitioners, and therefore assessment of a domain or domains of interest that focus our work makes sense. This could be symptom-based, such as with high-risk alcohol or drug choices, depression or anxiety symptoms, exercise, diet, or it could be focused on positive psychology concepts like resilience, character strengths, or life satisfaction. Or it might target the elements a practitioner views as essential within a broader theoretical model. For example, the practitioner might view a symptom focus as an initial entry point into exploring a behavioral avoidance pattern related to an underlying, unresolved causal factor (e.g., complex trauma, loss, or attachment issues). Third, there may be a measure of readiness to change included in assessment. These methods span from traditional psychological measures like the University of Rhode Island Change Assessment (URICA; McConnaughy et al., 1983) or Stages of Change Readiness and Treatment Eagerness Scale (SOCRATES; Miller & Tonigan, 1996) to staging checklists, readiness rulers, or metaphors (e.g., acorn to new growth to sapling to mighty oak). Fourth, and circling back to where we began, all these measures are secondary to the MI practitioner's tasks of engaging with the client, and specifically the dual tasks of creating comfort and safety and understanding the bigger picture of the client's life. For the purposes of our work together, we will use two readiness rulers, as brief, assessments for readiness to change.

In addition, because this is a book about developing MI practitioner skills, we have also included a link to a measure for assessing current MI skill level at the end of this chapter. This is a simple self-assessment to help focus our attention on areas where we might need to invest energy and effort, as well as recognizing areas where we already feel capable in our MI skills. This assessment would not be a part of a client experience with an MI practitioner, but it may be something we would encourage trainees to use as part of their learning within this text and more broadly.

The *How*: Identifying My Challenge for the SP/SR Process

Overview of the Exercise

This is a book about self-practice and self-reflection, and we need a focus for that self-practice. Within MI, the initial focus in our work with clients is a starting point, and this frequently evolves as the work progresses. We expect such will be true here as well. As a result, we begin by considering the challenges we all experience in life, both personally and professionally, and recognize that these may change as we work together through this book. There is a series of questions to guide this exploration.

Structure of the Exercise

While a practice partner might be helpful for a follow-up discussion, the initial part of this process is meant to be done in an individually directed manner. That is, we consider and explore these areas on our own.

We encourage an uninterrupted time and a quiet place for this process, a location where work can be done undisturbed. Once situated, let's begin by taking some time to think about our experience as a practitioner or factors in our current life situation. Reflect on the difficulties that sometime arise, the events that distress us, or the challenges that push us to do better. Perhaps we find ourselves behaving in ways that bother us, don't reflect our best selves, or don't represent the person we wish to be. Or perhaps we find ourselves in circumstances where we simply wish to do things better or differently. Maybe we feel trapped in these situations and aren't sure how to proceed. Again, these may be personal rather than professional situations.

If focusing on our practitioner-self, the work might target struggles with particular clients, situations, or work-related relationships (e.g., colleagues, supervisors, supervisees). It could be situations where it feels we're unable to make progress, against what seem to be insurmountable headwinds. Maybe our targets are situations where we feel stress, anger, or frustration. Maybe our supervisor wants us to see more clients and move them along more quickly, yet we feel overwhelmed with our current caseload. Or perhaps a particular kind of client or supervisee proves always to be a challenge. In general, good subjects for targets are people, things, or situations we ruminate about, avoid, or dread; places where we feel insecurity.

It could also be a combination of the personal and professional. For example, emotional regulation might always have been a challenge, and it appears with certain types of people, including clients. So, we might choose to work on this issue for both our personal- and professional-self in addressing this challenge.

Finally, embedded in our focus—personal, professional, or both—we expect to explore the value of MI to our work. This *inside out* experience is intended to grow our MI skills, consider the challenges in handling particular situations or deploying concepts, and build confidence in using skills and strategies in a more intentional and directional manner. The bridging questions will assist with this process.

If there is a follow-up discussion with a limited-practice partner, the practitioner's focus is about creating a safe environment and being curious about what the partner discovered and identified through these processes, as well as clarifying the partner's thoughts. ***Listening*** and ***open questions*** will be the tools employed to understand why these areas of challenge are important to the partner, but there is no expectation to interpret the materials, offer insights, or build motivation. The goal is to engage the person.

Traveling Companions: Examples with Takeshi, Quincy, and Sam

Takeshi's challenging problem is a lack of confidence in his therapy skills, particularly in relationship to people he views as more experienced in life than himself. He finds himself feeling anxious whenever he works with someone who's 10 years (or more) older than himself, and this leads him to be tentative and feel incompetent. He does feel more confident in his CBT skills than he does in his MI skills, which is why he's working through this book. He is a 24-year-old cisgender, straight man of Japanese descent who is currently a graduate student in clinical psychology.

Quincy's challenging problem is her rising feelings of burnout, her discouragement, her tendency to quickly judge, and increased irritability with clients and colleagues. This has led to feelings of dread about taking on new clients, confrontational tactics with clients, and withdrawal from or sharp reactions to colleagues. As a reminder, Quincy is a 38-year-old, cisgender, straight woman of African descent who works as an alcohol and drug (AOD) counselor. She has been introduced to MI and has not yet embraced the approach in her work.

Sam's challenging problem is her ambivalence about retirement. She loves her wife Debra and feels pushed by her toward a retirement she isn't ready to embrace. Sam, in her sixties, is a cisgender, gay woman of European descent who suffered a back injury about a decade ago and has shifted her successful therapy practice to address client's health concerns (e.g., managing chronic pain). As part of this, she learned MI and has become increasingly proficient in its use. She would like to become more nuanced and expert in her work.

Self-Practice

➤ ***In the following space, make a list of some of the specific challenges or problems you currently face in either your personal or professional life.***

____

____

____

____

____

____

____

____

____

____

Reviewing the challenges or problems just recorded, consider which you would like to be the starting point for working through these modules. Perhaps it is an issue that links some of the challenges listed, or it may be a very specific challenge that has been with you for some time. In selecting a challenge, choose something that falls within a moderate level of threat. That is, on a scale of 1 = virtually no threat to 10 = extreme threat, choose something that falls in the 5–7 range. We strongly recommend against selecting a problem that is too intense, defined as one that would lead you to recommend treatment for someone else experiencing that same issue. Of course, consistent with an MI approach, we also recognize this is your decision and you know yourself best. In the SP/SR tradition, experts recommend against choosing unresolved trauma, major relationship problems, or other situations that would cause you significant distress if not resolved by the end of the SP/SR process.

➤ ***Once you've selected your starting challenge, describe it in the space below. This description doesn't have to be lengthy but should include enough detail to clarify the issue in your mind.***

___

___

___

___

___

___

___

___

___

➤ ***Now, considering the area you've selected, on a scale of 1–10, how important is it to you to make a change in this area right now, where 1 represents not at all important and 10 equals extremely important?***

___

➤ ***What led you to choose that number versus one 3 points lower (e.g., a 5 vs. a 2)?***

___

___

___

➤ ***What would it take for you to move up one place in importance (e.g., from a 5 to a 6)?***

___

___

___

➤ ***Now that we've considered importance, let's consider confidence. On a scale of 1–10, how confident are you—if you decided to change—that you could change in this area, where 1 represents not at all confident and 10 equals extremely confident?***

___

➤ ***What led you to choose that number versus one 3 points lower (e.g., a 5 vs. a 2)?***

___

___

___

➤ *What would it take for you to move up one place in confidence (e.g., from a 5 to a 6)?*

Self-Reflection

➤ *As you considered the challenges in your life, what did you notice about how you experienced that in your body? What reactions did it elicit? What feelings emerged? What thoughts accompanied those feelings?*

➤ *What was the process like as you selected a target for this work? Did something immediately pop to mind, or did you find yourself* sifting *to select the right one? What drove that process for you?*

➤ *How did the idea of possibly sharing a challenge with someone else fit into the picture of your decision making? How did your body react? What emotions did it engender? What thoughts went through your head in the selection process?*

➤ ***The readiness rulers (e.g., importance and confidence scales) can be a simple assessment tool, but they can also be used to evoke change talk. Early on, this could feel like a subtle form of pressure to begin moving toward change, if handled with pressure rather than curiosity. What did you notice about this as you completed these simple assessments? Why?***

What If: Applying Skills to My Current Context

Bridging Questions to Practitioner-Self

Now, let's shift the focus and begin crossing that reflective bridge. We designed these questions to help us bring the insights from personal self-practice into our work with clients.

➤ ***How might these experiences, in thinking about an area of challenge and the intention of talking about it to someone else, be useful in considering your client's experiences of talking to you? What did you learn about that process? Why does that matter?***

- ***In considering your experience with even this brief assessment process (i.e., the readiness rulers), what do you want to be mindful of in asking participants to complete assessments and in your review of these materials? How might this affect your discussion about the results with them? Why?***

- ***How did this process of undergoing some self-examination influence how you might do your initial assessment with clients? What do you think might need to be different? How will you implement that?***

- ***What are your main takeaway messages from this SP/SR experience in relation to your understanding of the process of formulating an area of growth . . .***
  - ***From a practical perspective?***
  - ***From a theoretical perspective?***

- ***What if you were to apply this process to other areas of your professional practice (e.g., in a role as a supervisor or trainer perhaps)? How might you apply your learning to this new context?***

➤ ***How has this exercise influenced your understanding of, or personal relationship with MI as a way of being?***

____

____

____

Final Thoughts and Applications to Other Settings

Earlier, we mentioned taking this as an opportunity to self-assess your MI skills to provide a baseline and perhaps a focus for your attention and work as you do your limited peer practice. You will find a copy of this assessment, MO 01: Nine Tasks of Learning MI, as well as other forms in this text, at the book's companion site *www.guilford.com/rosengren2-materials*. We also recommend repeating this measure at the completion of the book so you can observe your progress, although you could also use it as a periodic assessment.

Also, we encourage limited partner practice as part of this book. When it is your turn to be the practitioner in this process, you might consider recording the session and coding it using one of the many coding instruments available for this work. You can find more information on coding instruments at the companion website. While this is not therapy and therefore does not fall under HIPAA regulation for American readers, it should be considered confidential material, and the recording should be destroyed once the review process is completed.

MI is used in many settings. By necessity, in this module, we've remained relatively broad in our discussion. Subsequent modules will offer more specific examples of how MI might be extended beyond the traditional therapy setting.

MODULE 2

Four Tasks of MI

Module Purpose

This module invites you to experience the ***four tasks of MI*** in relation to the area of personal/professional change and growth identified in Module 1. By the end of this module, it is our hope that the experience of the intentional practice of ***engaging*** and ***focusing*** generates thinking around how the four tasks can be used as a guide to structure an MI conversation without being linear or prescriptive.

The *Why*: The Tasks of MI Help Us Understand What, When, and Why to Do Something

As MI practitioners, we need to understand how we move through both an individual session and through the arc of a treatment episode with a client. By comprehending this movement together, we better understand the nuances of *Why* we are doing things at particular times and not at others. Miller and Rollnick (2013) described four concepts, which they referred to as processes initially, and offered general guidance on how we might use these ideas to help us in this work. In the most recent edition of their MI book, Miller and Rollnick (2023) have refined these ideas and described these as ***four tasks*** that pose implicit questions to clients:

- ***Engaging:*** Should we take a walk together?
- ***Focusing:*** Where shall we go?
- ***Evoking:*** Why will we go here?
- ***Planning:*** How will we get there?

Miller and Rollnick (2023) refer to MI as a flowing conversation. There is not a specific blueprint, but instead a conversation that will unfold between us. Understanding why we're doing things at a particular time helps guide us to choose what to do and how to do it in the moment.

The *What*: What Are the Tasks and What Tools Accompany These?

Miller and Rollnick (2023) view these tasks as the embodiment of MI. That is, these ideas encompass and integrate the ***spirit of MI*** and the techniques of MI (e.g., ***OARS+I***), which we will discuss in subsequent modules. Together, the relationship and technical elements form a structure for *What*, *How*, and *When* to do things. Principles of MI articulated by Miller and Rollnick previously (1991, 2013) are integrated into the tasks.

The tasks imply linearity. That is, we begin with engaging and then, once that is accomplished, we move to focusing. After we know what is important, then we move into the differential attention to change and sustain talk in evoking. Once motivation has been solidified and initial commitment reached, then we move into planning. It's a simple, easy-to-understand, four-step plan, which is, of course, not accurate. People do not just move in one direction through these tasks. Nor do they move in a straight line. Rather, it is an evolving interpersonal dynamic that may often involve a movement back and forward both within and across the four tasks. For example, a person who has suffered a traumatic loss and a subsequent loss of safety and identity may cycle in and out of engaging with the practitioner and the therapeutic process, with what is most important currently, and reasons for changing or protecting the status quo. As a result, other metaphors have been introduced. Sometimes it is presented as a hill or mountain where the first three tasks represent the hard climb up and the fourth reflects the trip down the other side. While this captures the relative effort exerted, it doesn't quite capture the bidirectional nature of the process. At other times, these are depicted as stairs, each task building on the prior level. This is how Miller and Rollnick (2023) describe the tasks in their most recent edition, and this does feel closer, though perhaps it removes an important part of the sequence—our moving up and down the stairs with the person. A better metaphor might be a dance done together moving up and down the stairs, with occasional jumps or falls to lower levels. The tasks are done in coordination with the other person, trying to move in sequence and rhythm, though succeeding only imperfectly. When done in a group, the process becomes even more complex.

With that dancing on stairs metaphor in mind, here are some short definitions and questions we might ask ourselves, drawn from Miller and Rollnick (2023), to see how we're fitting—as practitioners—within this stair dance.

Engaging is the first task and focuses on this implicit question, *Should we take a walk together?* We aim to provide a safe, comfortable environment within which people can explore difficult realities within their life. This does not mean they are comfortable with the issues or challenges in their lives, but they are comfortable exploring them with us. They feel welcomed and safe within our presence and thus decide they're willing to walk with us. As part of this task, we seek to understand the big picture of their world, as well as how the current issue, desire, or challenge fits within it. In this manner, we learn their areas of strength and resources, which can be called on in later tasks. This task happens at the beginning of either a treatment or a helping process, but also each time the person reengages in this process. To help us assess where *we* are in engaging with our clients, we might pose these questions to ourselves:

- How comfortable am I in this conversation? Where do I experience this is my body?
- What am I doing to help increase the client's comfort?
- In what ways does this feel like a partnership?

- How accepting am I of this person?
- Am I feeling compassion toward this person?
- What am I picking up as important to this person?
- How is the current issue or challenge impacting on this person and why?
- What strengths and resources do they have that I may need to work (later?) to evoke with this person?

Focusing, the second task, asks, *Where shall we go?* We look to understand what is important to the person both in this moment and in the big picture of their life. This necessitates that we be present in the current moment while retaining awareness of what this person wants beyond this moment. Once we understand these things more clearly, we can begin to move forward. It is also when we might begin to weave our agenda into that process.

Our agenda is often dictated by the context of our work together. Thus, someone working in a hospice setting will have a different agenda than a person working in a physical rehabilitation setting than someone employed in an alcohol and drug treatment center. There is a balance that we seek in working within our role with each client. Our agenda is transparent, not transcendent. It is secondary to the client's autonomy.

Miller and Rollnick (2023) observe that sometimes the goals are ***clear***, straightforward and the path seemingly apparent. At others, the long-term objective is clear, but many paths exist to get there. We assist the client in ***choosing***. Finally, there are times the goals are not clear, and our task is to help the client ***clarify***.

Questions we might ask ourselves in the moment with clients (i.e., self-reflecting *in action*):

- Do I understand what matters to them and why?
- Have I communicated my understanding of what matters to them?
- Are my aspirations in line with what matters to them?
- Are we dancing or wrestling together in our movement toward a common goal/purpose?

The third task, *evoking*, asks, *Why will we go there?* Together, we're exploring and perhaps discovering people's reasons—their *Why*—for change. We listen for, and seek to cultivate, more ***change talk*** and soften ***sustain talk***, all the while supporting the client's autonomy to choose. Helen Mentha (2020) notes that sustain talk is already getting lots of oxygen in clients' lives. Our aim is to give the change talk a little more oxygen. Of course, we cannot do this until we understand what is important to them through the focusing process. After we have elicited it, we seek to consolidate it and, if the client is ready, move toward commitment to an action. Questions we might pose to ourselves in the moment (i.e., self-reflecting *in action*) include:

- How well do I understand the client's reasons for changing?
- To what degree do I understand how important these reasons are for this person?
- Why now?
- What is giving them confidence in their ability to instigate and/or implement change?
- What is telling me if they are moving toward commitment?
- How is the desire to fix this issue (i.e., the ***fixing reflex***, Modules 18 and 19) pulling me?

Finally, the *planning* task asks, *How will we get there?* We can also think of this as evoking the client's *How* for change. Not surprisingly then, a series of questions might help guide our journey through this task. How might they go about doing it? What are their thoughts and ideas about making this change? What has worked for them in the past? We work with clients to develop plans that fit with their lives and skills, and what they're willing to do. It always starts with the client, and this is where our expertise can be helpful. To be clear, these are questions intermixed with a great deal of listening, ***summarizing***, ***affirming*** of capacity, and offering ideas when appropriate and with permission.

Questions we might pose to ourselves about planning include do I understand:

- How they think they would begin?
- How they might use their strengths, skills, and knowledge?
- What additional information might be helpful to evoke or exchange to assist in planning?

The tools to accomplish these tasks will be described in the remaining modules. While the basic skills remain the same, there will be different emphases at different times. For example, offering small bites of information can be helpful for people as they consider working with us during engaging. They need to know what we have to offer before they can decide if this will be a safe and comfortable place to try to accomplish their aims; that is, that they do want to walk with us. Information exchange will also be an important part of the planning process, though the nature of what and perhaps how much to share will be different.

Our intent will vary in our use of these skills as we move through the tasks. For example, ***reflective listening*** will be used to communicate our understanding of the person and their situation, and to help them feel safe during engaging. In focusing, it will be to understand what matters deeply and why. In evoking, we will sharpen awareness of change talk and solidify motivation through what we pay attention to in the conversation. In planning, we will reinforce commitment and consolidate plans, as well as organize information through our listening. Similarly, ***open questions*** will be broadly focused in engaging to help understand the big picture of the person's life and might ask specifically for areas of strength or resources. For example, *Where do you feel you're doing okay in your life right now?* In focusing, the questions will be designed to elicit what matters, which can be done directly or indirectly. For example, *What might a perfect day for you look like?* With evoking, the questions begin asking for change talk in a more specific and intentional manner. Notice how this question asks for statements of ability, *When your coach says you're not ready, what experiences tell you she's wrong in her assessment?* Finally with planning, the questions might begin with a more general focus, *What have you thought about doing?* However, there is not a hard rule, as a more specific question might fit some time-limited contexts better, *What's one or two small things you think you might be able to do now to help yourself feel healthier?*

The remaining modules will help deepen your understanding of concepts, as in the *MI* spirit, tools like *values* clarification, and skills such as *OARS+I*. As we move deeper into the book, some modules—like Module 22: Building *My* Plan—are specific to a task. However, in general, we should remember the dancers on the stairs. We will need to move fluidly among the skills, stepping lightly together up and down the stairs, as the client moves toward change.

The How: SP/SR on the Experience and Value of Engaging and Focusing

Overview of the Exercise

For this activity, you will need a limited-practice partner. Indeed, the activity is built around the start of limited practice together. Much as what happens in an initial encounter with a practitioner, this session will open with some discussion of the roles and expectations of this practice. Then the process will move into engaging and possibly into focusing.

Structure of the Exercise

While the work done together will focus on the challenge or area of growth identified in Module 1, we recommend that you do not narrow your attention to this initially. When in the role of practitioner in this practice, we encourage you to instead begin with making this a safe and comfortable environment for your partner. Ironically, if you already know each other well, this might be harder as you already have some boundaries, even if unspoken, about what will and will not be discussed and this work may press against those. We might assume we know everything there is to know about our partner. This situation requires us to look with fresh eyes and listen with keen ears to what we think we already know and discover what we don't.

The questions posed here are designed to guide and focus the conversations. However, like MI, they are not a specific blueprint. Use them to help find your way into the conversation and to keep the conversation on track. Utilize the skills you've already learned about MI and in this instance focus on the global intent of the tasks—engaging and focusing. Below is a general structure you may find helpful. As will be true in every module, listening and summarizing are assumed to be used well between questions; without this, it may feel more like a highly structured interview or even an interrogation. Even though the term *interviewing* is used to describe this approach, we need to remember that it is simply a particular way of talking with people about change and growth to strengthen their own motivation and commitment (Miller & Rollnick, 2023, p. 3).

Here is the flow of the conversation:

- Welcome the person into the practice space.
- Elicit their understanding of how this work is to proceed.
- Discuss boundaries for this work.
- Elicit what is going well in their world presently.
- Work to understand the big picture.
- Listen for values and goals.
- Introduce the area of challenge or growth.
- Be curious without an intention to solve.

Traveling Companion: An Example with Takeshi

Takeshi will help us illustrate this exercise. Recall that he is a 24-year-old, cisgender, straight man of Japanese heritage working on his doctorate in clinical psychology. Stress and high expectations have been ongoing issues. He is a strong student and shows promise as a counselor. He feels some frustration about his clients' lack of change at times. He sought out MI training at the suggestion of his supervisor and sees the value in it, though he doesn't feel as confident in this approach as he does in CBT.

➤ ***What is your understanding about the nature of this work we will be doing together?***

This is an opportunity for me to do some personal work. Feeling confident and managing frustration in my clinical work are both areas I'd like to grow. In terms of this work, my understanding is that we'll be meeting regularly to go through these modules together. You will be my "therapist" and then I will be yours. We're not supposed to have anything too dark or too deep as our focus.

➤ ***What boundaries or limits make sense to you as we begin this work together? How should we handle things like discussions out of this setting?***

Well, the obvious I suppose. We keep this information confidential. I can share about my process and issues with others, if I choose, but you cannot. The same is true for you. I think it makes sense to limit our discussion of these issues to this "limited-practice" space, but I think we should be able to talk about MI outside of here. Yes? I don't know. What do you think?

➤ ***What do you hope might happen because of this practice?***

Well, it's two levels, right? I get some insight about myself and become more confident and feel more capable in my work. But, I also want to understand how to do MI better. By doing this process, our professor said we should gain some insight into what helps and what doesn't. I'm hoping it will help me to "get" MI on a deeper level I suppose.

➤ ***What concerns do you carry into this practice?***

Same ones I always do. Will I be any good at MI as a practitioner? Am I going to be helpful to you? I also worry about feeling exposed when I share my stuff. It feels embarrassing and we do spend a lot of time trying to be competent, and let's face it, we do compete for things like assistantships and scholarships. It feels a little risky, even though we know each other, and I like you.

➤ ***Let's step back and look at the big picture of your life. Where are things going well in your life presently? Where are you having some success?***

Overall, I think I'm doing okay. My grades are good. I'm making good progress in my requirements at school, though sometimes it feels a little overwhelming. I get along well with my parents, though my mom can be a little much at times. Still, I like seeing them and spending time together. I've always been able to make friends, and while it's harder in graduate school, I feel like I'm still connected. In terms of my therapy work, I'm pretty good at the diagnostics and creating plans. I think I have a pretty good handle on what CBT is and the tools we can use within it.

➤ ***If you're willing, please tell me a story that captures some important parts of who you are.***

In high school, as part of senior year symphonic orchestra, we had an option to play a featured solo as one of the performances during the year. It was never a question that I was going to do this. I expected to do it. My parents didn't require it, but they do expect me to push myself. It's funny because not everyone did it, but it never even entered my mind not to do it.

I chose a tough piece because, well, why not? I practiced almost every day until the show in February. I've done a lot of recitals, so I'm pretty used to performing, but that night we had a guest violinist from the local symphony, and it just made me anxious. Like really? Tonight? But once we got tuned, and then I walked back out on stage, it's just like I dropped into the zone. Position, breath, first note, and away we went. I know it sounds like bragging, but I crushed it. Only a couple of things I wished I'd done better. I got a standing "O" from the crowd and that was cool, though you know, it is just a bunch of parents and other kids who know me, but still it felt good.

➤ ***What is the area you want to focus on in this work?***

I want to feel more like I did during that violin solo in my work with clients. Like I know this stuff and can just drop into it. Not worry about, "Am I doing it right?" "And why aren't they doing the homework?" I just want to be confident that I know my stuff and I'm doing it as well as I can. I also know that I tend to feel a little weird around guys who are older than me, and I want to figure out what's up with that.

➤ ***What makes this important to you now?***

If I go back to the violin, it's like this: I know how to play the notes, but putting it together with confidence and feeling is when the music really happens. I feel like that is sort of where I'm at with my skills. I'm competent, but I want to be great, and I feel like it's the little nuances that matter. And this is the time to learn.

➤ ***How does this fit into the big picture of your life?***

Well, as you probably guessed, I don't do things part way. If I'm going to do it, I want to do it well. It is the vocation—being a therapist—I didn't start out to do, but I like it and that means I want to do it well. School is my focus now and while there are lots of other parts to school, this is the one—doing therapy—I feel most unsure about. So, this is a big thing for me right now.

Self-Practice

Your task is straightforward. Engage with the questions. If you're doing this in a self-directed manner, write out your answers as though you were talking to your limited-practice partner. Make your answers reflect your authentic voice. If you're working with a limited-practice partner, have a conversation using these questions as prompts. You might consider writing down your answers before the conversation and then just talking—not reading—about your thoughts with your partner. To be clear, not just asking questions but also ***responding with listening statements are essential.*** Offering small bits of information might be helpful as well.

➤ ***What is your understanding about the nature of this work we will be doing together?***

____

____

____

____

____

➤ ***What boundaries or limits make sense to you as we begin this work together? How should we handle things like discussions out of this setting?***

____

____

____

____

____

➤ ***What do you hope might happen because of this practice?***

____

____

____

____

____

____

➤ ***What concerns do you carry into this practice?***

____

____

____

____

____

____

➤ ***Let's step back and look at the big picture of your life. Where are things going well in your life presently? Where are you having some success?***

____

____

____

____

____

➤ ***If you're willing, please tell me a story that captures some important parts of who you are.***

____

____

____

____

____

➤ ***What is the area you want to focus on in this work?***

____

____

____

____

____

➤ ***What makes this important to you now?***

____

____

____

____

➤ ***How does this fit into the big picture of your life?***

____

____

____

____

____

Self-Reflection

Normally in the self-reflection portion of the module, we will not include the thoughts of the traveling companion. This is because we want this area to reflect ***your thoughts*** about the process and not be matched to a model for the "correct" responses. However, we are aware that an initial model can be a useful guide for the kinds of reactions one person might have to these questions. Below you will find Takeshi's responses to this module. However, you will not typically find these in future modules.

➤ ***What did you notice in your body as you started talking about the nature of this limited practice?***

I was tense. My hands were a little damp, and I just felt a bit physically uncomfortable, which is weird because I was looking forward to this and I know and like my partner a lot. But this put us in a different role and it's like when I sat down, it was like, "Oh crap, this is strange." But, then I felt myself relax as we worked our way through those and pivoted to where things are going well.

➤ ***What emotions accompanied this process for you?***

I was nervous, anxious, and I guess excited. I've been curious about what this would be like and what I would discover. I guess hopeful, too, as it might help me get better in my clinical work and my MI skills, and that's really what I am looking for through this whole thing.

➤ ***What specifically was helpful in this process? What was not? Why?***

Well, it's funny—because I know about asking for strengths to begin and I looked at the questions ahead of time—but still being asked about what's going well really did help me think about those things. As I did, I had this thought, "A lot of stuff is going well," which is weird, because if you'd have asked me how I am doing, I would probably have said, "Meh, I'm okay." It really did give me a boost.

What didn't help . . . when my partner stayed on the surface with her listening. It just felt like it didn't go anywhere. It felt more like a technique. When she went deeper, it didn't. It seemed like she was really understanding me—or at least trying to.

➤ ***What value did you experience in having your partner understand the big picture of your life? Why is this important in the process?***

It's surprising to me because my partner and me are classmates. We spend a lot of time together—talking, sharing ideas, talking about our worries, but this was a whole new level of sharing. I feel like I revealed more of myself in this discussion than I had across many others. I feel ready to move into some of my challenges and fears.

Okay, now it's your turn. Please find a quiet space where you can do this writing. This is meant to be done alone and not necessarily shared with your partner. Keep in mind the difference between private and public reflections noted in Chapter 5.

➤ ***What did you notice in your body as you started talking about the nature of this limited practice?***

➤ ***What emotions accompanied this process for you?***

➤ ***What specifically was helpful in this process? What was not? Why?***

➤ ***What value did you experience in having your partner understand the big picture of your life? Why is this important in the process?***

What If: Applying Skills to My Current Context

Bridging Questions to Practitioner-Self

These questions are designed to help you bring the insights from personal self-practice into your work with clients. Again, to assist you in the process of learning self-reflection in the context of the bridging process, we're offering some of Takeshi's thoughts in this module to see and feel what these might be. Future modules will not offer this kind of example information.

➤ ***How does this experience help you understand the process of engaging with new clients? What about with current clients?***

I definitely felt the power of spending the time engaging. It helped me to lean into the process of this work and feel connected with my partner. I am very aware of how I often want to focus on the problem area quickly because that's why the client came in. But noticing how this session felt, beginning with "rules and roles," I noticed the tension, even for something I wanted. I can imagine better how that feels for my clients, especially those who are very ambivalent or even in precontemplation. They don't want to be here, but someone sent them. It certainly fits a lot of the men I've seen. I'm betting that my tension in combination with their tension is creating a lot for us to overcome.

➤ ***How might you integrate this learning into how you begin with new clients? What about with current clients?***

Well, that's not a big leap. I think rules and roles are helpful, but I'm also aware that the less time spent there, the better. Just enough to fulfill legal requirements and then let's get into the other stuff. By other stuff, it's clearly better to start with the big picture and strengths. The focus will emerge, but we will both be better situated to explore it if we take that time. I think even a short statement about that would be helpful. That's for new clients. For returning clients, I think it's about being more intentional about how I begin the session. It sets the tone and I'm aware of how my answer would've been "meh" if my partner asked me how I was doing. I'm thinking that I wanted to choose an intentional question to begin, "What went well this past week?" Or "Where did you have some success?" Or maybe "Where are you seeing some improvement and why?"

➤ ***What changes might you make?***

I need to slow down and do more listening. I've been way too quick to jump into planning when clients are still deciding if this is a safe place and what their agenda is for this work. I know in my MI class they talked about if we slow down it might actually go faster, and I am very aware of that today. By jumping to the CBT tools, I thought I was helping the client move ahead, but I was actually getting in the way. So, my plan is this: Slow down.

➤ ***How has this exercise influenced your understanding of or personal relationship with MI as a way of being?***

I am aware that it is not just a matter of slowing down. I feel like I need to do techniques. If I'm honest, it's doing things to people, instead of being with them. That makes me uncomfortable to say, but I think it's true. It's part of this performance thing where I want to do things well and know what I'm doing. I need to practice just being with people. It deepened my understanding of what way of being means, even though my practice isn't there yet.

Now it's your turn. Again, find a quiet place to write. These questions are designed to help you bring the insights from personal self-practice into your work with clients.

> *How does this experience help you understand the process of engaging with new clients? What about with current clients?*

> *How might you integrate this learning into how you begin with new clients? What about with current clients?*

> *What changes might you make?*

> *What are your main* takeaway *messages from this SP/SR experience in relation to your understanding of the four tasks of MI . . .*

- *From a practical perspective?*

- ***From a theoretical perspective?***

➤ ***What if you were to apply this process to other areas of your professional practice (e.g., in a role as supervisor or trainer perhaps)? How might you apply your learning to this new context?***

➤ ***How has this exercise influenced your understanding of or personal relationship with MI as a way of being?***

Final Thoughts and Applications to Other Settings

A great deal of deliberate practice can be done to target skills to the different tasks. Rosengren (2017), for example, provides opportunities to use the same sentence stems to create open questions and reflective listening statements across all four tasks. We might think of this as the *How* of MI. This book asks us to focus on another question, *Why*. Why here, why now, and why in this way? Through the process of experiencing the skills as a recipient, we come to know why a reflection done to understand more deeply and clearly during engaging may feel more powerful and useful than a reflection done to emphasize the importance of a change. We can also experience how techniques or strategies can feel out of step with our readiness. For example, how a question can feel like a subtle form of pressure where a reflection does not. MI may be done in situations where there will be a single contact. Or where there are contacts spread over long periods of time, like health care providers doing annual physicals. In these settings, the four tasks might need to be accomplished all in that session. Or it might become clear the person is not ready to make a change or is choosing a route that we are troubled by. Future modules will give more guidance about how to navigate these situations, but for now it is sufficient to note the goal is not to reach the "finish line" of planning. Instead, the aim is to help clients move toward their goals, which at times might not match our aspirations for them.

MODULE 3

Partnership

Module Purpose

This module invites you to experience the value of ***partnership*** in supporting people through change and growth. We conceptualize partnership as attitudinal (e.g., our view that clients are equal and active partners in the process) and behavioral (what we do and how we do it). By the end of this module, it is our hope that by reflecting on a current experience of an important but challenging partnership, you will experience how the combination of these attitudinal and behavioral elements interacts and can at times become out of balance, and what restores them to a more equitable footing in a genuine partnership.

The *Why*: Partnership Creates a Foundation

Within MI, there are two primary components that writers and trainers will articulate as core (Miller & Rose, 2009). The heart set of MI, known as ***MI spirit*** and that we review in Modules 3–6, and the mindset or technical skills of MI, which we explore in Modules 7–22. The skills are the *doing* of MI and the spirit is the *being*. We cannot have MI without both parts being present.

MI spirit, in turn, has four elements: ***partnership, acceptance, compassion, and envisioning (PACE).*** We will explore each with the present module focused on partnership. All these elements have an *attitudinal* as well as a ***behavioral** component.* These components differ in their observability. Behavioral components tend to be more externally observable, and thus by recording and reviewing our work, these can aid us in ***reflection** on action*. That is, because they are *external* and measurable, they are more *accessible* to self and others. Yet, the attitudinal aspects, which are perhaps more difficult to access, may be more important as they tell us more about our *intention* as a practitioner. Still, research suggests we can tap into intention via the use of recordings as prompts (Jefferis et al., 2021). We'll discuss this more later.

Partnership recognizes the value and necessary contributions of the parties involved in the therapeutic relationship. MI views the parties as coequals, even though the experience brought by each to this encounter is quite different. As practitioners, we arrive at this session with a learning and experience history that structures our understanding of the nature of problems experienced by clients. We also have theories as to essential elements that will assist them in change processes, and knowledge of methods to intervene successfully. Indeed, it may *feel* as though we understand the nature of the problem and know the solution after a short amount of discussion with a client. On the flip side, clients bring a learning and experience history of themselves. They know their experiences, needs and values, life contexts, and motivations better than we do. While their view will be incomplete and they may benefit from the additional views a practitioner might offer, the client is *the* expert in all these areas. The MI practitioner recognizes and respects the essential roles of each partner and embodies this partnership by being curious and using a style that assists the client in moving in the direction of the client's aims, goals, and values. However, this does not tell us what partnership looks like in practice.

The *What*: Attitudes and Behaviors for Enacting Partnership

Since there are both attitudinal and behavioral components, we'll address both together, recognizing the behavioral component will be easier to observe. The attitudinal component includes recognizing that the client is a capable and equal partner in this process, so we want to ask for their ideas and thoughts about where to begin our work, how we should work, and what would be useful for them. When we encounter problems, we work together to solve them, and this begins with finding out what they've considered, tried, and know about what works for them. We look for and note strengths and capabilities in clients instead of deficits and limitations. It's about what the client can do, not what they can't. Finally, there will be points of disagreement along the way, and we will need to engage productively around these. As we see in later modules, we'll want to offer information and feedback (including concerns), but how we do that is critical; most importantly, client views are what ultimately matter in this circumstance. They will be enacting change, not us, so they will need to decide. As suggested above, there is not one single behavior that corresponds to partnership, but rather a cluster of attitudes and behaviors that reflect its presence. Moreover, its absence is observable on rating scales like the ***MI Treatment Integrity Scale*** (***MITI***; Moyers et al., 2016).

Unlike other communication and counseling methods that have specific techniques associated with their use, MI is primarily *a way of being with* clients, using skills that are common to many therapies. Thus, by necessity, the self-practice techniques identified here are meant to capture not only specific techniques but also the quality of these experiences. Indeed, some of these experiences are not "MI" per se, but instead are focused on catching this quality of the MI interaction. Having said that, these practice exercises could be used by an MI practitioner with a little forethought and alteration to fit a client situation. The exercise that follows is an example of this process.

Finally, a word about language conventions. In this book, the word "skill" is used to denote a discrete behavior. It includes actions like producing reflections or open questions. Techniques or strategies refer to a larger combination of skills and/or structured activities. Thus, reflective listening contains a combination of skills such as asking ***open questions***, producing ***reflections***, offering ***affirmations,*** and creating ***summaries***, and so it would be a technique. Similarly, an exercise in this book may draw on a particular skill or skill set. A readiness ruler would be a technique used by many MI practitioners, within which skills—asking for ***change talk*** by the nature of the follow-up probe and responding with reflections—are emphasized.

The *How*: SP/SR on Becoming Aware of a Relationship Imbalance

Overview of the Exercise

Batman and Robin evolved from comic book pages to camp TV series to larger-than-life superheroes on the cinema screen and are often referred to as the Dynamic Duo. While it's true they have unique skill sets, it seems that Batman is nearly always the person in charge. Several years ago, when D. B. R. was doing a training with a dear friend and training partner, the training partner quipped, "I feel like Robin to your Batman." The partnership was unbalanced in the training work. This shift in relationship happened unintentionally and unconsciously as D. B. R. focused on getting tasks done. By identifying the imbalance, the partner created an opportunity to restore the relational balance.

In our work with clients, this relational balance can also become unequal. This can be due to a gradual shift, something specific about this client, a general belief or attitude we bring into our work with clients. For example, we may prematurely focus on task orientation as we view it as valued "intervention work," perhaps exacerbated by the health or social care system that we work within, at the expense of a relational focus. It might also be inevitable that at certain times the balance may shift. However, our general aim, as MI practitioners, is for the client to have more control, autonomy, and self-determination as they progress through the work with the practitioner. Within that framework, our first task is to recognize any inequality in the relational balance. However, this can feel a bit nebulous as we try to decipher the balance. Perhaps it's made easier when we think in terms of the Batman and Robin metaphor.

This exercise involves a review of an important partnership we have presently. This relationship might be with a client, a fellow professional, or someone in our personal life. Using the Batman and Robin metaphor and a series of questions, we will explore the relational balance and whether it has shifted.

Structure of the Exercise

This activity works well when done in a self-directed manner. However, it can be done as a discussion with a limited-practice partner.

If you do this as a discussion, when in the role of the MI practitioner, we encourage you to be curious in your follow-up to the questions. Keep in mind this idea of partnership and how the two of you can explore this task together. It is not an interrogation, but an exploration. The questions posed here are meant to guide and focus your conversations. However, like MI, they are not a specific blueprint. Use them to help find your way into the conversation and to keep the conversation on track. Use the skills you've already learned about MI to be a partner in this exploration. Bear in mind that becoming aware of a relationship imbalance may feel uncomfortable for your partner, so it is essential to create a safe place for this to occur. Below is a general structure you may find helpful. As will be true in every module, empathic listening and summarizing are assumed to be inserted in between questions.

Here are some Dynamic Duo balance questions:

- Who is driving the Batmobile and who is riding in the passenger seat?
- When you and the client are not sure what to do (about the Joker, e.g.), how do you talk about it? How does this get resolved?
- How are decisions made, especially when you disagree?
- What does your fellow caped crusader bring to this process? What do they do better than you and why?
- How does trust play into what you're observing here?

You might observe there is a playful quality to these questions. Batman and Robin? Really? This is in part personal style, and it's also a reflection of the quality of the work. This is serious business we're engaged in with clients but that does not mean all moments need to be somber. Indeed, if part of the goal is to create a safe and comfortable environment within which clients can explore difficult realities, then a bit of gentle humor and playfulness can help us in that endeavor (Fredrickson, 2009; Sarink & García-Montes, 2023). Indeed, researchers have even found that introducing humor into robots' programming in health care increases feelings of safety and experiences of empathy for patients (Johanson et al., 2020). Just to be clear, humor is more than jokes and laughter; it is finding the amusing and playful.

Traveling Companion: An Example with Quincy

Quincy is a 38-year-old, cisgender, straight woman of African descent who works as an AOD counselor. Growing up in a vibrant community, she has strong family ties and a foundation of giving to others. She was feeling some burnout with substance use clients and has taken an MI workshop, but it hasn't found its way into her work. Because of her feelings of burnout, she sought personal support and decided to find a therapist skilled in MI to learn more about the process. Q's therapist asked her to consider these questions in relationship to a client whom she was struggling with. Here were Q's answers:

➤ ***Who is driving the Batmobile and who is in the passenger seat?***

Oh, yeah. I have most definitely been Batman and have been doing all the driving. It didn't used to be this way, but I don't trust their driving to get us where we need to go. With this recent client, I felt like she's just too new in the process and her brain's still too impaired to let her drive.

➤ ***When the two of you are not sure what to do (about the Joker, e.g.), how do you talk about it? How does this get resolved?***

We've been meeting Jokers all over the place. It's interesting because I don't feel particularly uncertain about what to do, but clients do. My response has been to tell them what to do, and that's what I did with this client. I felt like she wasn't seeing the road ahead, and my job was to show her so she can change. I guess I resolved it. I'm recognizing now that it might not be such a good idea.

➤ ***How are decisions made, especially when you disagree?***

I've been making the decisions because I feel like I must. I've viewed disagreements as her denial about the consequences of her use. It's funny because I don't see myself as a particularly confrontational counselor—I'm always kind, compassionate, and respectful—but as I am thinking about this . . . I am seeing that respect and partnership are not the same.

➤ ***What does your fellow caped crusader bring to this process? What do they do better than you do and why?***

I am realizing that I haven't really been thinking about my clients as fellow caped crusaders. More like they're the Joker and I need to round 'em up, not be fooled, and helping them see the error of their ways. I hate to admit it, but I think my tendency would be to say they lie better than I do. Yuck! Do I really think that? If I take a step back, I think I've been focusing on me and my thoughts and feelings, not on them. If I stop for even half a second, I know they have courage, maybe more than me, to come to the agency and do this work again and again. I also know they are good problem solvers, though I wouldn't agree with their solutions always. They're also tough. Their situations demand this of them, so they must rise to the occasion, or they never make it back. All of that is true for my client. She's also funny. She's always got something to say, and she's quick. Even when I feel frustrated with her, I laugh.

➤ ***How does trust play into what you're observing here?***

I guess part of what I am seeing here is that I haven't really trusted my partners. I feel like I've been burned and so I am being self-protective, which is getting in the way of my work. I think it's their lying and that is wearing, but I'm also not stepping up. I am not putting myself out there, and as a result, I am not connecting with people like I did before. I know rapport and alliance are important, and it seems like I've been undermining it.

Notice as Q reflects on these questions, there are some issues that are quite challenging for her. In MI, we refer to these as *motivating **discrepancies***. Motivation can be both going toward something we desire, as well as away from something we do not want. Our framing of it might determine how we view what happens next, not the nature of the original discrepancy. The importance of the other elements of MI spirit, like acceptance and compassion, become important in this unfolding process.

Self-Practice

Think about an important relationship in your life where you've been struggling. This could be at work or in your personal life. If it is connected to the area you've chosen to focus on for this book, all the better. Then answer these questions.

➤ ***Who is driving the Batmobile and who is riding in the passenger seat?***

➤ ***When the two of you are not sure what to do (about the Joker, e.g.), how do you talk about it? How does this get resolved?***

➤ ***How are decisions made, especially when you disagree?***

➤ ***What does your fellow caped crusader bring to this process? What do they do better than you do and why?***

➤ ***How does trust play into what you're observing here?***

Self-Reflection

Please find a quiet space where you can do this writing. This is meant to be done alone and not necessarily shared with your partner. Keep in mind the difference between private and public reflections noted in Chapter 5.

- ***What was your experience when thinking about your role as part of the Dynamic Duo? What did you notice in your body? What feelings did you experience? What thoughts did you have?***

- ***How do these experiences reflect your bigger life experience with relationships at work (e.g., colleagues, clients) or in your personal life (e.g., partners)? In what ways are they the same or different? Why?***

- ***What specifically was helpful in this process? What was not? Why?***

What If: Applying Skills to My Current Context

Bridging Questions to Practitioner-Self

These questions are designed to help you bring the insights from personal self-practice into your work with clients.

➤ ***How does this experience help you understand*** **partnership** ***with new clients? What about with current clients?***

➤ ***How might you integrate this learning into how you begin with new clients?***

➤ ***How might this experience be helpful in your work with current clients?***

➤ ***What unique contextual elements do you need to consider in your circumstance? How might this experience assist you in making partnership work in your setting?***

➤ *What did you learn from this that you'd like to remember?*

➤ *What are your main* takeaway *messages from this SP/SR experience in relation to your understanding of the concept of partnership . . .*

- *From a practical perspective?*

- *From a theoretical perspective?*

➤ *What if you were to apply this process to other areas of your professional practice (e.g., in a role as supervisor or trainer perhaps)? How might you apply your learning to this new context?*

➤ *How has this exercise influenced your understanding of or personal relationship with MI as a way of being?*

Final Thoughts and Applications to Other Settings

Of course, your work might also be done in groups. Here, we might have to shift our metaphor. The Avengers, perhaps? The same principles will apply to not only individual members of the group but also to the group as a whole. For example, it's not uncommon for group counselors to slip into a circumstance where interactions flow through them and not between group members. This wagon wheel therapy—where everything flows through the central hub—can begin with counselors' good intent to either communicate understanding by reflecting client statements or create momentum in the group by their active participation. Unfortunately, it has the same effect of a partnership differential—the counselor is driving the Batmobile or Heli carrier, as the superhero case might be.

In brief encounters and different contexts, partnership might look different. A dental hygienist, physical therapist, surgeon, sports coach, and probation officer all have different roles, responsibilities, skill sets, lengths of contact, frequency of contact, and contexts that must be considered. Yet, partnership remains essential in all these situations, even with the surgeon. At times, it can be easy for us to observe the differences in our situation from others and believe this justifies a lack of partnership. Being alert to this tendency can assist us in avoiding its undermining effect on our work with clients, as can understanding *why* it's essential to be partners can help us remain alert.

MODULE 4

Acceptance

Module Purpose

This module invites you to experience what it is like to feel accepted by another and how this supports the process of growth and change. As in Module 2, we also consider nonjudgmental acceptance as a combination of attitudinal and behavioral components. By the end of this module, it is our hope that through reflecting on a personal experience of nonjudgmental acceptance with another person or animal, we deepen our appreciation of and value for warmth, genuineness, empathy, and curiosity as essential components of moving through the early tasks of change.

The *Why*: Acceptance Creates Conditions for Change

In Module 3, we noted ***MI spirit*** has four elements: ***partnership***, ***acceptance***, ***compassion***, and ***envisioning*** (***PACE***). This module will specifically focus on acceptance, though as noted previously, these elements blend into each other. There are not hard boundaries. Again, each of these elements has an attitudinal as well as a behavioral component.

Acceptance gathers several important concepts, but its core is quite simple. ***Nonjudgmental acceptance*** is a powerful healing factor (Rogers, 1961; Miller & Moyers, 2021) and extends well beyond therapeutic relationships to include coaching, leadership, education, parenting, and so on (Rollnick et al., 2019). Miller and Moyers (2021) note that effective therapists, across modalities, are characterized by *warmth*, *empathy*, acceptance, and their ***affirming*** of clients' capacities and abilities to make their own decisions. Embodying these ideas means truly viewing clients as having *absolute worth*, which on its surface can seem easy and trite, but may be challenging in practice—especially when they engage in behaviors that place both themselves and others in jeopardy.

Acceptance, and its associated components, also fit research from Ryan and Deci's theory of motivation (2017) that asserts *relatedness*, *competence*, and *autonomy* are *basic psychological needs* that we all need met, just like biological needs for air, water, and food. Relatedness reflects the degree to which we are connected to others and feel we matter to them and they to us. Competence is the ability to act effectively and make a difference in our environment. Autonomy is not independence, but rather the ability to act in a manner that is consistent with our beliefs and values. The degree to which these basic psychological needs are met in helping relationships determines our client's sense of internal motivation for a change, even when it's initiated by an external source (e.g., an unexpected change in health). More generally, the degree to which these are met in life determines our well- or ill-being (e.g., Ryan & Deci, 2000, 2017).

The *What*: Attitudes and Behaviors Associated with Acceptance

In practice, this means we view our clients with interest and curiosity, while respecting their knowledge of themselves. We focus our attention on them and engage with warmth and genuineness. Behaviorally, we communicate this interest through our core skills of ***questions***, ***affirmations***, and ***summaries***, but with a particular focus on listening well (Miller, 2018). The client is the focus, and while our aim is to be nonjudgmental and communicate unconditional positive regard, this is expressed behaviorally by our ***listening reflectively***. We actively look for strengths and capacities, rather than focusing on deficits and limitations. We look for *what* the client can do, rather than what they cannot. Then we help them notice these strengths by emphasizing the qualities through affirmations, reflections, and summaries. The perspectives offered by us may lead to a new felt sense, emotion, thought, or view. While it might be new, clients recognize it as true and genuine. This process offers clients a new sense of capacity and competence. We might also follow up with questions designed to explore these things further. An example of this with an angry, defiant teen might be, *You're someone who knows your mind, has a keen sense of justice, and is willing to speak her mind when you feel unfairly treated. I'm guessing there have been times you've used those capacities to help achieve something difficult. What's an example of when you did that?* Our aim is to have the client envision a way to achieve their hopes and goals, and see a path forward they feel capable of following.

The *How*: SP/SR on Exploring a Prior Experience of Acceptance

Overview of the Exercise

In the movie *Dead Poet's Society*, Robin Williams plays poetry teacher John Keating who strives to bring his young, preparatory school charges fully into the experience of being alive and finding their own thoughts and voices. When shy, reserved Todd Anderson fails to do the poetry assignment, Keating brings him to the front of the room. The process is not to shame Mr. Anderson, as Keating calls him, but instead to draw forth the abilities that he's observed in his young student. He does this through a series of interactions where he demonstrates acceptance, even as he gently challenges—*Mr. Anderson believes everything inside of him is worthless, and embarrassing, but I don't think so*—and then asks him to complete tasks, *Give me a barbaric yawp*. The upshot is that Mr. Anderson discovers within himself a capacity he had neither known nor embraced. You can find this video by searching YouTube for "barbaric yawp."

Mr. Keating's methods dovetail with an activity often employed by MI trainers. Originally developed by Dr. Carolina Yahne, this activity asks participants to think back over their life and identify a teacher, coach, mentor, or someone else who cared deeply for them and who saw possibilities they did not see in themselves, and positively encouraged them to become more than what they were at that moment. This person is someone who positively encouraged them, not someone who scared them into compliance. A series of questions are then posed to the participant being trained as part of a flowing conversation. It is this activity that we will do.

Structure of the Exercise

This activity can be done in a self-directed manner. However, we believe it is most powerful when done with a limited-practice partner.

If you do this as a discussion with a limited-practice partner, when in the role of MI practitioner, we encourage you to be curious in your follow-up to the questions listed below. These are simply meant to initiate the conversation and to explore certain avenues that might prove enlightening. Your careful listening and attention to elements of the MI spirit, both in terms of your stance toward your partner and in the description of the favorite teacher/coach/mentor, are what help this activity create depth and meaning.

Keep in mind the communication of your acceptance in the form of your warmth, genuineness, and empathy. As in Module 3, this is not an interrogation, but a curious exploration. The questions posed here are meant to guide and focus conversations. However, like MI, they are not a specific blueprint. Use them to help find your way into the conversation and to keep it on track. Utilize the skills you've already learned about MI and be especially attuned for feeling reflections and affirmations. This session can have a warm glow as your partner recalls this favorite person who helped them become more than they believed might be possible.

Also bear in mind that for some people with traumatic histories, it can be difficult to identify anyone who fell into this category, or they may focus on a negative person who positively influenced them, *I never wanted to be like that person so I. . . .* While there is no doubt that such people can have a profound impact, they are not the focus of this activity. The underlying aim is for us to recognize how we have encountered acceptance and how that influenced us positively.

If unable to find anyone that fits this bill, you might want to perhaps consider an animal with whom you have shared a special relationship. Many of us have experienced meaningful and accepting relationships with animals—horses and dogs are common examples. Of course, there is always the possibility that this might not be the right activity for you or your partner.

Guiding Questions

- What is the name of this person/animal who saw more in you than you thought possible or with whom you shared a special accepting relationship?
- What was their relationship to you?
- What did they see in you, or how did you feel around them?
- How did they communicate/demonstrate their interest, caring, and support?
- What did this lead to in the short term?
- How about in the long term?

Traveling Companion: An Example with Sam

Sam will assist us with this exercise. Recall that she is a White, cisgender woman of European descent who has been a successful counselor for many years. Fifteen years ago, she injured her back and because of that experience has shifted her private practice to health-focused care. She became interested in MI as part of the learning she did post injury, engaged in a variety of training and learning, and has recently been considering ways to advance her expertise. She had a cancer scare last year, and her wife is encouraging her to retire. Sam is ambivalent about making such a change, and this has become a point of contention between them.

Sam decided to talk about Mrs. Haddid, a widowed neighbor who had lived next door when Sam was a girl.

➤ ***What is the name of this person who saw more in you than you thought possible or with whom you shared a special accepting relationship?***

Mrs. Haddid. You know I'm not even sure I know her first name.

➤ ***What was their relationship to you?***

She was my next-door neighbor when I was growing up. She was always there. Her husband died before I can remember. She was just my neighbor, but she was often out in the yard working in her garden, and she would always say hello and ask [me] about things. Unlike other adults, she seemed generally interested in my answers. She wasn't just asking polite social questions. She wanted to know.

➤ ***What did they see in you, or how did you feel around them?***

When I got older, she asked about my plans. What I wanted to do, stuff like that. She knew I was curious, and she fed that by asking questions about what new things I was learning. She always said, "I don't know what you're going to do, but you're going to be the boss." I remember asking [her] if that was because I was bossy, and she laughed. I remember it clearly. It just stuck with me. She said, "No. You just are always thinking about how things work and wondering why things go a certain way. You always seem to have another way and that way makes sense." I just thought I was a pain in the ass because I was always challenging people.

➤ ***How did they communicate/demonstrate their interest, caring, and support?***

She never talked down to me. No matter my age, she just talked to me like I was a person, not a kid. She asked questions, but more importantly she really listened to the answers. Like what an 8-year-old or a 12-year-old had to say mattered. When I was a teenager and was a real pain in the ass for my parents, she never lectured me or took their side. She just listened, and often it seemed to calm the storm when I was worked up. Not that she always agreed with me, but she never treated me like, "You'll see when you're a little older and more mature." She also pointed out things maybe I didn't want to see but knew were there. Like, I still loved my dad even though he drove me crazy with some of his rules. She was also the one who noticed my restlessness when I was working for my parents.

➤ ***What did this lead to in the short term?***

In the short term, I just felt like I had somebody in my corner and that I could trust myself. It's not that my thoughts and opinions were always right, but that I didn't have to doubt them. They were good thoughts.

➤ ***How about in the long term?***

In the long term, Mrs. Haddid is the reason why I became a therapist. I might have made it out of the family business, but her noticing and reminding me about finding my answers was just the window I needed to open. Once that fresh air came in, I knew it had to change. Not that it was easy—because it wasn't—but I knew I could trust myself and obviously she was part of that. It helped me go out on my own.

Self-Practice

Your task is straightforward. Engage with the questions. If you're doing this in a self-directed manner, write out your answers as though you were talking to your limited-practice partner. Make your answers reflect your authentic voice. If you're working with a limited-practice partner, have a conversation using these questions as prompts. To be clear, it is essential to not just ask questions but also to respond with listening statements and affirmations.

➤ ***What is the name of this person who saw more in you than you thought possible or with whom you shared a special accepting relationship?***

➤ ***What was their relationship to you?***

➤ ***What did they see in you, or how did you feel around them?***

➤ ***How did they communicate/demonstrate their interest, caring, and support?***

➤ ***What did this lead to in the short term?***

➤ ***How about in the long term?***

Self-Reflection

Please find a quiet space where you can do this writing. This is meant to be done alone and not necessarily shared with your partner. Keep in mind the difference between private and public reflections noted in Chapter 5.

➤ ***What did you notice about your emotions as you considered this person? How did this show up in your body?***

➤ ***What did you notice about your thoughts as you considered this person? Why do you think these thoughts came up?***

➤ ***Was it difficult to identify this person/animal? Remember the experience? What made it so?***

➤ ***What qualities of this person/animal stand out for you? Why do they stand out?***

➤ ***If you did this as limited practice, in what ways did your partner's presence influence this process? What specifically did they do? Why did it matter?***

➤ ***People often feel a sense of gratitude when they reflect on this person/animal. Does the same happen for you? If so, what does the expression of that gratitude seem to require of you?***

What If: Applying Skills to My Current Context

Bridging Questions to Practitioner-Self

These questions are designed to help you bring the insights from personal self-practice into your work with clients.

- ***How does this experience help you understand*** acceptance ***with new clients? What about with current clients?***

- ***How might you integrate this learning into how you begin with new clients?***

- ***How might this experience be helpful in your work with current clients?***

- ***What unique contextual elements do you need to consider in your circumstance? How might this experience assist you in making acceptance work in your setting?***

- ***What qualities of this person/animal do you want to carry into your work?***

- ***Thinking about your clients, what would you need to do to make acceptance more available when you're next in session?***

- ***What are your main* takeaway *messages from this SP/SR experience in relation to your understanding of the concept of acceptance . . .***
  - ***From a practical perspective?***
  - ***From a theoretical perspective?***

> ***What if you were to apply this process to other areas of your professional practice (e.g., in a role as supervisor or trainer perhaps)? How might you apply your learning to this new context?***

____

____

____

> ***How has this exercise influenced your understanding of or personal relationship with MI as a way of being?***

____

____

____

____

Final Thoughts and Applications to Other Settings

Acceptance can be one of the most challenging elements for MI practitioners. It is not that we are unsupportive theoretically, but rather in its practical applications our own emotions and concerns can interfere. The higher the emotions, the harder it seems for us to be accepting. We want to slip into the ***fixing reflex*** to prevent harm or costly mistakes. Time pressures create a similar trap.

The shorter the time available for an encounter, the more pressure we can feel to tell the person what to do. This is especially troublesome for people who work in circumstances where time is short, contacts are infrequent, and consequences are high. Yet, the underlying dynamics of acceptance remain in place in these settings as well. Still, we will at times engage in ***directing*** or offering concerns, as we'll discuss in Module 16. Our first response should be ***guiding*** and only veering from that for conscious and intentional reasons.

Finally, as in Module 3, this exercise of naming an influential person in our life is not an activity typically done with clients. Instead, it's an opportunity for us to remember an experience that often contains elements of the MI spirit, in particular acceptance. The intention, therefore, is that this activity supports the reader's self-reflection of their own experience of acceptance and how they might demonstrate it. However, this activity could lead to an interesting exploration with a client about experiences they've had and strengths they can build on. At the same time, some clients might struggle to find someone who positively influenced their life. This is powerful information for us as practitioners and suggests both what a client might need from you and how different, potent, and perhaps risky this MI conversation might feel for them.

MODULE 5

Compassion

Module Purpose

This module invites you to consider what ***compassion*** is and to then have an experience of compassion using a *loving-kindness meditation.* By the end of the module, we hope you have a deeper understand of how it feels to receive compassion and how it assists us when we are challenged in the process of growth and change. This exercise also reminds us that we all experience, including in our work, variations in our ability to feel and extend compassion to some people and we can work to change this situation.

The *Why*: Empathy and Compassion Are Essential

It hardly seems necessary that we talk about the importance of ***empathy*** and ***compassion*** in the context of a helpful relationship; they seem like givens. Yet, Miller and Moyers (2021) note that therapists differ in empathy and this difference matters. Specifically, it is an essential ingredient for effective therapists, and low empathy in therapy can be toxic (Moyers & Miller, 2013). In addition, Zaki (2020) argues that empathy is not a trait that has a fixed quality, but instead is something that we are born with an initial level of, but then is influenced by our attitudes, environments, experiences, and choices. Empathy can grow over time, as well as recede.

Gonzales-Liencres et al. (2013) define empathy in a very specific manner, "to form an embodied representation of another's emotional state, while at the same being aware of the causal mechanism that induced this emotional state in another" (p. 1538). There are three elements Gonzales-Liencres and colleagues identify as part of this definition. First, there is a feeling component where we recognize the emotions of another and may even experience similar feelings. For example, Jayce is feeling heartbroken, and I have a sense of what that might feel like that. Second, a thinking component allows us to draw conclusions about why the person is feeling what they are. Jayce just lost a loved one unexpectedly, which might be the cause of the broken heart. Third, we recognize a distinction between the other's experience and our own.

Jayce is heartbroken and I might hurt for her, but my hurt is separate. Two different underlying neuroanatomical structures underlie these emotional and cognitive components (Miller & Moyers, 2021).

Compassion then flows from this experience of empathy. Miller and Moyers define compassion as a "desire and intention to alleviate suffering and facilitate others' wellness and growth" (2021, p. 5). At its core, compassion requires that we recognize and have an experience of others' distress (i.e., empathy) and then act in a manner that prioritizes clients' autonomy, interests, and values, as we work *to alleviate suffering and facilitate their wellness and growth*. Empathy provides the experience, while compassion is the movement to action as a result.

The *What*: Attitudes and Behaviors of Compassion

Of course, the challenge lies in determining what "acting in a manner" means. An excellent attorney might operate in the best legal interests of a client, but it is easy to imagine situations where this doesn't operate in the best emotional and psychological interests of that same person. A divorce attorney fighting over assets and parenting arrangements at the behest of the client is one example. Previously working in a civil commitment setting, D. B. R. observed attorneys arguing for their clients' right to be released, unmedicated, from a civil commitment into a world where they had no place to live, no resources to support them, and serious delusions that placed them at risk for harm of themselves and others. The lawyers were clearly working for what their clients desired, yet it fell short of alleviating their suffering or promoting their long-term autonomy and values.

This situation also points to the opposite perspective, where we as practitioners believe we know what is in the best interests of clients and then might act in a manner that limits choice and autonomy. While it might feel clear when there is an issue of imminent harm to self or others, there are many points further back on this continuum where practitioners might feel it is their responsibility to act to alleviate suffering, but it is not clear this facilitates the other's growth and wellness. Over time, there is a risk this leads to a paternalistic approach where we believe clients cannot be trusted to find solutions. Whether gently or harshly, we begin to press for *our* solutions.

Somewhere between these two perspectives, either blindly pursuing client desires or pressing for the adoption of our views, lies the wide avenue of compassion. To step into the avenue and their journey, we recognize that it takes courage. Engaging with the pain and struggle of another not only opens us to their suffering but also our own. We must be willing to engage with this discomfort to begin understanding their experience. It is also sitting in the uncomfortable "not knowing position." That is, we must tolerate the uncertainty of where the client is going to take us and sit in the genuinely curious position of trying to understand their position, the feelings attached to it, and how these fit within their value system, beliefs, goals, and so forth.

Once we've embraced that demand and rallied our courage, we observe that body, feeling, and thinking components have roles to play in this understanding. The relative value of each depends on the circumstance, but most importantly our understanding translates into a commitment to act to alleviate suffering, support growth, and enhance wellness for the other. Simply put, this is about them, not us.

Compassion-focused therapy (CFT) has many insights to offer us in this area. We recommend *Compassion-Focused Therapy from the Inside Out* (Kolts et al., 2018) for a more in-depth exploration of compassion, its components, and developing capacity in this area, as well as Steindl (2020), a text created by a highly skilled MI practitioner and trainer. We will take a more circumscribed approach to the description and practice of this concept, focusing primarily on compassion for others, knowing there are other important concepts (e.g., compassion for self) and additional practice resources available.

Tools for compassion, like those of the other ***MI spirit*** elements, are overlapping. It begins with fostering a belief in the value and importance of empathy and compassion. Listening deeply with curiosity and genuineness to understand the experience of another, holding it gently without judgment, and communicating the depth of that comprehension. Intentional questions, depth in ***reflective listening***, and targeted, well-organized summaries are all essential; so, too, is the cognitive understanding of the reasons for the struggle and the metacognitive ability to maintain awareness that the client's struggle is theirs and not ours (Gonzales-Liencres et al., 2013).

The *How*: SP/SR on Exploring the Experience of Self-Compassion and Other Compassion

Overview of the Exercise

There are multiple ways in which we can focus on developing compassion. We will begin the process by using a *loving-kindness meditation* that comes from Buddhist traditions of Metta and focuses on cultivating kindness and nonromantic love. There are variants of this meditation, their usage typically influenced by our familiarity and ability to sit in meditation more generally. We will draw from one of the simpler approaches. It begins with a focus on directing loving-kindness toward us, then moves to someone we know well and love, to someone we know less well, and finally to someone we find difficult. The intention of this meditation is that this loving-kindness will then extend out to all beings. Indeed, some Metta meditations conclude with this specific focus and intention.

Structure of the Exercise

In terms of this process, unless your limited-practice partner is experienced in this area, we recommend doing this as a self-directed activity and using a guided meditation. We recommend this one: *www.youtube.com/watch?v=sz7cpV7ERsM* from the University of New Hampshire's Health and Wellness Center. It is about 13 minutes long and will gently guide you through the four steps. In this process, you can choose to focus on someone from your private life or from your work as a practitioner. Do this in a comfortable location where you are unlikely to be disturbed. If this video is unavailable, we recommend a quick internet search for other loving-kindness meditations, such as those produced by Christopher Germer, for example. We recommend selecting a briefer video, 10–30 minutes long, for those new to meditation because of the challenge associated with the practice of meditating.

For some, this will be an unfamiliar practice. If you find your mind wandering, gently bring your attention back to the meditation. Similarly, if you find yourself being resistant to the process, simply be aware of the process and curious about it. We cannot force ourselves to be compassionate, but we can explore what gets in the way. From a cautionary perspective, we recognize that for some practicing loving-kindness through guided meditation can be an emotional experience, and for others even triggering of past adverse events. If you anticipate or find that this exercise is too uncomfortable or distressful for you, we recommend that you consider returning to it another time, should you feel able.

Traveling Companion: An Example with Takeshi

Again, Takeshi is a 24-year-old, cisgender, straight man of Japanese heritage working on his doctorate in clinical psychology. Stress and high expectations have been ongoing issues. He is a strong student and shows promise as a counselor. At times, he feels some frustration about his clients' lack of change. He sought out MI training at the suggestion of his supervisor and sees the value in it, though he doesn't feel as confident in this approach as he does CBT.

Takeshi did the loving-kindness meditation focused on three graduate school colleagues.

➤ ***What was your experience as you read the materials and thought about doing it? Where did you feel it in your body? What feelings accompanied these sensations? What thoughts did you have?***

I was skeptical. I had an immediate reaction to it, wondering what it had to do with MI. I know folks are hot on mindfulness and so I can see there might be something worth knowing here, but I was skeptical. I also know that sitting and doing nothing can make me anxious. In my body, I noticed tension. Not tension like before a test, but I just felt a little on guard. Emotionally, I wasn't exactly anxious, but think I sighed. I debated whether I was going to do it. I think I did the psychological equivalent of an eye roll, but then decided this was about stretching myself to get better, so I ought to do it.

➤ ***What was your experience of doing the meditation?***

I found my mind wandering quite a bit to begin. I couldn't quite get comfortable, then I was focused on what the person was doing and how they were doing it, and then when we got to the part of saying things in our head, I always seemed to be out of rhythm. But then that all began to slide away and next thing I knew I was just listening and not really caring about those things. My mind did wander then a few times, but I was able to bring it back. I tended to be a little self-critical of that at first.

➤ ***What happened in your body, feeling, and thinking?***

I notice how hard it was for me to relax at first and then how good it felt when I started breathing easily. I could feel the tension sort of seeping away. But I also noticed that when I started thinking critically, it came right back. I had to refocus myself, but it was easier. It's funny, but the harder I tried, the worse it was, and the less I tried and just did, the better it was. It was a little like Yoda said, "Do or do not, there is no try." My feelings went along with these things. I couldn't quite create all the things the person described. But, I could feel the warmth in me as I said the words and extended it out to others, and how much easier that was with the person who I related to easily than with others. But it felt important to do with the others.

➤ ***How did you feel afterward?***

Definitely more relaxed and more connected. Like I'd taken this deep breath and let out all this tension. I also felt more peaceful, and I have to say it, more compassionate toward all of them, especially my colleague Cyn. I'm unsure exactly what changed but saying the words—may you be happy, may you be peaceful, may you be well, may you be loved—changed my internal orientation. Like I was really focusing on them.

➤ ***What did you notice about your emotions as you considered these different people? How did this show up in your body? How about your thinking?***

With the first person, Michael, who's been a good friend and colleague, I just sort of felt even closer to him. It felt solid in my body before and it's still solid. I guess I thought I really like Michael. With the person I didn't know as well, I thought of this person who works in the clinic, Alicia. I don't know her well, but she's always been pleasant and helpful, and I felt like I had more curiosity about her life. I know she's a single mom, and I just wondered more about what happens away from the clinic. I just felt relaxed toward her or maybe like I was leaning in somehow. The person I struggle with is Cyn. That was interesting, because I've felt like she was just kind of self-focused and at times she's been abrupt with me. When I was doing the meditation, I felt myself softening toward her, as though a guard came down. Like I was feeling her struggles a little more and feeling more gently toward her. I was probably less tense, too, and more curious about why she is the way she is. Overall, I came away feeling pretty good and definitely feeling more loving.

➤ ***What did you rediscover in this process?***

First, how much skepticism and tension I carry all the time. I was not even aware of it until I started to relax. Yet, I know it's there. Second, how much my thoughts, especially the harsh ones, influence my sense of peace and balance. Of course, I know thoughts are important as part of the CBT process, but it's always a bit shocking to see how easily they slide in and influence me even though I should know better. LOL, just like that. Third, I recognized again how easy it is to stay locked in my world and not step out into the world of the other—really. It's likely courtesy compassion, but not the depth that this work demands, and it reminded me of how important it is to be intentional.

➤ ***Was it helpful to do this activity? Why?***

Actually, it was. It was really helpful. I like to think of myself as a compassionate person, but I realized that can really vary by the person. I'm not sure I wanted to know that, but in some ways I already did. By being aware of it, I can work on being more compassionate with people I struggle with. I also realized that my thoughts and attitudes are at play here. I mean I thought it was about them, but it's really about me, isn't it? I also see more clearly my closed attitude about doing this meditation could've really gotten in the way of my learning something important. I see this in clients, but I hadn't seen it so clearly in me.

Self-Practice

Do the loving-kindness meditation, thinking about three people from either your personal life or your work context. Remember to select someone you know well and love, someone you know less well, and finally someone you find difficult. To maintain a consistent focus, we recommend not intermixing these two areas—personal and work—for this exercise.

Self-Reflection

Please find a quiet space where you can do this writing. We recommend doing it immediately after the meditation. This is meant to be done alone and not necessarily shared with your partner. Keep in mind the difference between private and public reflections noted in Chapter 5.

- ***What was your experience as you read the materials and thought about doing it? Where did you feel it in your body? What feelings accompanied these sensations? What thoughts did you have?***

- ***What was your experience of doing the meditation?***

➤ ***What happened in your body, feeling, and thinking?***

➤ ***How did you feel afterward?***

➤ ***What did you notice about your emotions as you considered these different people? How did this show up in your body? How about your thinking?***

➤ ***What did you rediscover in this process?***

➤ ***Was it helpful to do this activity? Why?***

What If: Applying Skills to My Current Context

Bridging Questions to Practitioner-Self

These questions are designed to help you bring the insights from personal self-practice into your work with clients.

➤ ***What clients do you find easy to have compassion for and why? Who is more difficult? Why do you think this is?***

➤ ***What do you think might be needed for you to feel more compassionate with challenging clients? Please explain why.***

➤ ***How might you use this process to help you prepare for your work with those clients you find difficult?***

➤ ***What lessons do you want to integrate into your work with clients, as you reflect on this experience?***

➤ ***What unique contextual elements do you need to consider in your circumstance? How might this experience assist you in making compassion work in your setting?***

➤ ***What are your main*** takeaway ***messages from this SP/SR experience in relation to your understanding of the concept of compassion . . .***

- ***From a practical perspective?***

- ***From a theoretical perspective?***

➤ ***What if you were to apply this process to other areas of your professional practice (e.g., in a role as supervisor or trainer perhaps)? How might you apply your learning to this new context?***

➤ ***How has this exercise influenced your understanding of or personal relationship with MI as a way of being?***

Final Thoughts and Applications to Other Settings

Loving-kindness meditation is not an MI-specific practice. However, it is a useful tool to experience what is meant by compassion for self and others. It may also be an appropriate activity for a client and then discussing the experience afterward. For example, it might reveal sources of struggle in compassion, which keep the person entangled in vertical ambivalence. The third person in this sequence will often be a struggle, so discussion and guidance about the person to select might be helpful, especially if there is a history of trauma. Difficulty with maintaining focus is common and should be explored with kindness and curiosity.

Working in brief settings, the ability to form connection, experience empathy, and express compassion may be even more immediate. Rapid engagement is something that coaches, health care workers, first responders, and mental health professionals all need to do at various times. It requires the practitioner be a careful observer and respond in immediate ways, sometimes nonverbally. To do this well requires training, a deep knowledge of the population being served or anticipation of what might be needed, a willingness to focus on the other and form connections, and the ability to express this in nonverbal and verbal ways. A look, eye contact, a smile, a gesture, tone of voice may be small but essential elements. Offering of tangible elements—a chair on which to sit, a hand to grasp, an arm to hold onto, a drink of water—might all be expressions of compassion in rapid engagement situations. Finally, verbal skills are often needed, though not always in the manner typically anticipated. See Box 5.1 (on page 114) for D. B. R.'s personal observation of a police officer doing this in an exceptional manner with a nonverbal person.

BOX 5.1. One Dark Morning

D. B. R.: While taking my daily, early morning walk, which at that time of year is in the dark, I came upon a bus and two vehicles pulled to the curb. Their hazard lights on, and their drivers out, looking into the middle of a dark street where stood a barefoot girl of 8 or 9 on this 53°F (11.7°C) morning, mumbling to herself. As the other drivers watched for vehicles, the bus driver informed me the girl wasn't responding and might have autism. I approached the girl, who was mumbling about the big machine and hopping from one foot to another. Unwilling to engage directly, she did respond to my encouragement to join us by the curb, which was when the police officer arrived.

After being informed about what we knew, the bus driver reboarded his bus and left on his route, while the other drivers went on their way. The police officer tried to engage the girl in conversation. It quickly became apparent that she was either unable or unwilling to provide answers. However, this did not stop the officer from observing her bare feet and thin pajamas. He noted it was chilly outside and invited her to sit in his car where it was warm, which she willingly did. He left the door open and went to the other side of the vehicle, where he told the girl he needed to make a quick call on his radio. Then returning to her side, he removed a small stuffed animal from the vehicle and asked if she might like to hold it. She snatched the bear and began softly kneading it. The officer spoke gently but did not press for information. He always told her what he was about to do before he did it. When the paramedics arrived, he asked if she might like to hop in the back of their vehicle where it was warm, and they would help find her way home, which she willingly did.

This officer had a noncommunicative participant in this interaction, but through understanding the context and what the girl might need, he was able to offer help in a manner that met her needs. Notice the little things he did. Inviting her in, offering her a tangible form of comfort, speaking to her gently and respectfully even while she did not outwardly respond, and recognizing that closing the door might help him manage the situation, but might frighten her. All these actions communicated his empathy and compassion, and it was a remarkable bit of community policing.

MODULE 6

Envisioning

Module Purpose

This module explores the role of ***envisioning*** and its relationship to hope within the change and growth process. We do this by inviting you to experience a visualization exercise that focuses on your developmental journey as a practitioner. By the end of this module, we believe the visualization exercise can evoke experiences of hope, capability, and seeing our possibilities, which we can then transfer into how we specifically work to produce hope and envisioning with our clients.

The *Why*: Importance of Hope, Capability and Seeing Possibilities

The fourth element of ***MI spirit*** has been given different labels over the years. Originally ***evocation***, this domain captured the notion that resources for enacting change lie within the client, both in terms of motivation and in solutions to problems. Our job as practitioners then is to call forth what is already present and assist the client in noticing, appreciating, and building on these elements. This idea did not eliminate the need for practitioners to introduce new ideas, see new connections, or offer new skills. It simply recognized the impetus for doing these things, and sustaining that effort must come from clients. The client is the engine for change, not us; our job is to facilitate this process.

As clear as that might seem, the use of similar labels to describe an MI process—***evoking***—and practitioner behavior—***differentially evoking change talk***—has led to confusion among writers, trainers, and practitioners as to whether these were the same things or different things. In the latest iteration of *Motivational Interviewing Fourth Edition* (MI-4; 2023), Miller and Rollnick use the term ***empowerment*** to describe this domain. The focus is on clients growing capacities to embrace and enact change in their lives, and the practitioner's role in assisting that process. The act of empowering is intended to give energy to an idea, belief, or action. The value of it seems clear, but there is also a concern hidden within this term for us.

The dark shadow within empowering is that *practitioners* have the power and they imbue clients with it. This view seems directly at odds with Miller and Rollnick's writing on this matter and more importantly their intent. While Miller and Rollnick (2023) emphasize they are using the second definition of empowerment, the first definition remains *to give power to*. This is NOT something practitioners give to clients, but rather something clients discover within themselves. The practitioner might help in the discovery, but the materials (e.g., capacity and wisdom) are already there. We can think of this like the seed that produces a new plant. The gardener doesn't create the life; it is already there. The gardener helps bring the conditions under which the seed and subsequent life will grow and flourish. There is a question to consider, and we will answer it a bit later: Who is the gardener in this process—the client, the practitioner, or both?

We believe a better term would be *envisioning*. It is a gerund of the verb "envision," implying an action, which in this case is to imagine as a future possibility, to visualize. Some clients already come with a clear image of what they want and simply desire assistance in finding a route. They already know their garden and what they wish to grow there; they just need help with the technical parts of creating their garden—what needs direct sun, nutrients, and regular watering. Others might need assistance in finding the right image. They want to grow this garden and don't know where to begin or how. At times, this might mean we visualize something as possible and assist the client in seeing that possibility as well. This envisioning is built on the strengths and capacities of *this* client, as well as our prior experience with other clients. There is an interactive process then, where we come to a common vision of something that may not exist presently but could. It is not something we *do to* clients, but something we do *with* them.

There is another important element underlying this, which will also come into play when we discuss ***change talk***. Specifically, the vision might be co-constructed. That is, the vision for the individual may not be explicitly formed at the beginning of the process, but through interaction with the practitioner comes into being; together, we create the vision. Ultimately though, it must be the client's vision that takes root, if it is to grow and be sustained (Wagner & Petty, 2022).

Hope, which Miller and Moyers (2021) identify as a characteristic of effective therapists, is a close cousin to these ideas. Hope builds from first imagining that something is possible and is strengthened by seeing methods to accomplish the steps toward the imagined possibility. At times, clients cannot see that possibility and so will need to borrow the practitioner's hope to begin. That is, our belief that things can change gives root to something within the client. Yet, if we help create an image of something new, but the client has no capacity or opportunity (Michie et al., 2011) to reach this imagined goal, the vision becomes something that feels unattainable and thereby risks generating feelings of disappointment, depression, or despair. There is a risk then that hope without self-efficacy—the belief that I can act effectively in this situation—can lead to defensiveness as clients move to protect themselves. We've unintentionally undermined rather than supported the client's motivation for something different.

The *What*: The Attitudes and Behaviors of Envisioning

The MI practitioner's role is a complex one, where in part we help client's build self-efficacy. It begins by modeling hope for clients, which provides vicarious learning. We draw attention to elements within the client that support hope, without becoming a cheerleader for it. These ideas intertwine with the ***fixing reflex*** and the value of ***affirmations***, concepts that we will pick up on later in this book. We note prior performance and accomplishments, and help clients observe these capacities within themselves. We encourage them to attend to physiological cues that support their internal sense of knowing (e.g., *It feels right when I think about that, I feel settled*). The practitioner uses both common tools—***open-ended questions***, ***reflections***, ***affirmations***—and more involved strategies—visualization, focused body awareness (e.g., *Where specifically do you feel that in your body*)—in a skillfully sophisticated manner.

Envisioning requires careful listening and attention to client values, experiences, and hopes. It demands our own dispositional optimism that change is possible and the careful nurturing of that for ourselves, as well as our clients. It also requires situational optimism for the specific challenges that clients face, and this is built by not only practitioner knowledge of resources and additional elements that might be helpful, but also by careful observation of the tools and capacities that clients have now, and that they have displayed in the past.

The practitioner is like a patient, experienced gardener who completes coursework and labs to become a master gardener. They then share this knowledge and experience with others. Master gardeners know the seed contains life, and life of a particular kind. A seed for a willow will never produce an oak, nor do they expect it will. They recognize and encourage the seed for what it is. They know the elements needed for new life and help clients learn to cultivate these things as it will be the *clients*' willows, oaks, peas, tomatoes, or daffodils that grow and need tending. But, in all this, the client is the gardener, not the practitioner. The master gardener offers input as requested, and with time their input becomes less and less.

The client will determine what is in their garden. We might help envision the garden and even help them see a garden is possible, or once was but is now overgrown or hidden, when they can't quite see it for themself. We will help them perceive the tools they have at hand, as well as those they might need to obtain. We may assist in providing information about conditions that assist with growth, but we also recognize the client knows this plot of land better than us. We might offer observations, ideas, or suggestions, but we know the client will decide which of these to follow. For it is the client who will do the hard work to bring that garden to fruition. The practitioner's role is to assist in that process.

The *How*: SP/SR on Your Envisioning Process to Become a Practitioner

Overview of the Exercise

We have already begun work thinking about envisioning. Indeed, envisioning is often part of what many favorite teachers and mentors do for us. In this instance, we will focus on the process that led you to become a practitioner, and we will use visualization to help us in this process. Typically, envisioning is forward looking. However, in this activity we are looking back. Notice—through the activities we reflect upon in this self-practice—how you came to envision yourself as a practitioner.

This process can be done as a self-directed activity, a limited partner activity, or a combination of both. The script below walks you through this visualization activity. We do not recommend reading the script and doing the visualization activity at the same time. Instead, pre-record the script on your phone, or have your limited partner pre-record it for you, or do it live with your partner.

Structure of the Exercise

Voice matters in this process. Whether it is done live or pre-recorded on your phone and played back to you, do not use your everyday voice. Instead, allow your voice to be more relaxed, gentle, calm, and paced than usual. Feel free to substitute your (or your partner's) name into the script.

Find a quiet place where you will be free of distractions and that helps you calm your mind. Feel free to add small accoutrements to this process if it is helpful, like candles, incense, or soft music. Provide a comfortable place to sit.

Here is the script:

> "Sit comfortably with legs uncrossed and hands resting in your lap. You can close your eyes if you feel comfortable. If not, simply find a place to let your gaze land on gently. Breathe in through your nose and out through your mouth. Breathing slowly and evenly. Focusing your attention on your breath coming in and then flowing out. Continue to do this five more times, simply attending to breath as it comes in and flows out. And then after the fifth breath, just continue to breathe naturally and easily, noticing sensations of relaxation flow over you.
>
> "Now, open a picture in your mind's eye. Visualize it opening in front of you. Eventually, focus on when you began thinking about becoming a practitioner or therapist or psychologist or social worker or whatever profession you have or are working toward. Just allow the image to form and be surprised by what you see. Take your time allowing it to come into focus. Breathing easily and comfortably. If there is not a specific time, allow your mind to open a period when this might have been. Notice where you are and who is there. Feel your body in that space. What is happening in this situation? Just notice what is happening. Take your time and breathe easily and comfortably.
>
> "What are the emotions that accompany you in this situation? Know that if these are strong emotions, you can touch them, but don't need to feel all the power they held back then. You can simply observe and know they're present. As the situation begins to resolve into a hazy cloud, what is the feeling that you were left with?
>
> "Continue to breathe easily in this warm, comforting place. Notice your breath moving in and out easily. Allow yourself to float here. Any sounds that come in simply drift in and out. And as you continue to breathe, allow your mind to open an image as you begin the process of becoming either a practitioner or your current profession. As these things come into focus, notice who is there encouraging you. What did they say? How did they say it? What did they do? What was useful, and what got in the way? What were your reactions in your mind to these things? What about your feelings? How about in your body?
>
> "Float in these things for a bit, knowing that if there are strong thoughts, emotions, or sensations, you can notice these, but do not have to embrace them fully or feel overwhelmed by them. And as you float, allow your mind to close this image and return to floating in the warm, comforting cloud. And now notice your smooth, easy breathing coming in and out, in and out, and in and out. Allow yourself to float here. Notice the feelings in your body as you float. Any sounds that come in simply drift in and out. And as you continue to breathe, allow your mind to open an image as you completed the process of becoming a practitioner or whatever your profession is. If you're amid this process still, imagine what it will be like when you finally complete those requirements.
>
> "You might imagine yourself at graduation being hooded. Feel yourself standing there. The sensations inhabiting your body. Or perhaps you're gathered with family or

friends celebrating. Or maybe you see yourself in your first treatment setting. Breathe easily as you notice the feeling of accomplishment. Wherever it is, notice your thoughts, feelings, and bodily sensations. What role does pride play in this day? Excitement? Notice these or any other emotions you might be experiencing. What thoughts accompany these things? What hopes do you have? What fears or concerns? How have you overcome them?

"And now as you slip back into the warm comfort of the cloud, know that you take with you these feelings of accomplishment and the strength it took to complete this journey. As you continue to breathe easily in and out, in and out, in and out. When you're ready, you can return to the present time and place, bringing with you all that you wish to bring and leaving behind any of those things you do not care to bring forward. You will feel refreshed and invigorated by recalling this journey and all you accomplished, and strengthened by the remembrance."

Traveling Companion: An Example with Quincy

As a reminder, Quincy is a 38-year-old, cisgender, straight woman of African descent who works as an AOD counselor. Growing up in a vibrant community, she has strong family ties and a foundation of giving to others. She was feeling some burnout with substance use clients and has taken an MI workshop, but it hasn't found its way into her work. Because of her feelings of burnout, she sought personal support and decided to find a therapist skilled in MI to learn more about the process. Quincy decided to ask her practitioner to lead the guided imagery with her at the end of a clinical session.

➤ ***Which approach did you decide to use for the visualization activity? How do you think that affected the experience?***

I decided to use my counselor, but I didn't want to write in front of her, so we did it at the end of a session. I just went to a coffee shop and wrote in it afterward.

I think using my counselor was good, though it felt a little weird at first because we hadn't worked that way before and I'm not sure I really believe in visualization as a method. It feels a little too touchy-feely for me. But her voice was calming, and I found it useful. It would have felt weird to be writing in front of her as long as I did, so I'm glad I went to the coffee shop. But that also meant I drove there and ordered a coffee, waited for it, and then found a seat, and put my earbuds in to drown out all the noise, all of which kind of moves me further and further away from the visualization and that experience, so maybe I should have just sat in my car. I feel a little more in my head now.

➤ ***What happened in your body, thoughts, and feelings as you began this visualization process?***

Well, like I said, I'm not a big fan of the touch-feely stuff, so I found myself feeling a little tense and maybe resistant to begin. It's like I didn't want to let go, even though I said I wanted to give it a try. Maybe it's control, maybe it's skepticism, or maybe it was me wanting to prove I'm right about this woo-woo stuff. Now, there's a thought; I hadn't considered that. I want control and want to be right. I'm not sure I like that insight—LOL. So, I guess those were my thoughts and maybe feelings, too. I don't think I felt worried or anxious—just a little tense and negative. Annoyed? In terms of my body, tension would describe it. I could feel it in my arms, legs, hands, and shoulder. I noticed it when my counselor told me to put my hands in my lap and I realized I was gripping them together. It was then that I started focusing on the breathing and trying to relax.

➤ ***In what ways did the process change as you moved through the visualization?***

Well, it most definitely changed, or I should say, I did. The breathing helped me to start to let go of some of the tension, and as that started flowing out, then it was like the skepticism went along with it. I stopped resisting and I wasn't particularly good at visualizing things, but I would get images and the things that my therapist would say, I'd notice. My attention wandered at times, but I didn't feel tense or like I had to do or go along with anything. I just sort of let it happen, instead of fighting it. I was certainly more relaxed by the time we got done. That felt good.

➤ ***What did you observe when you opened your mind to first becoming a practitioner?***

Well, that's the weird part. I couldn't quite see it, but I could. Anyway, it was like I remembered being a teen and hanging out with friends, and they would tell me things. Not like gossiping, but more like because they felt like they could, and I felt good because I felt like I was being helpful. A lot of my friends would give advice—you should do this, don't let him do that—but I tried not to do that. I don't know why exactly I didn't give advice other than it seemed like it was more about the other person if I didn't. Anyway, friends would say, "You should be a shrink" so I started thinking about it.

➤ ***What was important in your making this decision to be a practitioner? What was your hope for yourself?***

That's pretty easy. I knew I was going to school, and I wanted to do something that would pay some money, but also let me help in the community. That was always big in my family. I felt like this was a way I could do some good and help some people. If I could do that, it'd be alright with me. That was my hope.

➤ ***What did you notice about your emotions as you considered this time in your life?***

I felt energy. Like when I started, I was skeptical and tense, and my energy was limited. But here, I felt young and hopeful. I don't want to say it, but maybe I was. I had this belief the world could be better, and I was going to help that. I felt excited. Now, I feel more jaded. Life has kicked my ass a few too many times to know anything is going to come fast or easy, or without a fight. But I remember the power of that belief—a person can make a difference in other people's lives, and if we can, we should. We can't fix every problem, but we should fix the ones we can.

➤ ***As you started the work of becoming a practitioner, who was there helping you and what did they do?***

There are a lot of folks in that group. Different people at different times, but it always starts with my parents. They believed I could, expected I would, and helped pay the bills for me to get there. There was Dr. Robinson. He was my undergraduate advisor in the psychology program, who encouraged me and helped me figure out tests and application processes, especially the essays. There was Ms. Christy. I know her from church and the Boys & Girls Club. I don't even know what her job was when I first started going there, but now she's the director. She's been there forever, but she seems to know every kid's name and talks to them all. She's kind of my hero and sort of like a second mom, in good ways and bad. She likes to tell me what she thinks I should do with my life, but I know she cares. She's always said, "You got the gift. Use it." In fact, that's what I heard in my head during the visualization. Ms. Christy said that. The only correct answer is "Yes, ma'am."

➤ ***As you completed, or look to complete, the professional training process, how does the role of practitioner fit into your identity, and how might that influence your work?***

Well, by the end, it was pretty core. It's who I am, not what I do. I think that's why I've been feeling a bit discouraged and burnt out. If it's who I am and I don't feel effective, what does that mean about me? So, if I step back, and that's been the whole point of therapy, it's to think about this issue.

This is core to who I am, and I've been allowing that to take me in directions I know aren't helpful. I've started to feel responsible for making other people's decisions and that's a problem. I'm only a little way in, and I can already see that. I can still have it be a core piece, but they have to tend their own gardens and my pushing or getting irritable with folks doesn't make them better gardeners. See, I'm paying attention! I feel sort of embarrassed saying it now, but it also feels like such a weight has been lifted.

➤ ***How might the role of practitioner, envisioning and avoiding the fixing reflex, fit together? What challenges or opportunities might these create and why?***

This goes right with what I was just talking about. I've seen my role as the one who provides the vision because clients can't see it. Instead of our doing it together, I'm trying to force them to see and accept mine. And while I think it's for lots of good reasons, my clients have been fighting it. Doing this visualization helped me realize that I knew this approach was a problem back in high school, and somehow, I just forgot along the way. Maybe because it was clear to me that it was life and death for some of these folks and so I couldn't just leave it up to them. I am just realizing that by my feeling responsible, I've let it cloud my thinking about what is helpful. I mean how would anybody like it if I walked into their garden and just started doing whatever I please, especially if they hadn't given permission. No wonder folks are pissed and lying.

➤ ***What lessons do you want to pull forward into your work with clients, as you reflect on the prior question, and why?***

I am thinking about getting a little sign for my office wall and the group room that says, "Whose garden, is it?" Beyond that, I have a few thoughts. First, I think the visualization exercise was helpful. Even though I was skeptical, I can see the value in it, and it doesn't have to be all touchy-feely. So, I am adding that to the toolbox. I don't know how I'll use it, but I am thinking maybe early when folks are thinking about how they'd like their life to be different. Second, I know that clients need me to help see possibilities, so I can't just abandon this process, but we need to work together. It needs to be their "vision" ultimately, but I love the idea that we work to see it together. Third, I know that being a counselor is who I am at my core, but I've forgotten some of the wisdom I had before I even started this process. People need me to listen and not just tell them what to do and how to do it.

➤ ***How might this idea of you as the master gardener and the client as the gardener help you envision the counseling work that you and clients do together? How has this exercise helped you to clarify this vision?***

I'm loving this image. It kind of makes me want to learn something about gardening. Like maybe I should do this as part of my therapy process. In the big picture, it helps me get right about what my role is. I am not the gardener in their garden. They are. I've seen these master gardeners out at these hardware stores. They sit and listen to people. Offer advice when asked. Get excited about what people tell them. They motivate people by being interested in them and in their gardens. They don't tell them they're screwing up. They will offer thoughts about what might be going on, when problems exist, but it's always the person asking the master gardener who goes home and does the work. There is joy to that work, and I can see it. That's what I want to have again.

Self-Practice

Do the visualization process described above. To assist in this process, we recommend you either do this with a partner or you read this script into your phone to create a pre-recorded visualization track you can listen to. If creating your own visualization recording, we recommend a calm, gentle tone paced for a peaceful stroll through these issues. Remember, the goal is to have you relax and see, not march and endure. If you record your own track, this will have the added benefit of giving you practice if you choose to do a similar process with clients. It will provide an opportunity for self-reflection about what helps and what gets in the way of this type of visualization.

Self-Reflection

➤ ***Which approach did you decide to use for the visualization activity? How do you think that affected the experience?***

____

____

____

____

____

____

____

____

➤ ***What happened in your body, thoughts, and feelings as you began this visualization process?***

➤ ***In what ways did the process change as you moved through the visualization?***

➤ ***What did you observe when you opened your mind to first becoming a practitioner?***

➤ ***What was important in your making this decision to be a practitioner? What was your hope for yourself?***

➤ ***What did you notice about your emotions as you considered this time in your life?***

➤ ***As you started the work of becoming a practitioner, who was there helping you and what did they do?***

➤ ***As you completed, or look to complete, the professional training process, how did or does the new professional role fit into your identity, and how might that influence your work?***

➤ ***Was this visualization process helpful in understanding the envisioning task? Why or why not?***

What If: Applying Skills to My Current Context

Bridging Questions to Practitioner-Self

These questions are designed to help you bring the insights from personal self-practice into your work with clients.

➤ ***How might the role of practitioner, envisioning and avoiding the fixing reflex, fit together for you? What challenges or opportunities might these create and why?***

➤ ***What lessons do you want to pull forward into your work with clients, as you reflect on the previous question, and why?***

➤ ***How might this idea of you as the master gardener and the client as the gardener help you envision the work you and clients do together? How has this exercise helped you to clarify this vision?***

- *What unique contextual elements do you need to consider in your own work circumstance? How might this experience assist you in making envisioning work in your practitioner setting?*

- *What are your main* takeaway *messages from this SP/SR experience in relation to your understanding of the concept of envisioning . . .*
  - *From a practical perspective?*
  - *From a theoretical perspective?*

- *What if you were to apply this process to other areas of your professional practice (e.g., in a role as supervisor or trainer perhaps)? How might you apply your learning to this new context?*

- *How has this exercise influenced your understanding of or personal relationship with MI as a way of being?*

Final Thoughts and Applications to Other Settings

Guided imagery, visualization, or self-hypnosis—however we choose to label the activity just completed—is not an MI-specific practice. However, it is certainly an activity that we can do with clients if we feel comfortable with the process. It is a practice with evidence to support its utility across a variety of settings (e.g., Hackmann et al., 2011; Ruano et al., 2022) and might be a specific method to assist clients in visualizing something new or different.

Some clients will report they're poor at visualization or have doubts about its utility, just as Quincy did; this is not a problem. Ask them to pay attention to their body sensations, feelings, and the thoughts that pass through them as they go through the process. Past trauma is an important consideration here and we might not be aware of our client's experiences; be mindful of how we engage in this process. For example, invite people to either close their eyes, if comfortable doing so, or to choose a spot they can comfortably focus on. The underlying theme is to invite, not command, and to cede control, allowing people to participate as they're comfortable. If it's uncomfortable for someone, then do something else. In this manner, we see this work as slipping into an MI-consistent way of being with clients.

MODULE 7

Creating Safety

Module Purpose

This module explores the importance of client safety within the change and growth process and specifically invites you to experience your therapeutic working environment from the client perspective. That is, looking through the client's eyes and experiencing all the thoughts, sights, sounds, tastes, noises, and the like that you might if visiting your workspace for the first time. By the end of this module, it is our hope that experiencing the working/therapeutic environment through the client lens will help to identify new opportunities for creating safety and/or strengthen areas of existing practice that you found helpful in this process.

The *Why*: The Role of Safety in Engaging

There are three basic elements within ***engaging***: ***creating safety***, ***seeing the big picture***, and ***opening possibility***. Like many things within MI, the boundaries between these areas are fluid. In research terms, we might say these elements share significant variance, but for our purposes, let's keep it simple—as we influence one area, it will impact the other two. In this manner, all three are essential and while logically the point of entry will be creating safety, we might just as effectively begin by doing good work in seeing the big picture. Undergirding all three areas is the importance of *being understood*.

Creating safety means we are building and holding a space for clients where they can explore difficult realities. That is, when clients feel the need to defend behaviors, they will. This is not a condition inherent to either a particular personality type or a psychological disorder—it is a function of being alive. When we feel under attack, our two common responses are to either attempt to flee or stand and fight. There is no news there, except that over the years we've pathologized this tendency, misunderstood that attempting to break through *denial* elicited a natural human response, and then misattributed this response to something inherent to this type of client and/or condition. We misread what was happening within the interpersonal dynamic; Carl Rogers did not.

Rogers (1980) through careful observation and research noted that when we accept clients as they are, we are creating psychological safety. Under these conditions, clients are more likely to change. Conversely, when we pressure them to change, they are less likely to do so. The 40 years of research on MI reinforces what Rogers began writing about in the 1950s.

The *What*: Tools for Creating Safety

We can think about creating safety as falling into physical conditions, practitioner behaviors, and strategies. Physical conditions refer to the space we meet clients within and, of course, we have varying degrees of control over what that space looks and feels like. In our work lives, these settings have varied from a personal space that could be painted and furnished as we pleased; to locker rooms; to volley courts, squash courts, poolside, rugby clubs, cricket clubs, golf clubs; to medium- and high-security psychiatric units; to children's services in a basement play center with toys, a sandbox, and two-way mirrors; to medium- and maximum-security prison settings, and emergency rooms. Our clients have arrived in formal dress, casual clothes, clothing made rough by living outside, sports attire, backless hospital gowns, prison coveralls, shackles, and occasionally disrobed. The physical environment in all these spaces influences the nature of our discussions, particularly at the beginning of a new relationship. Of course, virtual environments add additional challenges and complexity to this process, including quiet and private spaces, freedom from intrusion, appropriate settings, lighting, and attire—to name just a few.

To the degree practitioners have control over their physical spaces, we encourage you to think through details like paint color, pictures on the wall, lighting, personal items, objects for clients to handle, and offers of hospitality. What works in one setting would not be appropriate in another. For example, when working with teens, hospitality items such as an electric tea kettle with tea options, a candy jar with treats, and a small supply of snacks were useful. While this was reasonable for hungry teens in D. B. R.'s setting, it would not have been appropriate in L. H. J.'s NHS weight management and bariatric surgery setting. Another element might include the use of music. The purpose of these things is to create a comfortable and welcoming environment, where the client controls choices, as the situation permits.

When we do not control the physical environment and/or it's particularly institutional in character, our efforts to create a welcome become even more important and will require flexibility and creativity within that setting. It is also a natural stepping off point for practitioner behaviors.

While physical environment matters, how we work is *the* critical factor. Rogers identified the importance of unconditional positive regard exemplified by being genuine, nonjudgmental, and warm (Rogers, 1961). These are the bedrock for the MI practitioner, though easy to misconstrue. Being warm is important, but if our natural personality is reserved, then it would be disingenuous to force that warmth. Perhaps for a reserved person, it appears in a wry sense of humor or a love of dogs; these then would be the authentic route to warmth's expression for this practitioner. Similarly, there are known cultural differences in the way in which warmth is expressed openly within group or individual settings. Unconditional positive regard means that we regard each person as someone of worth and value, which is unearned but instead bestowed by virtue of their being a fellow human. At a practical level, this can be quite hard at times when we work with clients who've engaged in egregious behavior toward others. Yet, the imperative remains, so we translate this into finding something we can genuinely connect with this client about. If we cannot, we might not be able to work effectively with that client and should consider referral to another provider or whether we should work in a different context.

The expression of these conditions mirrors those things we discussed in the ***MI spirit*** area. Listening well is at the core. Asking ***open-ended questions*** that invite conversation is also important. Offering small bits of information that answer clients' explicit or implicit concerns rounds out the tools in this beginning process. Explicit concerns might be factors like how long we will talk, with whom we will share this conversation, and what happens to any notes. Implicit questions might be like these: How does this therapy process work? How do we work together? Can you understand me? The specifics of these skills will be discussed further in future modules, and combining these into strategies will be addressed in Module 7. The essence of such skills is captured in a beautiful quote from MINT colleague Helen Mentha (2020, p. 10):

> Be someone good to talk to.
>
> If you offer appointments, be someone worth going to see. If you do home visits, be someone you would want to let in the house. If you see mandated clients, be a relief.
>
> When we need help, we want to see someone who can see the best in us, is curious about our experience and values our point of view. Someone who is safe to talk to, who is clear that their opinions and hopes come from them and doesn't expect them to be ours. Someone who can laugh at themselves and doesn't see the encounter as a test of their own worth or competence, or a test of ours.

As clients enter this space, they are trying to sort through a new role, *How to act with this person in this setting*, as well as consider the receipt of support for the issues that are bringing them in. Be mindful of this first task as you welcome them.

The *How*: SP/SR on Exploring How We Welcome People into Our Space

Overview of the Exercise

For this activity, we will use a combination of direct experience and imaginal practice. The aim is to have an experience in our setting and our manner within that setting from the client's vantage point. Then to use this information to consider what might enhance our client's sense of safety and welcome. This is an exercise most likely to be done in a self-directed manner. However, it could be done with a limited-practice partner. Their role would be to use the instructions to guide you and deepen the experience.

Structure of the Exercise

This exercise has three parts. After each part, there are questions to answer. We encourage you to find a comfortable space to write in and to then return to the next part. This is an activity we recommend be done in one "sitting." We provide a shortened description of the process immediately below.

The process begins with *in vivo* work. We invite you to enter your primary or usual space where you work with clients. Choose a period to do this when you aren't pressed for time. Sit in the space where clients often sit, not in your usual spot. Just sit quietly and notice the space and your reactions. Use all your senses. Answer the first set of questions.

Now, go outside the room, think about being a client either in therapy or visiting your workplace for the first time. Imagine your body. Notice your sensations. Attend to your senses, your feelings, and your thoughts. What thoughts might you have about the treatment process and about your concerns that bring you here today? Imagine you've met yourself and now are being escorted into this space; enter the room and pay attention to what you notice. What does it feel like as you sit down? What do you want from this practitioner as you sit down? What would be helpful for you? What would make this person someone good to talk to? What don't you want?

As you sit in the client's space, let your mind roam. What comes up? You might have clear images in your head, or it might be physical (somatic) experiences in your body, or thoughts running through your mind. Try not to judge and instead just allow them to float through and be curious about what you observe. It might be that you can really see these things, or the experience might be more like a film running in your mind. When you feel that imaginal process has run its course, exit the room. Answer the second set of questions.

For this last part, start from wherever you as practitioner begin the process of meeting a new client for the first time. If you're seated at a desk reviewing case materials, begin there. If it's rushing from the bathroom to be on time, begin there. Where you typically start in meeting someone new, begin there. Recall a client you recently started with. Engage all your senses. Again, attend to your body, your feelings, and your thoughts. Reflect on the questions offered later in the self-practice. Then enter your space and sit where you sat with that recent client.

Give yourself a moment to recall the situation. What do you remember seeing? How did you open the conversation? Where was your focus? What were you feeling? What was happening in your body? Now take a moment to answer the third set of questions.

Traveling Companion: An Example with Takeshi

As a reminder, Takeshi is a 24-year-old, cisgender, straight man of Japanese heritage working on his doctorate in clinical psychology. Stress and high expectations have been ongoing issues. He is a strong student and shows promise as a counselor. He feels some frustration about his clients' lack of change at times. He sought out MI training at the suggestion of his supervisor and sees the value in it, though he doesn't feel as confident in this approach as he does CBT.

As Takeshi is relatively new to the counseling process, he has not built a routine that is well established yet. However, he is thorough in his review and preparation for seeing clients and aware that he might be focusing more on his anxieties than on the clients to begin. He works in a psychology center clinic where the therapy rooms are shared with other graduate students and must be maintained as they are. It does include a one-way mirror from which all student sessions are video-recorded for supervision purposes.

Part 1

➤ ***What did you notice as you sat in your client's chair? What drew your attention? Was this surprising to you?***

I was aware that I didn't sit in the client seat except when occasionally having supervision. Because this is shared space and the sessions are video-recorded, they are set in standard ways, and I hadn't really considered how that arrangement works for clients. When I came in, I immediately noticed there was nothing personal in the space. The focus over the "counselor" was the one-way mirror, and I found my attention kept drifting back to that. The colors in the room were warm enough, and the seat was comfortable. The overhead lights are warmer than most, but it still doesn't feel like someone's personal space. It feels like a clinic and I'm under observation. There is basically one nature picture on the wall. It feels like hotel or hospital art. What surprised me was the view from that client chair generated some of the same feelings I have in my chair—anxiety, uncertainty, maybe a little fear—like what if I screw up? That's where I started, anyway.

➤ ***What was quieting and comforting? What was disquieting and discomfiting?***

Well, the color on the walls was quieting. I'm glad it wasn't institutional white. There was carpeting on the floor and that also made it feel different than a doc's exam room. I'm glad there was a picture on the wall and the nature was nice. It seemed like it provided some room to breathe. The chair was comfortable. More comfortable than the counselor chair. There is an end table with tissues.

What wasn't comfortable is the lack of other "human" touches. Also, the fact the one-way mirror is directly in my line of sight. I felt fixated on it. Who's back there watching, what are they seeing, what are they thinking? Am I being assessed, tested, judged, is anyone laughing at me or being sarcastic? What are they saying to each other, do they care, are they being compassionate and professional?

➤ ***What sensations did you notice in your body as you sat? What feelings and/or thoughts?***

I felt anxious to begin. I could feel tension in my shoulders, and my feet and hands were restless. But as I sat longer, I became more relaxed and seemed to sink into my thoughts. The chair felt comfortable, and I felt my body relax as my thoughts began to drift. The tension sort of ebbed away. I think I kind of covered my feelings and thoughts in the last answer.

Part 2

➤ ***What sensations did you experience in your body as you stood outside the room and thought about how this client might be feeling?***

This was interesting, as I again felt anxious. But the focus was different now. It was less on the space and more on the person and what we were going to do. It's like the space mattered, but I wasn't thinking about it. My tension was about sharing things with a stranger and all kinds of questions about that. Would I like this person? Was this a bad idea? Are they going to judge me? Is there something really wrong with me? All these things amped up my anxiety, so I again felt tension in my back and shoulders as I entered the space.

➤ ***What did you observe in yourself and the room as you sat down? How was it alike and different from what you noticed before?***

Now, this was interesting. I was focused on the chairs and where should I sit. It was like I was trying to figure out roles and how I was supposed to be as a client. Like, what's my job here? Once I sat down, then I noticed the room more. I noticed the Kleenex and wondered if I was expected to cry—not happening! I saw the mirror and, of course, the counselor had told me about videoing the sessions so he could improve his skills, so I wasn't surprised. He didn't seem nervous about it, so I wasn't. I was more focused on the counselor chair and what we were going to do.

In terms of the alike or different, I noticed that I looked at things in a different manner when I was in the client's shoes. What I thought would be a focus was not, or not nearly as much, as what was going to happen in the therapy process. I was also aware of how much I was trying to figure out my role as a client. That was curious to me.

➤ ***What would make this practitioner someone good to talk to?***

Given how focused I was on my role, I was aware that it had to do with helping me understand my job and how the therapy process would work. I also wanted to know if this was someone who would understand me. Would they get me? I expected they were generally trustworthy because of the role they were in and what the confidentiality forms stated, but that didn't mean I was immediately ready to share everything. I wanted to get to know them and suss them out to see what they were like. I also wanted to know if they could help me. I didn't want to share all my vulnerabilities and tell them all my inner thoughts and then have them say, "Well, sorry. This isn't the right place for you." I was holding back the deeper stuff.

➤ ***What didn't you want?***

I didn't need someone I could go have a beer with. I didn't want a friend. I also didn't want someone who had no clue about what to do. I wanted to have some confidence they could help me. But I also didn't want them to tell me what to do or that this was going to be easy because I'd already been trying and that would make me feel like an idiot. I wanted someone who really understood the issues and understood me, and I guess proved it by how they responded. Saying, "I understand" or "I've seen this before" might be a little reassuring, but it wouldn't feel like real understanding. I wanted to feel their understanding through the way they were with me, not simply the words they were saying. The words alone can seem trite. I didn't want some standardized phrases like you see in the rubbish movies about therapy, "And how did that make you feel?" Anyone who understands and gets the feeling would never have to ask me that question. They would know how I feel and would tell me.

Part 3

➤ ***Where do you begin this process, and what do you notice about how you feel as you anticipate this first meeting?***

All our records are now electronic, so it begins with my reviewing the forms the client has completed. The way our clinic is set up, there is an inner core of six offices with video cameras set up inside a shared internal space. There is a hallway around those therapy spaces and then rooms on the outside where we can do work, prep, and supervision. These are the rooms where I usually go to prep. I've typically, carefully, gone over all these materials the night before if the client has completed them, so the day of the session is just a review or a refresher. But sometimes, these forms don't come in until right before, so I am reviewing as I wait for the person to arrive. When this happens, I feel less well prepared and more anxious. In general, I feel anxious before most first meetings—performance anxiety or impostor syndrome, like I want to do a good job, but I feel like a fraud—like I really don't know what to do.

The last person I saw, it was all these things. Materials were late arriving. The person was older than I am, so I thought they might see me as a young punk. It was also working in an area I feel less knowledgeable about, chronic pain and depression. At least having reviewed the forms, it gives me the illusion of having more control. I guess it's making me think more about the importance of my ability to sit with uncertainty a bit more.

➤ ***What caught your attention as you met this person for the first time? What did you focus on?***

Well, I noticed this was a rugged, outdoors sort. Good-looking with a beard, flannel, and fleece. Like he would know his way around a vehicle and could fix things in his house—a man's man, so to speak. He had a strong handshake. He rose like his back was stiff but didn't complain. Frankly, I felt a little intimidated by him, and this made me feel more anxious and maybe a little concerned. I think I was focused on my reactions rather than on him to begin. That kind of bothers me to think about it.

➤ ***How did you address psychological safety as you began the conversation either in your office or your workspace?***

He was kind of a take charge guy, so he immediately began asking questions and addressing his concerns. It felt like he was trying to use humor to take the edge off things and to put himself a bit more at ease. He said things like "Well, it looks like this is probably my chair." "Not exactly homey." "So how does this work, doc? I don't see a couch, so I suppose I'm not going to lie on one and tell you about all my dreams or how I want to marry my mom." It's interesting because when he started doing that, I felt on a little firmer ground. Like, I know what needs to happen here.

So, I just started with a question my supervisor taught me, "What do you know about how all this works?" Most of his ideas were from bad TV, but he had some ideas about what he did and didn't want. I spent a lot of time just listening and offering some information.

I went on a little too long at one point, but it was just like I couldn't quite stop myself. I thought about it afterward. It seemed clear that anxiety contributed to that, as well as my desire to feel knowledgeable with this guy who was a little intimidating. The cues to stop were there; Lord knows, I felt them, but I didn't stop. So, next time, be aware of the tendency and then use the cues.

➤ ***What did you discover about your workspace as you worked through these different parts?***

Well, I'm aware of how impersonal it feels. I'm wondering if there are some ways that I can make it feel just a little more comfortable or homey for people. Like flowers would be great, but that's not very practical. A fern? I'm not sure, but something that just adds a little warmth to it.

At the same time, I am much more aware that it's about how I help the person feel in this space. They're really focused on themself, their role, and me, so I need to focus on them, not me. I need to provide some info if they need it. Just be aware of my cues that I'm focusing on me.

➤ ***What changes might you make based on these discoveries?***

Well, I guess I jumped ahead a bit in my last answer. I think something small and tangible in the space would help it. It needs to be something I can either transport easily or leave within the clinic. I'm thinking about a couple of small things for handling I could put on the end table, and which I could carry in my backpack. I need some wipes or something to clean them, and of course, they'd have to be easy to clean.

In terms of creating more welcome or safety, I think the focus needs to shift. I've been worried about my work as a therapist when we start. I need to shift that and be fully focused on the client, and what this person needs. I'm thinking I'll use that anxiety I have as a cue to focus my attention on the client's anxiety and uncertainty and to slow things down. I'm going to tell myself "Less is more" if I feel I am starting to talk too much. Then I need to focus on hearing their concerns and addressing those, as well as how the therapy process works.

➤ ***What lessons did you learn about your process*** **prior to** ***and as you meet new clients? What might need to shift or change for this to be a better experience for you or clients?***

I'm aware that I feel much more relaxed when I can review the materials the night before than when I'm rushing the day of therapy, but I also don't have much control over that process. It's making me see this could also be acting as a bit of a safety blanket, which may be getting in the way of learning to tolerate a little bit more uncertainty and flexibility. I think making sure I have a pause between clients is important. Sometimes I'll have clients scheduled all afternoon and that makes it hard to not feel a little rushed with someone new, so maybe I can be strategic about what time slots I put new people into. Like, I schedule them as the first client of the day or the first client after lunch. Then I think I need to be deliberate about focusing on the client and I probably just need to develop a routine—like a quick moment of breathing—where I check in with myself and then turn my focus to them. I don't want to ignore my feelings; I just don't want them to be the focus.

➤ ***Once your clients are in your space, what can you do more to be a person who is good to talk to? What might you need to do less of?***

I think I've been a little too task-focused. "Let's get down to business and solve this problem!" I cringe thinking about that, but I think that's been my underlying focus. I think I need to pay a little more attention to the interpersonal factors, and once those are in place, the tools will fit.

Related to those comments, I also need to slow down. My sense was by getting to what my client wanted they would feel like the session is helpful, but I'm thinking it's more nuanced than that. By slowing down, I'm meeting what they need first, which then will let the second part—the tools—feel more natural and the client will be ready to use them. I feel like I'm jumping the starter's gun a bit.

I've said this already, but I think it's worth making this the third leg of this stool, I need to shift my focus to the client. I know that should be obvious, but it's also easy when anxious to worry about my side of the process, instead of putting my focus where it needs to be—it's about the client!

Self-Practice

We invite you to set aside 20–30 minutes for the *in vivo* and imaginal parts of this practice, and at least another 15 minutes for the writing portion. If it's easier, you might use your phone to record the introduction part of each section and listen rather than reading as you come into that space. You might also use your phone to record your thoughts and then write these down afterward.

Again, choose a time where you will not feel time pressure. We recommend closing the door when in your therapy/practitioner space, so you won't be interrupted. If you begin this process outside of your office and have concern about how others might perceive what you're doing, make the obvious, obvious. Just tell them you're working on an activity to help deepen your knowledge about creating safety as clients begin treatment and that includes understanding how this process works for you.

The practice has three parts. After completing each part, answer the questions for that section. While you can bring along this book, we recommend reading it before entering that part of the process and then just focusing on your sensations, feelings, and thoughts, and images as you move through the time. Of course, taking a quick peek to see if that jogs anything further is something we all do, but in general, our aim is to be fully present in each part. Once a part is complete, retire to a quiet space to answer the questions.

Part 1

The process begins with *in vivo* work. We invite you to enter your primary or usual space where you work with clients. Choose a period to do this when you aren't pressed for time. Sit in the space where clients often sit, not in your usual spot. Just sit quietly and notice the space. Let your eyes wander around the room and notice what they might focus on. Notice any sounds or smells. What do you find quieting and comforting? What is disquieting and/or discomfiting? Notice the sensations in your body as you sit here, what do you feel, where specifically do you feel it? Be curious about your body. Where are points of tension and relaxation? What feelings do you notice? Now imagine seeing yourself in a video in the room; what does that show? How do you see yourself on the video? Now, exit the room. Answer the first set of questions.

- ***What did you notice as you sat in your client's chair? What drew your attention? Was this surprising to you?***

____

____

____

➤ ***What was quieting and comforting? What was disquieting and discomfiting?***

➤ ***What sensations did you notice in your body as you sat? What feelings and/or thoughts?***

Part 2

While outside the room, think about being a client in therapy for the first time. Imagine your body. What do you notice in your hands? Feet? Chest? What smells are present? Any tastes? What sounds are you hearing? What are you seeing? How are you holding yourself? Now, pay attention to the feelings you might have—fear, anxiety, dread, hope—comingled. What thoughts might you have about the treatment process and about your concerns that bring you here today? Imagine you've met yourself and are being escorted into this space; enter the room and pay attention to what you notice. Notice any sounds or smells. What does it feel like as you sit down? What do you want from this practitioner as you sit down? What would be helpful for you? What would make this person someone good to talk to? What don't you want?

As you sit in the client's space, just let your mind roam. You might have clear images in your head, or it might be physical (somatic) experiences in your body, or thoughts running through your mind. Try not to judge and instead just allow them to float through and be curious about what you observe. It might be that you can really see these things, or the experience might be more like a film running in your mind. When you feel that imaginal process has run its course, exit the room. Answer the second set of questions.

➤ ***What sensations did you experience in your body as you stood outside the room and thought about how this client might be feeling?***

➤ ***What did you observe in yourself and the room as you sat down? How was it alike and different from what you noticed before?***

➤ ***What would make this practitioner someone good to talk to?***

➤ ***What didn't you want?***

Part 3

For this last part, start from wherever you begin the process of meeting a new client for the first time. If you're seated at a desk reviewing case materials, begin there. If it's rushing from the bathroom to be on time, begin there. Where you typically start in meeting someone new, begin there. Recall a client you recently started with. Bring the thoughts, feelings, and physical (somatic) sensations you had to mind in anticipation of meeting this person. What were you wearing? How was your energy? What thoughts were you having? When in the day was it? Were you hungry or thirsty? Once those recollections are available to you, then move to the space where you met this individual. Recall the thoughts, feelings, and sensations there. What was your immediate reaction? Were they what you expected? What did this person look like? How did you greet them? What do you recall of the conversation? Then enter your space and sit where you sat.

Give yourself a moment to recall the situation. What do you remember seeing? How did you open the conversation? Where was your focus? What were you feeling? What was happening in your body? Now take a moment to answer the third set of questions.

➤ ***Where do you begin this process, and what do you notice about how you feel as you anticipate this first meeting?***

____

____

____

____

____

____

➤ ***What caught your attention as you met this person for the first time? What did you focus on?***

____

____

____

____

____

____

➤ ***How did you address psychological safety as you began the conversation either in your office or your workspace?***

What If: Applying Skills to My Current Context

Bridging Questions to Practitioner-Self

These questions are designed to help you bring the insights from personal self-practice into your work with clients.

➤ ***What did you discover about your workspace as you worked through these different parts?***

➤ ***What changes might you make based on these discoveries?***

➤ ***What lessons did you learn about your process*** prior to ***and as you meet new clients? What might need to shift or change for this to be a better experience for you or clients?***

➤ *Once your clients are in your space, what can you do more of to be a person who is good to talk to? What do you need to do less of?*

➤ *What are your main* takeaway *messages from this SP/SR experience in relation to your understanding of the concept of creating safety . . .*

- *From a practical perspective?*

- *From a theoretical perspective?*

➤ *What if you were to apply this process to other areas of your professional practice (e.g., in a role as supervisor or trainer perhaps)? How might you apply your learning to this new context?*

➤ *How has this exercise influenced your understanding of or personal relationship with MI as a way of being?*

Final Thoughts and Applications to Other Settings

We've focused our practice on a new client, yet engaging and creating safety are not one-time activities. That is, once done, they're always accomplished. Rather, they are something renewed upon each meeting. While the time and effort may diminish with repeated contacts, the need remains present. As we grow in experience as a practitioner and have repeated contacts with a client, it can be easy to lose our focus in this area. We need to remain intentional about creating safety and welcome each time. Perhaps we need to amend Ms. Mentha's message to *be someone good to talk to . . . today.* Perhaps as a corollary, we might add, *With each repeat encounter, reinforce this as an ongoing, iterative, and deepening interpersonal process in relationships.*

In brief and single meeting settings, establishing safety may be even more important, as the relationship will not have an opportunity to evolve. Therefore, we need to rapidly engage and to create this safety. In nontraditional settings, where privacy is limited, our ability to hold space with and for the other person becomes more challenging. Eye contact, physical contact, voice tone, gestures, and demeanor all matter. Attending to client needs in a tangible manner, like the police officer in Module 5 who noted it was cold and offered the warmth of his cruiser, assists in creating safety. Informing people what we're doing and why makes us more predictable and trustworthy. Acknowledging the limits of the situation and identifying our aim in the situation. Finally, moving at the speed and readiness of the client becomes even more essential, so our close attention to them is magnified. We need to talk to them, not at them.

When time is of the essence, we are at even greater risk of falling into the ***time trap***, which Miller and Rollnick (2023) identify as the pressure to rush or hurry. The unfortunate consequence of this trap is that as we press to move quickly, we fail to listen, and things take even longer as a result. Miller and Rollnick (2023) also identify three other traps, including the ***expert trap*** where we try to convince people of our authority and try to fix the problem for the person. A subset of this area is the ***assessment trap*** where we gather lots of information so we can solve the problem. The ***persuasion trap*** involves us trying to convince someone of why they need to change. The ***wandering trap*** involves our just listening to clients and never finding a focus. All these traps interfere with engagement and undermine safety for the client.

For example, earlier we observed Takeshi needing to feel expertise in relationship to his older male client and how this caused him to focus on himself and not the client. These traps are common and, as happened with Takeshi, our reflection on action (after the fact) can help us become more prepared to reflect in action (when it's happening) by learning from the cues we identify in our self-reflection process.

MODULE 8

Seeing the Big Picture

Module Purpose

This module encourages you to consider the whole person, rather than the presenting problem. We refer to this as *seeing the big picture* and invite you to experience it by guiding you through a series of written activities designed to explore the different facets of you, not just the area of growth and development that you have identified. By the end of this module, it is our hope that you have either a deeper understanding or appreciation of your value as a whole, autonomous, and capable person and, through that lens, then see your clients in a broader context. We hope this affirms the importance of understanding the person, not just the problem or challenge, and how this bigger view aids in finding strengths, capacity, and motivation for change.

The *Why*: Seeing the Big Picture Helps Us in Several Ways

Often in the work we do, it is easy to become locked into *why* the person is coming to see us. It makes sense that we would, as this is what we do at our agency, program, or practice—treat addiction, increase healthy behaviors (e.g., physical activity), decrease unhealthy behaviors (e.g., smoking), assist with eating disorders, ameliorate anxiety, relieve suffering from depression, or learn to move forward with a cancer diagnosis. Its why people see us, so it makes sense that we would "get down to business" and address the problem. Yet, this could make us slip into ***focusing*** before we have done the work of ***engaging***.

Of course, taking a history is a typical part of the intake process. Doing this, depending on the nature of our setting, we might find out about the client's family background, education, work, drugs and alcohol use, relationship, and spirituality. The aim of this process is to provide a context for understanding the individual and the context for the presenting problem. This is part of understanding the big picture, though it is easy to slip into a mindset of trying to find the origins of the current issue or problem.

MI, in this circumstance, is a *strength-based, whole-person approach*. There are several reasons for this approach. To begin, it helps us maintain perspective—we look beyond the presenting problem to see the person. We respond to the person first and the presenting issues second. We don't become so narrowly focused that we fail to see and prize the person in front of us. Using our garden analogy, this is seeing the whole garden for what it is or could be, even when it might be hidden at present. It is seeing the elements that are present, the soil conditions, the available light, and not just the weeds or a specific corner of the garden.

Seeing the big picture also helps us make a *shift from negative emotions to positive emotions*. There has been a growing literature about the value of emotions (Fredrickson, 2013a, 2013b; Stifter et al., 2020). Indeed, experiential tools have been developed to enhance therapeutic work with emotion (e.g., Hilton & Murphy, 2023). Negative emotions serve us well. They alert us to danger and motivate us to attend and respond to them. But such emotions carry a cost, as they're designed to mobilize us in the short term, not the long term. For example, they trigger constriction of our visual field, release stress hormones (e.g., cortisol) designed to save us in times of danger, and lead to bodily changes (e.g., reduced blood flow to extremities, increased blood pressure). Clients either entering treatment or seeking support with behavior change are typically awash in negative emotions.

Positive emotions function differently. They cause our visual field to expand, which permits seeing new opportunities. They release hormones like oxytocin that help connect us to others and increase blood flow. These emotions allow us to broaden and deepen our social connections, as well as our awareness of resources (Fredrickson, 2009, 2013a, 2013b). By *seeing the big picture*, we can attend to not only what is challenging in the client's situation, but also strengths, capacities, and what is going well.

Unsurprisingly then, *seeing the big picture* includes intentionally looking for the strengths, goals, dreams, and motivation of clients. This is not an exclusive focus on what is right and well, to the exclusion of what is challenging. Instead, it is tuning our ears to hear and notice all factors, even as clients fill us in on their lives. We hear the melody of the song, even as we listen to the lyrics. Through our ***reflective listening*** and ***summaries***, we will demonstrate our understanding, as well as aid the client in seeing these things, too.

Of course, to accomplish these tasks, we need to look at the whole person and the attitude we hold toward them. We view our clients as capable and autonomous, and our job is to be curious, seek to understand, and then help to draw out these capacities so the client can build on them, as well as for both of us to understand the dilemmas and challenges at hand. In MI, we do not assume we know either the problem or the solution to it. Instead, as we carefully work together, we come to a conjoint understanding of the challenge and then discover the approach that makes sense for this client.

The What: Tools for Seeing the Big Picture

The techniques we use flow from these ideas. It begins with focused, positively framed, ***open-ended questions***. Examples of these questions might be:

- What is going well in your life right now?
- Where do you feel like you're either having some success or at least holding your own currently?
- In the day-to-day rhythm of your life, where do you feel like you're doing okay?
- If I were to ask someone who knows you well, what would they say are one of your best qualities?

These questions, particularly when used to open a conversation, can not only begin to shift the emotional tenor of the discussion from negative to more positive emotions, but they may also inoculate people through a self-affirmation process to discuss more difficult parts of their lives (Sherman et al., 2000).

Directly recognizing and commenting on client strengths are another technique. Later, we will talk in more depth about ***affirmations***, which serve this function, but for now it's enough to simply listen for and make note of these for clients. There is a more subtle form of affirmation that is also present in this type of encounter—we prize the individual for who they are. By providing our curiosity and interest, and listening to their stories, we communicate they have worth and value beyond the matter that has brought them to us.

Finally, there are specific strategies we can use to *see the big picture.* One of these is just to state directly what we want to do.

> *I know we need to talk about* _________________________. *However, before we do, I'd really like to understand a little more about you and what's happening in your life. If you don't mind, fill me in about your circumstances. I know that's vague, but I want to leave a wide-open space for you to start.*

There are other approaches we might deploy. For example, we might ask, *What's important for me to know about you as we start our discussion today?* Another strategy might be to tell a story and ask a question.

> *Recently, I was reading a book where the author referenced the Quaker tradition of naming their children with character virtues. Their children might be given names like Patience, Peace, Serenity, Perseverance, or Courage. I thought that was interesting, and it made me think what my virtue name would be. I could think of a few that might be right, but the one that I kept coming back to was Determination. I'm curious. If you were to choose a virtue name, what might yours be?*

The answer to this would, of course, be followed up with curiosity and exploration.

The *How*: SP/SR on a Writing Exercise for Revealing Our Big Picture

Overview of the Exercise

For this activity, we will tell our autobiography in five different *chapters*:

- Just the facts
- Just the roles and tasks
- Just the strengths
- Just the hopes and aspirations
- Just a story about a day off

We prompt each chapter by asking different questions.

Structure of the Exercise

There are five chapters to be written/explored in this exercise. We encourage you to find a comfortable space to write and to do this activity in one *sitting*. This could be done as a self-directed activity, where answers are written in response to the questions. This approach might allow a deeper, slower, and more focused self-exploration based on the question posed.

A limited partner practice would involve using the chapter questions to guide the exploration, though this will require the partner to follow up, staying within the theme of the questions for a particular chapter. We encourage writing answers to the questions, prior to engaging in discussion with your limited partner practice. Share your answer and then explore these with curiosity, staying within the frame of that particular chapter. For example, in "the facts" chapter, just explore the facts. The aim is to see and feel how the exploration of the big picture influences our understanding of it.

Traveling Companion: An Example with Sam

Recall that Sam is a White, cisgender, gay woman of European descent who has been a successful counselor for many years. Fifteen years ago, she injured her back and, because of that experience, has shifted her private practice to health-focused care. She became interested in MI as part of the learning she did post injury, engaged in a variety of training and learning, and has recently been considering ways to advance her expertise. She had a cancer scare last year, and her wife is encouraging her to retire. Sam is ambivalent about making that change, and this has become a point of contention between them.

Chapter 1

➤ ***Write about the big picture of your current situation, sharing just the facts: name, age, city/town, village you reside in, relationship status, sexual orientation, gender identity, children, living situation, job, income, pets, and the like.***

My name is Sam, and I am 64 years old. I live in LaConner, Washington, which is in the Skagit Valley where there is a huge tulip festival each spring. I live with my wife, Debra. We've been married since shortly after the marriage equality legislation went into effect in Washington state. I am a lesbian, cisgender woman. Debra and I own our home, or at least the bank does and we're paying it off. We have a black lab named Sheba; she is our baby. No kids. Debra is retired from her job and loves the freedom to garden, craft, hike, and travel. I am still working. I have a therapy office attached to our home, which has a separate entrance. I try to limit therapy to 3 days a week so I can do paperwork on the fourth, and then Debra I are free to travel. We also like to bike, kayak, and camp. Since we're getting older now, we do less backpacking and more "glamping" in a little trailer that we bought and Debra restored.

Chapter 2

➤ ***Write about the big picture of your life through the lenses of your roles and the tasks that accompany each of those. For example, what is/are your role(s) at work and what tasks are you responsible for there? If you're in a relationship, what is your role in that relationship and what tasks are you responsible for in that.***

I'll start with work. Well, obviously I am a therapist, so my job is to provide psychotherapeutic services to my clients. Tasks include treatment planning and case conceptualization, planning possible session content, etc. But it also includes learning new techniques by attending continuing ed events and conferences, reading books, doing some online coursework, and I have a consultation group that meets once or twice a month, depending on the season and need. I used to do more journal reading than I do now. Scheduling is done by me, though I do use an after-hours service; sometimes I wonder if that's worth it. I do use a billing service, so there is preparing the materials for them. As a small business owner, I do my own accounting, bill paying, and the like, using a software program. I also pay estimated taxes. I do use an accountant to help me with filing my tax returns.

At home, Debra is the handier person, so she does home repair and maintenance. We both garden. I have tended to be the primary cook, as I am a little more creative in that department. We do maintain a vegetable garden, and I love to use what we've grown. Debra is the early riser, so she handles morning dog duties, including taking Sheba for a walk. I handle evenings, and we typically do a walk together, although sometimes Debra gets stuck with that if I have late clients. Housekeeping is shared but tends to fall more my way as Debra takes care of other tasks. I handle the money, pay bills, and maintain contact with the financial analyst. I tend to be the more social of the pair, so I maintain the social calendar and do the planning. If we have guests, I do the primary meal prep, and Debra is the sous chef and does clean-up. I interact more with the neighbors. Debra plans the camping outings or the landscape jobs, those sorts of things.

Chapter 3

➤ ***Talk about your big picture strengths. What do you do well? What would friends, family, or coworkers say they admire or appreciate about you? You might think about these in terms of circumstances, like what do I do well at work, school, home, with friends.***

I guess I got a little ahead of myself in Chapter 2 because I already started talking about these things, though I think I can add a little more depth and context. I tend to be warm and nurturing, and confident in who I am. It was not easy growing up as a lesbian at a time when that was not well accepted, but I decided that I would be myself. I think people appreciate that about me. There is no subterfuge or hidden agenda. What you see, is what you get.

Because I am comfortable in my own skin, I think people can be comfortable in theirs. I am genuinely curious about people, and I love hearing about them and their stories. I think my training has made me a pretty good listener, though I do make a distinction between "Sam at work" and "Sam at home." I can listen well, without being a therapist with friends and neighbors. But I am the kind of person who'll have a conversation with the postal carrier, the cashier at the grocery, and the person browsing in a shop. We have a lot of tourists come through our town in the spring and summer, and Debra tends to become annoyed by how difficult they make it to get around and to accomplish chores. She gets grumpy. I get a kick out of them and am happy to answer their questions, take a picture of their family, and have a conversation. It's not that I never get annoyed—shopping can be a real pain in the summer—but on balance I lean into it.

I think that is one of the things my friends would tend to say about me: I tend to be pretty happy and upbeat. I laugh easily and often. I tend to look for the best in people and I can see it. It doesn't mean that I don't see or hear about the worst in people. I do. I'm not Pollyanna. I just believe we have a choice. For me it's also a form of spiritual practice. It's like looking for the light in others, and by nurturing it, we nurture it for ourselves, too.

Chapter 4

➤ ***What were your hopes and aspirations for your life? What are those hopes and aspirations for right now? What are your hopes and aspirations for a few years down the road?***

Oh, that's a big question. When I was young, I wanted adventure. I wanted to travel and see the world. I just knew there was more out there. It's like living next to Mrs. Haddid. She came from the Middle East, and it's like I wanted to go see all those vibrant colors like she wore and smell those spices that she sometimes used. I wanted to hear those voices in languages that I didn't know. To meet people and have conversations about interesting things was what I was after. I wanted a big life, which meant that I didn't just want to work in the family business. That was my parent's dream. Not mine.

My aspirations for now . . . well, I want to keep doing what I'm doing. I love my wife and my life. I get to have these interesting conversations now. What I learned is that travel is great, and I love it, but I didn't have to go to exotic places to meet interesting people. I just had to be willing to talk to people and really listen to their stories. Early in my life, I think I was too impatient to hear those things. Now, I love when Debra tells me about her trip to the hardware store or when a friend talks about a visit to her mother. There's juice there if I let myself really be present. So, I want to walk the dog, garden in our little plot, sit on the patio and laugh with friends, see my clients, and help them find their way.

A few years down the road, I hope my health will still be good and I can still be physically active. I'm at the point in my clinical career where I don't have great ambitions for doing something marvelous. I just want to continue to get better at my practice. I believe learning MI has helped me become better already and so I look forward to refining that skill. The person who trained me has suggested I consider becoming a "MINT trainer," though I haven't really looked into it seriously yet. I guess I am of the mindset that if you're not learning, you're dying, and I'm not ready to do that yet. Becoming a MI trainer might be fun to do. It would certainly stretch me.

Chapter 5

➤ ***What do you like to do on Saturdays or your day off? Provide details about the things you do, and what makes them something you*** **like** ***to do and not just something you have to do.***

Well, this would depend on the time of the year. During the spring, when the daffodils are up and later the tulips, I love getting up early with Debra. We grab a cup of coffee, throw the bikes on the Subaru rack, and scoot over to the flower fields. Then we just ride down the lanes as the sun comes up. It's often brisk and damp, but it is spectacular when the sun hits those fields. We're out before all the traffic starts arriving from the cities, and it's just us, the farmers, and the pickers. It's our own little slice of heaven.

As people start arriving, we drive back to La Conner and grab a booth at one of the coffee shops, order a pastry or some eggs and potatoes—we did just earn it, right—and enjoy the coffee and the town before it's flooded with folks. We take our time, and then go home and take Sheba for a short walk, and then we're ready for the rest of our day. Sometimes it's gardening. Other times it's another project. Sometimes it's going to the San Juan Islands or the mountains for a hike. It just feels like we get to choose our adventure. Then we would come home. Plan a meal. Invite some friends over, sit under the Edison lights around the fire ring, and talk and laugh—that sounds about perfect to me. Of course, not every Saturday is like that—the toilet does need to be cleaned and those floors won't mop themselves—but that's what I do love when I get to choose.

For this module, we have also included some of Sam's self-reflection answers as they might be helpful in thinking through your own answers.

➤ ***Please read back over the five chapters in this exercise. What do you notice as you do? What do you experience in your body? In your feelings? In your thoughts?***

There is a definite deepening of the story, of my story. It's like we started from the outside and worked our way in. Of course, I sort of jumped ahead, so I might have blended it a little, but I can see it. More importantly, I can feel it. It's like I catch a little more emotion—including a little more positive feelings—as we move through it. I also felt a little inspired, like I want to have that Saturday this Saturday and so I found myself thinking about talking to Debra. I also realized things I hadn't before. Like I wanted a BIG LIFE and I thought I knew what that meant, and now I am realizing that I did that, just not in the way I thought I would. I also have reaffirmed what I love and what I appreciate about myself. The things I want to nurture and be more of.

➤ ***Each of these chapters tells a different part of your story. They all have value and provide access to a different facet of you. What was the value of each for you?***

This is a tough question. "Facet" is a good word because it seems like each asks some aspect of this question, "Who are you, Sam?" None of the chapters is the full answer. They all contain a piece of the truth, but none are the whole truth. The first one gives me the "deets," like the kind of thing you'd find on a Wikipedia page. To see those and to recognize—that's not all of me. Then the same thing with roles and tasks. I chose two big areas—work and home life—and realized there were lots of roles within the roles, and lots of tasks. I also realized that it's easy to begin prioritizing and seeing myself only in those roles. And, of course, those aren't the only roles. I play the role of the neighbor who loves Halloween, and we didn't even talk about that. Thinking about strengths took me on a whole different path. It's like looking in the mirror and seeing the best version of me. The me I like. Hopes and aspirations were fascinating because it took me on a journey of time and thinking about the thread of my life. The last one was just so unexpected and delightful. In talking about what I loved to do, it revealed something about who I am and what brings me joy and amusement. It inspired me to do something.

➤ ***Was there one chapter that seemed to capture you best? If so, in what ways?***

I don't think so. It's a bit like taking a picture of the Skagit Valley during the four different seasons and asking, which is the real Skagit Valley? They'll capture different things and there might be parts that feel more pleasing, but they're all Skagit Valley. So, too, all are me.

➤ ***As you think about your work with clients, how do these chapters reflect your usual ways of discovering the big picture? What strikes you about that?***

It seems as plain as the nose on my face that I've been only focusing on a facet or two. Finding out the details and the roles, primarily. While that's a start, it feels quite limited, and it doesn't feel like that will build a sense of connection like the other three might. I'm thinking about how I integrate this more intentionally into my work.

➤ ***What might be the value for you and for the client in altering how you see the big picture for your clients? What benefits might accrue?***

The details of a life feel relatively impersonal, even though they can be quite personal in nature, like gender identity. It seems to be a very cognitive exercise in information gathering. As we move into roles, we might get a little more affect, but it seems like this might be the tension about tasks and the demands of the person's life. Important to know about, but perhaps more targeted to negative emotions. Like it's tiring just to think about. It's in the last three that we start to turn the tide to some more positive emotions. It almost feels like this might be a far better place to begin and then work our way backward. Thinking back to the questions and strategies suggested in the beginning of this module, these seem like they would fit there.

➤ ***What are some specific things you might do to alter your approach? How will you assess if these are effective?***

I'm thinking two things. First, how I begin my first session has been focused on information collection and some sharing. "Let's review the paperwork," "Here's how we work," etc. I'm thinking that needs to change and be more intentional about finding other facets that reveal some of their strengths and start us on a positive note. People need hope. I know I did. But it must come from some place authentic, and it seems like that's what this does.

Second, I think I'm going to spread these things out. We often think of clients like onions where we peel back layers, but I like this idea of facets. Like a diamond, where we can only see certain parts at a time. I want to be more intentional about looking at those, but not doing it all at the beginning.

Self-Practice

Please complete each chapter before moving onto the next. Allow the process to unfold and see what you discover. This activity might require more paper and time than others. Give it the time you need. For those who prefer to talk rather than write, you might consider recording your answers, then listening back, and noting the most salient or poignant elements. Use extra paper as needed.

Chapter 1

➤ ***Write about the big picture of your current situation, sharing just the facts: name, age, city/town, village you reside in, relationship status, sexual orientation, gender identity, children, living situation, job, income, pets, and the like.***

Chapter 2

➤ ***Write about the big picture of your life through the lenses of your roles and the tasks that accompany each of those. For example, what is/are your role(s) at work? If you're in a relationship, what is your role in it? What tasks are you responsible for in either role or both?***

Chapter 3

- ***Talk about your big picture strengths. What do you do well? What would friends, family, or coworkers say they admire or appreciate about you? You might think about these in terms of circumstances, like what do I do well at work, school, home, with friends.***

Chapter 4

- ***What were your hopes and aspirations for your life? What are those hopes and aspirations for right now? What are your hopes and aspirations for a few years down the road?***

Chapter 5

➤ ***What do you like to do on Saturdays or your day off? Provide details about the things you do and what makes them something you*** like ***to do and not just something you have to do.***

Self-Reflection

➤ ***Please read back over the five chapters in this exercise. What do you notice as you do? What do you experience in your body? In your feelings? In your thoughts?***

> ***Each of these chapters tells a different part of your story. They all have value and provide access to a different facet of you. What was the value of each for you?***

> ***Was there one chapter that seemed to capture you best? If so, in what ways?***

> ***Was it difficult or easy to do this process? What made it so?***

What If: Applying Skills to My Current Context

Bridging Questions to Practitioner-Self

These questions are designed to help you bring the insights from personal self-practice into your work with clients.

> ***As you think about your work with clients, how do these chapters reflect your usual ways of discovering the big picture? What strikes you about that?***

➤ *What might be the value for you and for the client in altering how you see the big picture for your clients? What benefits might accrue?*

➤ *How does this help you understand how to focus at the beginning of a client encounter and questions to use early in MI?*

➤ *What are some specific things you might do to alter your approach to engaging people? How will you assess if these are effective?*

➤ ***What are your main* takeaway *messages from this SP/SR experience in relation to your understanding of the concept of seeing the big picture . . .***

- ***From a practical perspective?***

  ___

  ___

  ___

- ***From a theoretical perspective?***

  ___

  ___

  ___

➤ ***What if you were to apply this process to other areas of your professional practice (e.g., in a role as supervisor or trainer perhaps)? How might you apply your learning to this new context?***

___

___

___

➤ ***How has this exercise influenced your understanding of or personal relationship with MI as a way of being?***

___

___

___

Final Thoughts and Applications to Other Settings

The tendency might be to think that *seeing the big picture* involves searching for a buried treasure, which we and clients unearth together. In some cases, that might be so. However, Rosengren (2017) has previously asserted there might be a co-creation that happens in this process. That is, as we carefully work in a trusting environment to understand, a mutually influencing process occurs. The result is a new idea or understanding, one that had not existed before, but which the client can then use to assist them in moving forward. Sam's realization that she is living a BIG LIFE could be discovery of buried treasure, but it could also be that through a process of responding to questions, she came to understand an idea that had not existed for her before: My life now is big, rich, and full of the things I wanted as a young woman. Much as happens in narrative therapy (e.g., Dallos, 2023; Monk et al., 1997), the psychological truth of this idea and the organizational power it provides create both a structure for the client and a pathway forward.

Such a process would require a great deal of care for practitioners. Hence, the importance of compassion and autonomy within the ***MI spirit***. We must be mindful that this is the client's goals, aspirations, and life. It requires that our empathy includes the capacity to retain our sense of self, to separate from our cognitive and affective understanding of what is happening for the client. It must be their narrative, not ours.

Within brief encounter settings, we often experience pressure to "get down to business" and focus on the presenting problem(s). This leads to the ***premature focus trap***, which happens when we move to focus and help solve problems before we understand the person's context, the resources they have available, and their reasons for undertaking a change. A health care example would be a patient seeing a surgeon for a knee replacement. The surgeon may enter with experience that tells them a combination of pain and/or loss of function is driving the request, so therefore, the focus should be on the logistics of the surgery, the recovery, and subsequent rehab. None of this, though, elicits the person's *Why*, their reasons for undergoing this arduous process, which will also be the reasons for sustaining effort when the situation becomes difficult. Again, time pressures and clear agency agendas can make it easy to overlook this process.

An ancillary challenge, fueled by many of the same dynamics, is the ***assessment trap***. That is, we ask a series of questions and then provide the client with the answer or solution to their problems. The client's agency and autonomy get lost in such a process. Again, brief encounters and setting dynamics can place us at greater risk of falling into these traps.

Recognizing these issues allows us to take a step back and ask ourselves, *What does this person want to accomplish, and why does it matter to them?* Simple questions can be helpful here. For our surgeon, it might be asking, *Why is having this surgery important to you? What are you hoping the outcome will be?* Stepping back to *see the big picture* might slow the immediate process slightly as some additional conversation will be required, but it will allow the subsequent process to move more efficiently and with increased likelihood of follow-through as the client's overall reasons for engaging in the process become either more internalized or strengthened.

MODULE 9

Being Understood

Module Purpose

This module explores what it means to be understood, and the challenge inherent in connecting with and understanding another with whom we disagree. Your self-practice experience invites you to have a conversation with someone with whom you have a different view and to feel the difference between listening to respond and listening to understand. The key aim is to utilize MI skills to help this person feel understood, while you explore the bodily sensations, feelings, and thoughts that accompany you in this process. By the end of this module, it is our hope that you will experience how we might help others feel understood, how easy or difficult this can be, and how this transfers into the process of supporting someone through change and growth.

The *Why*: The Role of Being Understood in Expanding Knowledge of Self

We are herd animals. As a species, we do best when we are interconnected; our brains are wired to release hormones that assist with this connection process and neurons that fire in a manner that allows us to anticipate and respond to the experience of others. It is no surprise then that we have a deep desire to connect with and be understood by others. Yet, *being understood* is a complicated business, which we all know from experience. But what do we mean by being understood?

Let's begin with a pragmatic definition. Being understood is the experience of thinking and feeling that another person comprehends our inner experience, as well as our outward manifestations. They know something of who we believe we are, which might include our thoughts, feelings, beliefs, desires, needs, motivations, strengths, and limitations. We might say things like "They know my heart" or "They get me." Of course, this knowledge is always incomplete, as so beautifully articulated by the Johari window (Luft & Ingham, 1961). See Figure 9.1.

Being understood at a superficial level involves information in the open or public area, but when people feel more deeply understood, that range of knowing expands outward into the blind spot, hidden area, and unknown, as depicted below.

	Known to self	Not known to self
Known to others	Open area	Blind spot
Not known to others	Hidden area	Unknown

FIGURE 9.1. Johari window model.

This experience of being fully understood, as suggested by Figure 9.2, is not one of just being more fully known by another but also by ourselves. We expand our self-knowledge. It is part of what makes this process of being understood so powerful and at the same time increases our sense of vulnerability. It is why the elements of the ***MI spirit—partnership***, ***acceptance***, ***compassion***, and ***envisioning***—and ***creating safety*** are so fundamental to the work, But, why does it matter?

Research and experience suggest many reasons why it matters to be understood; here, we will focus on four. To begin, being understood decreases defensiveness (Miller & Rollnick, 2023). That is, when people feel heard and understood, there is a decreased need to defend behavior against either real or perceived attack. However, as we proceed through the book, we will deepen this idea and note that consistently asking for, and exploring, thoughts that sustain the status quo may not always be helpful; this approach may further entrench the person's thinking and defensiveness (e.g., *Why don't you think you need to change?*). The aim then is to understand these things and then assist the person in thinking beyond them if that is part of their goals and values.

This brings us to the second reason why being understood matters—it increases connection and trust (Miller, 2018). Being understood gathers the ingredients of a strong relationship: connection and trust. These characteristics help to cement a growing bond, which in turn allows people to feel we have their best interests in mind. It is the manifestation of empathy and compassion we discussed previously (Rogers, 1980). With decreased defensiveness and increased connection and trust, we move into the third reason why being understood matters—it permits consideration of new possibilities. We are literally more open and can see possibilities that previously were either unavailable to our awareness or we see them in a new light (Fredrickson, 2013a, 2013b). We find solutions to our problems in the leeward side created by such a relationship and this permits us to turn back into the wind when ready. Finally, when done well, being understood moves beyond the specific context or issues to understanding ourselves more

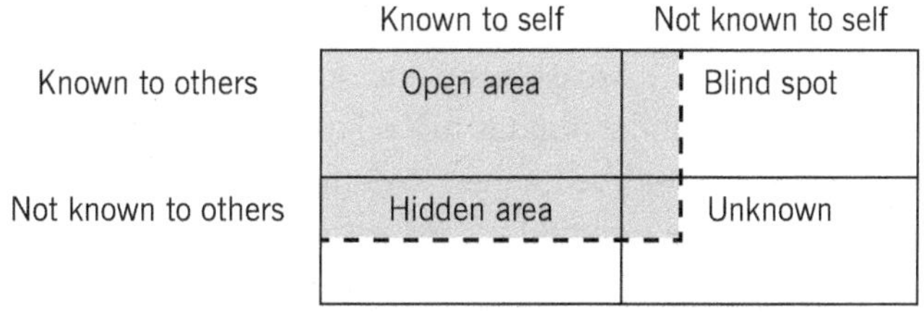

FIGURE 9.2. Johari window: Being understood.

broadly. We see the whole person, including our strengths and capacities, as well as our foibles, and have a better sense of how those create the mosaic that we are. This also permits us to bring more resources to addressing the challenges that life presents. These factors create a virtuous cycle that increases the power of each individually (e.g., Kellerman & Seligman, 2023).

The *What*: Tools of Being Understood

Having discussed the *Why* of being understood, we move to the *What*. The obvious answer is listening. While listening is common, listening well is not. It requires more of us than happens typically in our daily conversations and often in our professional encounters. It begins with decluttering our minds.

Often in everyday conversations, our brains are filled with the myriad tasks, thoughts, and beliefs associated with that day and this encounter. Here's how those thoughts and beliefs might work with Henny, our disgruntled friend:

> *Henny always complains about the city government and the nature of politicians. I've heard this before, and it goes nowhere. I know what her complaints are and what she's going to say; I also believe that I know why she says them, based on her prior complaints. She starts and I nod and say, Uh-huh, but my mind begins to wander, What time do the kids need to be at that dental appointment today? What did I need to pick up at the store? Should I do that before or after we go to the dentist?*

As this process unfolds, we've missed what Henny is saying. The same process can happen for us as practitioners. For example, we might think the following:

> *Henny often moves into complaining mode, but never quite sees how this mode fits into her pattern of being stuck. We need to get her to step back and look at the big picture of how this is working or not working for her. It's a maladaptive pattern and it keeps her dissatisfied, but also allows her to vent emotion.*

This is a reasonable conceptualization, yet we have not heard what Henny's telling us. This falls in the category of *listening to respond*. There are several common patterns that happen in listening to respond. To begin, we assume understanding what someone means, instead of checking the accuracy of our understanding. Then we often wait our turn to share our thoughts, views, or stories. While doing this, we are less involved in hearing the other, but rather are preparing our remarks. Finally, we might be formulating our rejoinder; that is, we are martialing our cannons to return fire about something we disagree with. This type of listening is common to everyday conversation, but in MI we ask people to do more—*listening to understand*.

Our first task in listening to understand is to declutter. We make space in ourselves to hear what the person is telling us. It could be likened to doing some spring cleaning; we make space for what the client has to say. The second task is we turn our focus onto the other. That is, as we declutter, we move from the thoughts, ideas, beliefs in our head, and turn our full attention to what the other person is saying. As we do this, we adopt a curiosity about what is being said; this is the third task. We don't assume we know, but instead hear what is being expressed by the client in this statement. The fourth task is to go below the surface of the client's words to understand them more fully and to help the client do the same. If we think about the Johari window, we're dipping into the elements that appear in quadrants 2, 3, and 4—what is private to the person, what it unknown to the person, and what is unknown to us both. With Henny, this might be her feelings of powerlessness and a desire to find ways to regain agency. We will not know until we test our understanding by offering it to Henny and she tells us how it fits. Throughout this process, we retain an attitude of curiosity. This approach precludes our being judgmental if we truly embrace it. We're trying to understand how these thoughts, feelings, or experiences come together from this person's point of view. Since this process often moves into areas unknown to the client as well as us, we discover her understanding of self together.

Listening well involves using ***reflective listening*** strategies (see Box 9.1). The mechanics of listening have been discussed in-depth elsewhere (e.g., Frey & Hall, 2021; Rosengren, 2017) and presumably in prior training, so they will not be covered at length here. If you feel that you need additional practice in these areas, we encourage you to pursue one of these resources. To recap ideas expressed in those texts, reflective listening involves making statements, not asking questions. The tone of voice drops at the end of each sentence. It does NOT require a lead-in, such as "I hear you saying. . . ." It can take multiple forms in response to a client statement.

Imagine a client says, "I tried therapy before, and I'm still stuck." We might stay on the surface of what the person says: "You've tried this before" or "You're stuck." Yet, reflections are most powerful when they go below the surface to explore thoughts, feelings, and beliefs that may be present: "You want to change. It's about figuring out how to get there." They may understate the emotional content to encourage more exploration: "You're a little worried we might not get to where you want to go." Or overstate it to help the client assess whether this is a position they indeed hold: "It scares you to think this might never change." They can anticipate a direction in which the client's thoughts might lead: "And so you're looking for something different from our time together." They can contain the client's ambivalence: "Part of you might want to protect yourself from disappointment in our work, and part of you feels hope that things could be better." All or none of these ideas might be accurate. The client's response will tell us if they are true and will lead to more exploration, if the client feels we are genuinely curious about their inner world.

Notice how this process of going below the surface allows us to expand the area that is known in the Johari window. In this manner, it also helps us to identify interconnections within the individual and potentially see the bigger picture of the client's life. This is an exploration, not "drilling down" to find the client's problem, challenge, or issue. We need to remain intentional about what and how we explore, looking for ways to expand rather than narrow our focus.

BOX 9.1. Elements of Listening to Understand

- Declutter our minds.
- Focus on the other.
- Be curious.
- Go below the surface.

In the example of our client statement above, this could be done by making a reflection like the following: "In this area, you're stuck, and that isn't true in all areas." Notice that here we are taking a guess, but the client will tell us if it is accurate.

The *How*: SP/SR on an Exercise in Being Understood by Working with a Challenging Other

Overview of the Exercise

For this activity, we want you to engage with someone whom you would normally have trouble listening to. We want you to use this encounter as an opportunity to practice listening well in a circumstance where your tendency will be to argue, dismiss, or attempt to dissuade another of a position or point of view. Your goal is to create for this other person the experience of *being understood*. Just to clarify, this does not mean agreeing with the other person, but rather being able to honestly say to yourself, *I understand why they might see it that way*. This activity will be done independently; that is, without your limited-practice partner.

Structure of the Exercise

For this activity, we want you to venture into the world for a conversation. Find someone with whom you disagree on a topic. If this is part of your area for growth, the conversation can be a helpful one, though make sure you're ready for it. If the conversation is above that 6 or 7 on your difficulty scale, choose someone else.

This may be someone you know or someone you encounter. Politics are an area that may be a rich resource, with many people we might choose from. This conversation may be challenging because your thoughts and beliefs will likely press on your intention to listen. The aim of this conversation is not to convince the person they are wrong, but instead to explore why they hold the position they do. The opening of this conversation is relatively straightforward and could sound something like the following:

> *You and I seem to have different views on that idea, I'm wondering if you might help me. I'd really like to understand better what you are thinking and why. My aim is not to convince you of anything or to make you change, but just to understand. Could we talk about this for just a couple of minutes?*

Keep in mind the four key ideas: Declutter, focus on the other, be curious, and go below the surface. Work to really understand and communicate to the person what you're understanding is. Give yourself a 15-minute goal; that is, you'll listen with great interest and curiosity for 15 minutes, before changing the focus or ending the conversation.

Traveling Companion: An Example with Quincy

Remember, Quincy is a 38-year-old, cisgender, straight woman of African descent who works as an AOD counselor. Growing up in a vibrant community, she has strong family ties and a foundation of giving to others. She was feeling some burnout with substance use clients and has taken an MI workshop, but it hasn't found its way into her work. Because of her feelings of burnout, she sought personal support and decided to find a therapist skilled in MI to learn more about the process.

Because we can't be privy to Quincy's conversation, we will instead take a look at her responses to the self-reflection questions.

➤ ***Who did you decide to talk to and why?***

I spoke to one of my coworkers; I'll call him Reg. He is someone who has an opinion about everything, and I find myself often getting annoyed when he starts jabbering about one thing or another, so typically I avoid him. This time I decided to choose one of the things that annoy me and start a conversation about it. I chose one that irritated me before so I knew it would challenge me to manage my feelings.

➤ ***What bodily sensations did you have as this conversation began? How did you manage these? What feelings and thoughts followed?***

I won't lie. I felt a few flutters in my stomach and kept rubbing the palm of my hand with my thumb. I was a bit nervous and a bit skeptical about Reg and the exercise. I kept thinking, "Really? Like, what's the point?" even though intellectually I knew this was a good thing for me to do. One of my challenges with burnout has been jumping to conclusions or being judgy. I figured this is the way forward. I guess that is one of the ways I managed it. Focusing on my self-talk and attitude. I did use "Be curious" as kind of a mantra. In terms of the nervousness, I handled that the way I always do—I told myself to be brave and then jumped in.

➤ ***What did you discover, were surprised by, or hadn't known before as you listened more deeply?***

Okay, do I really have to say this? I guess I do. I found out that Reg had some things to say, if I listened. He normally gets loud when I challenge him, but when I listened, that changed. He had thought through some of these ideas and had some reasons to back up why he thought the way he did. As he talked, I realized there was more substance to him than I'd given him credit for. Also, as he talked, he also softened some of his positions. I could see these positions weren't as hardened as he usually presented and that he was drawing on some stuff from his childhood that bothered him. I didn't know much about his family or some of his experiences, and he shared some details.

➤ ***How did your big picture of this person broaden because of more careful listening?***

He was a 3D person in a context rather than just this cartoon, this opinionated guy. I could see how it tied together with his past and how it might influence his work. I also got a sense for his caring for folks that I had missed. I'd just heard a lot of "People need to pull themselves up by their bootstraps," without really understanding what that meant to him. I could also see how he felt like folks were missing something important and that this put clients at risk. I understood that better, even though I don't agree with him.

➤ ***What were some examples where you felt as if you listened particularly well? Try to be specific in recollecting what the person said, what you said, and how this impacted the person.***

Here's an example. He said people need to be accountable. Normally, I would argue with him, but instead I said, "You want people to see their power to choose." And he said, something like "Exactly, instead of blaming others for their problems, I want them to take responsibility." What was interesting is there was kind of an energy when he talked then. Like someone understood and he wanted to tell me more—which he did.

➤ ***At a global level, how did this person react to your listening? What specifically did you notice? Why is this important?***

Really well actually. It's like he still had the fire, but it was more contained. More like passion for the subject, than being argumentative with me. It also felt like a barrier, or something, was lowered between us—at least a bit. Like he let down his guard when I let down mine. Like my listening told him I was interested in him. He's been a bit more friendly, and I've felt friendlier toward him.

➤ ***How did your attitudes, thoughts, and/or feelings change because of this listening process?***

Now, that is the interesting part to me. I just said we felt more friendly and that's important from a work relationship perspective. We're clearly not going to be best friends, but I also feel like I understand him better. While I disagree with him, I find myself being a lot less judgy. I also find myself being more open to listening to what he has to say. Now, he isn't a client, so I kind of wish he would listen to ME, but that hasn't happened yet.

➤ ***What challenged you in this listening process? Why, when, and with what do you find yourself internally disagreeing?***

The biggest challenge were my emotions. When we hit on an area I felt strongly about, I'd find myself starting to build counterarguments. I also needed to pay attention to my body and my nonverbals. I told myself to relax and not do things like shake my head or grit my teeth! I really had to remind myself not to jump in and respond but to intentionally listen to understand, to be curious, and to go below the surface. My clutter—thinking I knew what something meant—was also a big obstacle, and I had to remind myself to stop assuming and—again—be curious.

Also, when he started getting passionate, I found myself starting to feel more emotional. When that happened, my tendency was to pull back or slip into disagreement.

➤ ***What might be useful to take from this practice and apply to your work with clients you find challenging?***

This turned out to be useful, so there are a lot of things I want to pull forward. First, reminding myself of the four parts of listening well really helped me, but especially staying curious.

Second, I recognize that my emotions tend to lead me away from listening. So, while they might be good for empathy, emotions can also be a distraction. I need to recognize when they're coming up and reminding myself to listen. Third, I am aware of how much more I understood about the person by listening to what they had to say and then taking it further. Focusing on his emotions not only helped with managing my own, but also let me see how his emotions and what they might evoke in others would help me work with Reg, if he was a client. Finally, and I feel kind of silly saying it, but I also noticed that I tend to ask a lot of questions, but when I stop doing that, I seem to get more and better information. For example, I heard what is core for Reg and how that lines up with what he says and does, and how knowing that, I can understand him better.

➤ ***What would be the benefit of these changes for the client and for you?***

Well, to begin with, the relationship is better. When that's better, I feel like there is more hope for something. With Reg, it's that we can get along. With clients, I would expect it's that they can achieve their goals. I also notice there was a lot less tension, so it felt like we had energy for other things—both of us. I also didn't feel drained at the end, even though listening is hard work. I also know that I felt more peaceful and centered, and I would expect the same would be true for clients. Not that everything is easy, but just like . . . things are safe? Well, that makes sense given the prior module, right? We create safety, and it leads to more safety and that leads to more calm.

Self-Practice

Again, the aim is to have a conversation with someone with whom you disagree. This may either be someone you know or a chance encounter. The aim of this conversation is not to convince the person they're wrong, but instead to explore why they hold the position they do. The opening is straightforward and could sound similar to the following:

> *You and I seem to have different views on that idea. I'm wondering if you might help me, I'd really like to understand better what you're thinking and why. My aim is not to convince you of anything or to make you change, but just to understand. Could we talk about this for a little bit?*

Self-Reflection

➤ ***Who did you decide to talk to and why?***

___

___

___

___

___

➤ *What bodily sensations did you have as this conversation began? How did you manage these? What feelings and thoughts followed?*

➤ *What did you discover, were surprised by, or hadn't known before as you listened more deeply?*

➤ *How did your big picture of this person broaden because of more careful listening?*

➤ *What were some examples where you felt as if you listened particularly well? Try to be specific in recollecting what the person said, what you said, and how this impacted the person.*

➤ *This exercise had you working to understand another person instead of having an experience of being understood. What did you observe about that change in focus? How did it impact you? Why?*

➤ *Did this exercise help you learn about yourself in terms of how you do or do not listen to someone you disagree with? Why or why not?*

➤ *At a global level, how did this person react to your listening? What specifically did you notice? Why is this important?*

➤ *When is a time you felt deeply understood by another unexpectedly? How did it affect you? Why was that significant?*

What If: Applying Skills to My Current Context

Bridging Questions to Practitioner-Self

These questions are designed to help you bring the insights from personal self-practice into your work with clients,

- ***How did your attitudes, thoughts, and/or feelings change because of this listening process?***

- ***What challenged you in this listening process? Why, when, or to what do you find yourself internally disagreeing?***

- ***What might be useful to take from this practice and apply to your work with clients you find challenging?***

- ***What would be the benefit of these changes for the client and for you?***

➤ *What are your main* takeaway *messages from this SP/SR experience in relation to your understanding of the concept of being understood . . .*

- *From a practical perspective?*

- *From a theoretical perspective?*

➤ *What if you were to apply this process to other areas of your professional practice (e.g., in a role as supervisor or trainer perhaps)? How might you apply your learning to this new context?*

➤ *How has this exercise influenced your understanding of or personal relationship with MI as a way of being?*

Final Thoughts and Applications to Other Settings

Being understood and the listening skills that accompany it will form a cornerstone for all that is to come. As a result, a single opportunity to practice these skills will be insufficient to build the capacity needed for this essential skill. Instead, think of this as the foundation on which we will scaffold other skills and continue to refine these. Our returning to these ideas is not a simple repetition, but instead an intention to deepen and broaden skills by adding reflection and refinement to this *Inside Out* process.

Earlier in this module, we discussed the Johari window and how to expand into quadrants 2, 3, and 4. As the practitioner, we have described our role as the master gardener for the client who is the gardener. The practitioner's job within the Johari framework may be to help discover what is already in quadrant 2 (blind spot), have the courage to connect and articulate what is in quadrant 3 (hidden) and perhaps, via this iterative process of discovery, more of quadrant 4 (the unknown) becomes known. There is also a parallel process for us as learners in using this process of self-practice and self-reflection—where we are the gardeners in our own development. We will likely find an SP/SR discussion group helpful in discovering and learning more about the method and ourselves. However, we may find particular benefit from a mentor, coach, or supervisor who can assist in expanding our own self-knowledge: of our blind spots, our hidden areas, and the parts that are unknown.

The master gardener and beginning gardener share the same tools (hoe, shovel, pruner) and the knowledge of ingredients for growth (water, sun, fertilizer, soil, seeds). However, master gardeners' experience and refinement in practice help them to see, understand, and respond with nuance. That experience and refinement are what we bring to clients, and what we work to develop here as learners of MI.

In brief encounter settings, it is a common experience for people to feel they don't have space for listening, Time is of the essence, and therefore, we feel compelled to tell people what to do. As we've noted, this desire to move quickly fails to attend to how motivation becomes more internalized, how the internalization of that motivation leads to better follow-through especially as things get difficult, and how important psychological needs like autonomy and competence are undermined. It is these factors that cause MI trainers to note that telling/persuading increases time in the long run as the change effort will take more attempts and contacts with us as the practitioner.

Having said this, we can set limits on how much time we will spend and take steps to focus our interactions. For example, we might say to a person with whom we're having a consultation:

> *We have 5 minutes before we'll be interrupted. What's essential that we discuss in that time for you?*

It is also important to be honest in our assessment:

> *We're not going to be able to take on all of what you have just shared with me now. What's one piece that we could address that would feel meaningful to you?*

By taking the time to establish these limits, we can then lean into our task of listening deeply, so people feel understood and can begin expanding their knowledge of themselves and move forward in their areas for growth or change.

MODULE 10

Opening Possibility

Module Purpose

This module explores the role of hope within MI, including its role in the transition from ***engaging*** to ***focusing*** and building awareness of capacity for change. By the end of this module, it is our intention that you experience how opening possibility through recollection of past experience, optimism, and careful listening can help to raise curiosity, self-efficacy, and readiness to change in clients.

The *Why*: Opening Possibility as a Path to Motivation

The previous three modules focused on ***engagement***. That is, these are about creating an environment where the client can feel safe with us, and we can see at least a snapshot of them situated in the big picture of their life. We work to communicate our understanding, which in turn creates an opportunity to explore the realities and challenges in their lives more deeply. Sometimes this is all clients need. However, for many clients this safe holding space is a relief, and it can also leave them mired in their current contexts. The next step then is about *opening possibility*.

Opening possibility is about *hope*. Positive psychologists, using the *broaden and build theory* (Fredrickson, 2001), place hope in the *positive emotions* category (e.g., joy, love, contentment). Positive emotions broaden our response capacities to the challenges of living and build our resilience, at least in part by strengthening our social connections. While *negative emotions* (e.g., regret, anger, jealousy, sadness) have their place—after all, they can save us from dangerous situations—positive emotions enhance our ability to respond when difficulties arise. They help us to see new possibilities and become more creative and effective problem-solvers. One interesting thing about hope is that it can occur without psychological safety being present. Other positive emotions (e.g., joy, awe, amusement) require safety. But this relationship might be more complicated than we know. For example, it might be that hope agency (i.e., the ability to reach one's goals) and not just hope pathways (i.e., many routes to reach an outcome) are essential for hope to have power (Chang et al., 2021; Li et al., 2021). One important aspect of positive emotions is that they often feel weak in comparison to negative emotions, but they are contagious. That is, our hope for clients can suffuse them with hope, which is consistent with the research on therapist effects that has consistently demonstrated therapeutic alliance influences favorable outcomes for clients (e.g., Bibeau et al., 2016; Flückiger et al., 2018; Hilton & Johnston, 2017).

Researchers in psychotherapy find that hope in the form of therapist optimism results in dramatically better outcomes for clients (Miller & Moyers, 2021), even when that optimism is based on nothing more than random assignment to a group of high potential responders to treatment (e.g., Leake & King, 1977). Conversely, pessimism has been associated with negative outcomes (Sandell et al., 2006). It is also clear counselors' beliefs in their intervention method also matter in terms of outcomes. Hope is not only an important ingredient for clients, but it is also essential for practitioners in being effective in their work. The first step in kindling hope for clients seems to be attending to hope in ourselves.

The *What*: Tools for Opening Possibility

Fortunately, the steps for enhancing client and practitioner hope appear to be similar. It begins with attunement. Specifically, becoming aware of what is happening within the client and us, and allowing ourselves to understand these thoughts, feelings, attitudes, and beliefs, and how they might fit together, as well as what is happening between us. Note that this does not require that we experience the same emotions as the client. While emotional resonance can clarify, it can also interfere when we fail to distinguish between the client's experience and our own. When we engage in our own process of becoming attuned, emotion can be both helpful and impair our ability to observe the interactions of these elements. It affects our ability to "know thyself."

The next step is careful listening. As we noted previously, listening is not just the process of hearing but entails communication of our understanding of what is being conveyed. To be helpful, it typically must go below the surface of what has been said and deepen the understanding. Again, this is true for clients and practitioners.

Part of this careful listening will be hearing exceptions and strengths. Sometimes this will require us to ask for these things; at other times it emerges naturally. For example, when someone says, "usually," "typically," "often," or "mostly," these words convey one type of occurrence is more prevalent, but another does happen. These words signal there are exceptions and invite our attention. Being curious helps in this process, though we can also structure our conversations to provide natural opportunities for these to surface. Beginning client conversations with positive, present-focused questions helps these possibilities to arise. A useful question for new clients is *What is going well in your life right now?* Or *Where are you doing okay?*

As we move past the big picture into exploring where clients struggle, speaking truth can be helpful in building hope. This is also where practitioner optimism stands front and center. Change is difficult, and people do change successfully—all the time. Because of the power of negative emotions, we tend to pay particular attention to those who do not change, but the data are clear: Evidence-based psychotherapy practices in general and MI have a powerful impact.

We have reasons to be optimistic. If our initial approach proves unsuccessful, we can shift to another strategy.

Finally, we need to recognize that people often need to borrow hope to begin. Indeed, it might be how you felt about learning MI to begin with. Here was a method you heard about but had no experience with. It would be normal to be skeptical, especially if you were required to attend training for which you had no time. Yet, here you are reading this book, so you clearly picked up hope somewhere along the way—there was a flicker inside you. Maybe it was a colleague you trusted. Or it was that first trainer, book, or video—something opened possibility in you.

Our clients are in the same position. Just as for us learning MI, if we try to convince them, we will only engender more skepticism. Cheerleading, genuine but superficial encouragement (e.g., *I know you got this!*), has its place, but it is not particularly helpful here. Instead, honesty and humility matter. The message we convey might go something like this:

> *We have something that we believe makes a difference. The data support that. While we are optimistic it could make a difference for you, you will have to decide. What do you think?*

The *How*: SP/SR on Using Past Success to Build Hope and Open Possibility

Overview of the Exercise

For this activity, we want you to venture into the world of your own struggle to change and to find an exception. That is, we want you to think back over your life to a time when you recognized a substantial change that had to be made. One you were not sure you either could or wanted to make, but somehow you were able to persevere and make the change. We will work through the six areas described below.

Structure of the Exercise

This activity can be done in a self-directed manner, though it might prove most productive if done in combination with a limited-practice partner. If done in a self-directed manner, then please answer the questions in the self-practice area. If done as part of a limited practice, use the questions to help guide the discussion.

When working as the practitioner, continue to use your strong listening skills. Be mindful of going below the surface to help your partner become more attuned. Keep in mind that attending to the body is often a helpful ingress to feelings and thoughts (e.g., *Where do you feel that in your body? How does your body communicate that particular emotion to you?*). Listen for and attend to exceptions. Our looking for strengths helps us see them.

Traveling Companion: An Example with Sam

Sam, who is a White, cisgender, gay woman of European descent, has been a successful counselor for many years. About 15 years ago, she injured her back and because of that experience has shifted her private practice to health-focused care. She had a cancer scare last year, and her wife is encouraging her to retire. Sam is ambivalent about making that change, and this has become a point of contention between them.

> ***Think back over your life to a time when you recognized a substantial change that had to be made. One you were not sure you either could or wanted to make, but somehow you were able to persevere and make the change. Describe the situation when you began.***

In some ways, this is easy to identify. It was back when I was working in the family store. My family relied on me to make the business work and I was good at it, but I felt trapped and knew I wanted to make a change. I loved psychology and helping people, but I just couldn't see how to do it. I'd leave my family in a tough spot and feel like I disappointed them. I'd also have to figure out which kind of degree to pursue, find the right school, think about moving, and pay for it all.

> ***As you think back to this situation, attune yourself to what was happening at that time. Close your eyes and imagine you are back there. Give yourself a few moments to recall what that situation was like. How did your body feel? What emotions did your body communicate to you? What emotions did you notice? What were your thoughts? What attitudes were influencing your thinking? How about beliefs?***

Oh, I haven't thought about this in a long time. There was this constant low-level tension. It wasn't like I was tied up in knots, just . . . more like, I'd notice I was clenching my teeth, or if I paid attention to my shoulders, I would take a deep breath, exhale, and just feel them fall. It wasn't like there was this constant unhappiness—I enjoyed the customers, the work, my family—I just felt like I was leaving stuff on the table. I wasn't using all I had to offer. Like there was a bigger world, and I was living a smaller life than I'd intended. I kept telling myself that it was okay, and it should be enough, but I knew it wasn't. I didn't want to complain to my parents. I was grateful for everything they'd done for me, but I also couldn't really tell them I wanted out—or at least that was what I thought. My attitudes and beliefs were this weird combination of family is the most important thing and they've sacrificed so you could go to college. It was hard when I came out as gay, but they were totally supportive of me and total allies whenever I needed them to be. They didn't take crap from anyone. So, I felt like I could tell them this really big thing, "I'm gay," but couldn't tell them I wanted out of the business. It would be a . . . betrayal of all they'd done for me.

> ***Now just take a moment to consider the things you wrote. What do you notice about how these things fit together? After you start to observe a pattern or essential elements, write (or offer) a brief summary that will put these things together in a way that helps organize them for you.***

I loved my parents and knew they loved me. Out of this came loyalty, which I began to feel as a burden. It tied me to their dreams and not my own. By doing that, I had misunderstood and misdirected the gifts of their love. It felt like loyalty and love were a leash that kept me within their dream, instead of a safety line that connected me no matter where my dreams would take me.

➤ ***Now think about the course of this change. How did it unfold? What happened? Who was there to help? What strengths do you observe in your earlier self? How did you use them?***

I sought out Mrs. Haddid. We talked and she just let me sort through my thoughts, though she was the first to say I was underestimating my parents' love for me. She noted how adventurous and risk-taking I was and that I had always been myself. Yeah, like all teens, I made some decisions my parents wouldn't have been happy about, but I also knew my mind. I didn't just go along with the group thing or what everyone else thought was right. I planted my own flags, and Mrs. Haddid noted how my parents had never once told me not to. They talked with me about what it might mean for me, but never said "no." It made me realize I had this inner compass and strength, and my parents respected and encouraged that. I came to realize they had never said I needed to stay with the family, I'd made that decision myself, and they were just happy to have me around and relied on me as I took on more, which is what I do.

My strengths are a strong sense of self, belief in my beliefs, trust in my judgment, willingness to connect with others and listen to their advice, and knowing I am a hard worker. Planning is also something I feel like is a strength. I also had courage and knew I would need to show some here and tell my parents, but I wanted to have a plan first. So, I reached out to some old college professors for their thoughts and asked them to put me in touch with people they thought I should talk to, which I did. I figured out the degree, the tests I needed to do to get in, identified schools, and put together a timeline. Then I talked to my parents.

➤ ***What spoke truth to you in this situation; that change was possible? It might have been an imperfect process, but when did you begin to believe that change could happen?***

Truthfully, it was when in talking to Mrs. Haddid, I realized it was me putting the limits on myself, not my parents. Once that weight was gone, then it felt like I could start to do all the other things. It was like suddenly I realized the betrayal was not in pursuing this dream for my life, but instead misjudging them and then failing to pursue my life. As I started talking to people and begin identifying tasks, I started to believe it could happen. I knew it would be challenging, but I'd always been willing to work hard. I knew it would be tough getting into school, so I would need to put the time and effort into studying for the tests, writing good essays, and creating polished applications. But again, those are things I'd done before, so I knew I could do them again.

➤ ***How did someone lend you hope in this situation? What impact did that have on you?***

That is an interesting question. Mrs. Haddid, my old profs, and the people I talked to, all were encouraging and hopeful for me, and I know that helped me stay afloat. Belief mattered, more than I originally thought. I mean, I probably would've done it anyway, even if they said, "Look this is really tough and you probably won't get in." But, having them hold hope for me was like tail winds in sails that pushed me along faster. They made a difference in my initial energy, which of course was important as I ground through all the tasks. And, of course, having the timeline in place and the confidence I could do these things made the conversation with my parents easier, as it felt like something real and not just a whim.

Self-Practice

- *Think back over your life to a time when you recognized a substantial change that had to be made. One you were not sure you either could or wanted to make, but somehow you were able to persevere and make the change. Describe the situation when you began.*

- *As you think back to this situation, attune yourself to what was happening at that time. Close your eyes and imagine you are back there. Give yourself a few moments to recall what that situation was like. How did your body feel? What emotions did you notice? What were your thoughts? What attitudes were influencing your thinking? How about beliefs?*

- *Now just take a moment to consider the things you wrote. What do you notice about how these things fit together? After you start to observe a pattern or essential elements, write (or offer) a brief summary that will put these things together in a way that helps organize them for you.*

- *Now think about the course of this change. How did it unfold? What happened? Who was there to help? What strengths do you observe in your earlier self? How did you use them?*

- *What spoke truth to you in this situation: that change was possible? It might have been an imperfect process, but when did you begin to believe that change could happen?*

- *How did someone lend you hope in this situation? What impact did that have on you?*

Self-Reflection

- *What did you notice in your body as you worked through this process? What feelings did you have? Thoughts?*

- *What stands out about what you did in this situation? How can that be useful to you now in working on the challenge you identified in Module 1?*

- *Think about a client who surprised you with how they changed. Perhaps this is someone who had long odds at the beginning, but somehow persevered. Or maybe it was someone who was quite difficult to engage or engaged with lots of pushback initially? What happened?*

➤ ***What parallels do you notice between your experience and what happened with this client?***

➤ ***How did your hope or optimism come into this picture? For example . . .***

- ***What helped or hindered this process?***
- ***What did your hope or optimism look like?***
- ***How would this be observable to the client?***
- ***How did you know it came into the picture?***
- ***How did you communicate your hope or optimism to the client?***

What If: Applying Skills to My Current Context

Bridging Questions to Practitioner-Self

These questions are designed to help you bring the insights from personal self-practice into your work with clients.

- ***What are some things you have done recently to help build your optimism for clients changing? What steps outside of the practitioner room do you take to build optimism?***

- ***Specifically, how might you convey your hope to clients without cheerleading? What might this look like or include? How would the client know, perceive, or feel this?***

- ***What are your main*** takeaway ***messages from this SP/SR experience in relation to your understanding of the concept of hope within MI . . .***
  - ***From a practical perspective?***
  - ***From a theoretical perspective?***

➤ ***What if you were to apply this process to other areas of your professional practice (e.g., in a role as supervisor or trainer perhaps)? How might you apply your learning to this new context?***

____

____

____

➤ ***How has this exercise influenced your understanding of or personal relationship with MI as a way of being?***

____

____

____

Final Thoughts and Applications to Other Settings

Opening possibility and specifically offering hope might seem like a long-term therapy task, something not necessarily done in brief encounters. Yet, many times in brief encounters, the route forward is unclear and clients look to us to provide possibilities and direction. How do we convey genuine and realistic hope? The challenge is to do this without engaging in the ***fixing reflex*** and/or moving quickly into cheerleading that change is possible. This process calls for us to give solutions and general encouragement, and it makes attention to thoughtful and focused efforts at listening even more important within our broader attempts to be helpful. A general axiom then—the less time is available, the more important is careful listening.

In matters like supervision, our ability to both envision the practitioner as an independent professional and recognize the areas in which they need to grow requires a balanced approach. We help practitioners see themselves within their zone of competence and still encourage movement into their zone of proximal development. We help supervisees attend to their strengths and use these as they move into areas of growth. A basic reminder as a supervisor is, instead of telling people what they might do, ask what they observe as the challenge and how they might address it. We can always help to either shape the response or offer, with permission, an alternative for consideration.

We now begin the transition from engaging into focusing. As clients begin to explore new possibilities, we work to understand what is important to them and why. It is not just that they can make changes, but instead whether these changes fit with what matters to them. Support for autonomy comes center stage as we move into the focusing process.

This also goes hand in hand with the recognition that opening possibility might overlap with readiness to change, but it is not the same. Before people will consider the possibility of change, they must believe it's possible; this is a necessary precondition. Yet, just because we believe change is possible does not mean we are ready to do it. We are just one step further on the path.

MODULE 11

Exploring Values

Module Purpose

This module explores how values influence our motivation, at times operating below our awareness, and how engaging them more directly can provide clarity in what makes our life the one we wish to live and initiates and sustains our efforts at change. By the end of this module, it is our intention that though an experience of a day that reflects your values you connect with the power of how life feels when it is in alignment with important things and how awareness of misalignments, carefully and nonjudgmentally considered, can provide energy, focus, and vision to consideration of alternative choices for our clients.

The *Why*: Exploring Values as a Path to Focusing

Exploring values is one of the ways we transition from ***engaging*** to ***focusing***. Clients have begun to feel safe, and the big picture of their lives is coming into somewhat better focus. They experience us as trustworthy in these discussions and, as they do, they become more willing to talk about what matters. This is always a highly personal process, even if clients consistently use the same language. For example, when one of us (D. B. R) was working with street-based drug users, they often endorsed *getting right with God* as a *very important* value in a value-sorting activity (whereby clients sort through values to identify ones that are most important to them). While there was great consistency in this selection—despite it being just one value out of a group of 100—the meaning of it was often quite different. Consequently, it was the start of a discussion where clients became more explicit about what the expression meant in their lives.

The reason for values sorting is not just deepening mutual understanding, but also to understand what drives and/or directs behavior (Schwartz & Sortheix, 2018). When people live in balance with their values, they often describe their experience in words such as "peaceful," "calm," "joyful," "content," "happy," "excited," "engaged." Yet, as we all experience, it can be hard to live consistently with our values. For example, D. B. R., as a person who lives with Type I diabetes, values healthy eating and regular exercise, yet at the end of a busy day, he appreciates relaxing in front of the television with a bag of chips and an entertaining show. When we become aware of this discrepancy between what we hold dear and the choices we are making, it can become a powerful motivator for change. But this is a difficult thing to see, it is not always straightforward, and it can be exposing and conflicting to look at it directly with another person; it requires that we feel safe and unjudged by them. Therefore, the engaging task is both an essential precursor to this exploration and remains important through any MI encounter.

According to Ryan and Deci (2017), *autonomy* also has multiple important roles to play. It is an essential part in externally motivated behavior becoming internalized and integrated by the individual. For example, a male teen is often not a voluntary participant in therapy and over the course of treatment may come to see how the choices he makes can more closely align with what he wants and values. The choice to change shifts from an external locus of causality (*I'm here because the school made me come here*) to an internal one (*I come because I don't want other people calling the shots in my life*). (See Table 2.3 for more information.) In addition, research indicates the more supportive someone is of an individual's autonomy, the more people turn to and rely on this other person for emotional support and to live more authentically as themselves, as well as to live in closer alignment with their ideals (Ryan & Deci, 2017). Thus, by encouraging another's autonomy in exploring values and examining their behavior without drawing conclusions, the more likely they are to find us useful in this work and make choices consistent with how they want to live. Not surprisingly then, when a discrepancy is noted, it is not our job to tell a client what needs to happen next, but instead we maintain our curiosity about how they understand this disconnection and how it influences them.

The *What*: Exploring Values

The exploration of values can happen directly or indirectly. The direct methods include asking straightforward questions about what is most important to an individual. While this approach can be useful, it may also be challenging for clients, and they often benefit from further structure to allow greater exploration of values. An example of directly asking with structure is to work with a client on a values card sort. The explanation of how to do this has been described elsewhere (e.g., Rosengren, 2017) so won't be repeated here except to note the client is given a deck of values cards and asked to sort these into unimportant, important, and very important categories. This task is then followed by a series of questions designed to engage the client in exploring these values and to consider their relationship to life activities.

We refer to these as direct activities as the client is clearly aware that we are talking about values. With the indirect methods, values emerge as part of the discussion and require the practitioner to be listening for and acknowledging them as they emerge. We offer three ways to approach this in the discussion.

The value of the first approach emerged as a serendipitous outcome in a listening activity developed for MI workshops. We asked participants to practice listening skills in pairs and gave them a prompt question, *What do you like to do on Saturdays or your day off?* A seemingly innocuous question, but what emerged over the years is how when people think about their free time, they do connect to what is important to them. As listeners worked to move below the surface of their partners' leisure activities, they discovered important values and activities, as well as the impediments to their living fully aligned with these things.

The second method is complementary to the first and just asks people, *How do you spend money when you have a little extra?* The particular focus is on discretionary funds, but this question also carries potential economic class-related issues to which practitioners need to be attentive. If this question is not appropriate for your situation, do not use it. Still, this question taps another tangible form of how people expend their limited resources, just as with time in the prior method, and helps us understand what matters to them.

Finally, we can ask clients about the people they admire. The person they identify may be important, but even more important are the characteristics they ascribe to this person. This typically reflects the aspirational values of who they want to be but might not feel in their life currently.

In these explorations, it is helpful to add phrases or questions that ask about *meaning*. That is, by adding the phrase "and what does that mean to you?," we deepen their exploration. It moves beyond simple description and their potential to make this process more impactful.

In all the indirect methods, there are opportunities for discussion of values to unfold naturally. It requires the practitioner to be attentive and to be listening below the surface and contributing observations. While we can offer possible connections, it will be most powerful if the client is the one drawing the conclusions, and particularly the meaning.

The *How*: SP/SR on Using the Review of a Day to Explore Values

Overview of the Exercise

For this activity, we want you to think about or discuss with your practice partner a recent day off where you spent the day engaged in activities you wanted to do, not those that you had to do. Unless ticking off items from your to-do list is your absolute favorite thing to do in the world, we don't want you to focus on that. Instead, think about when you can set the course for a day—or even part of a day—how do you like to spend your time in that free space? Think about how such time starts. Who, if anyone, is with you? How does it unfold? What do you notice? What sights, sounds, smells, or touches are present? What thoughts or feelings accompany this time?

Structure of the Exercise

This is a session we believe is enhanced by your working with a partner. However, if you're doing it as solo work, imagine a time when this happened recently and play it back in your head as if it's a movie and savor the experience of that time. Then write your answers to the questions.

If you're working in a limited-practice setting, use the self-practice questions to guide the discussion. Work to deepen this information through careful, curious listening. Pay attention to what lies underneath the words and activities and reflect these to your partner. Listen for and notice values. ***Affirmations*** are helpful in this practice as well.

Traveling Companion: An Example with Takeshi

Takeshi will help us illustrate this exercise. In this activity, we will provide Takeshi's responses to not only the self-practice but also the self-reflection. Use this as a guide to check the depth of your self-reflections.

Recall that Takeshi is a 24-year-old, cisgender, straight man of Japanese heritage working on his doctorate in clinical psychology. Stress and high expectations have been ongoing issues. He is a strong student and shows promise as a counselor and is feeling some frustration about his clients' lack of change at times. He sought out MI training at the suggestion of his supervisor.

➤ ***Imagine you have a day or at least part of a day to do as you wish, not tasks for work, school, or family. How would you spend your time? You might think back to a time when that happened recently and describe that time.***

This is a hard activity for me because I am so task-oriented and feel like I always have been. I always seem to be under pressure to get something done. But, if I slow it down, then I guess the contrast becomes clearer.

You'd think I might like to lie around, but that makes me feel anxious. So, it is an active day still, but the pace feels a little more self-directed. It's the things I want to do, instead of having to do.

So, here is what a Saturday might look like. I get up relatively early, like 7:30, and I go for a run someplace where I like to run—like down by the lake. If I've gotten my act together ahead of time, I arrange for one of my friends to meet me there and then we do like a nice easy 30- to 40-minute run. We're talking the whole time. Then afterward, we stop and grab a bagel and a coffee, sit outside if the weather cooperates, and watch people go by for an hour or so. Then I head home. Normally, this would be when I do some housecleaning, but since I am spending the day doing what I want, I'd just make sure the house is tidied up and the kitchen is clean. It feels better to me when it's neat. I'd have some music going. Then I'd shower up—no shave today, because well, it's my free day. I'd call my buddies and we'd arrange to meet at the park for some pick-up soccer later in the day. Then I'd hang out on my balcony, with another cup of coffee, and read for an hour or so—something I wanted to read, maybe even a novel, instead of something for school—then I'd put on my soccer gear, grab my cleats, and head down to Pike's Place Market. I'd grab a hum bow [Chinese meat- or veggie-filled bun or pastry] and sit in the park and watch the ferries and the sailboats on the Sound. Then I'd grab some flowers for my mom—she loves flowers—and I'd swing by my parents' house on my way to the park. They'd be working in the yard, and we'd chat for a bit. I'd help my dad with something in the yard he needed a second set of hands for, then I'd be on my way to the park.

The soccer would go on for a few hours. It's co-ed, so men and women. People talking trash, playing hard in spurts, laughing, and just having fun. Then we'd hang out for a while afterward and talk, maybe go to a pub and have a pint. Then I'd go home, and shower and we'd meet up for some late dinner and maybe clubbing. If it's a really good night, maybe I'd meet someone interesting that I'd spend the evening talking to, dancing with, and get her number. Maybe have a couple of drinks—nothing too much because I don't like getting sloppy. Take a rideshare home or walk if it's close by. That is a day I'd love.

➤ ***As you consider this day, what immediately grabs your attention?***

There is a lot going on. I said that being active is important and I am aware that there is only a little in the way of the slow or contemplative, but a lot of moving between places and movement within places. I like being engaged in my life and not just watching it flow by.

➤ ***What role do people play in this day?***

It's interesting because I've always thought of myself as being a bit more introverted, but it's clear that people play a big role in how I want to spend my time. Of course, people play different roles. Like my parents provide a foundation, or a touchstone. But, my soccer friends are more about play and camaraderie.

➤ ***What was an unexpected discovery, as you considered this day?***

It's interesting that I included my parents. Sometimes I feel beholden to them and begrudge the time I spend with them, but I realized it wouldn't feel like how I wanted to spend my day off if I DIDN'T see them. I just want smaller, manageable doses, not the entire day. Doing something limited with or for them makes me happy. I just don't want to spend the whole day weeding their garden or rebuilding a retaining wall.

➤ ***As you sift back through this day, what is important to you and what underlying values do they seem to reflect?***

Earlier I mentioned activity. Physical activity and health are clearly important. I do the running and the soccer, the walking, and even the dancing because it feels good to move. So, much of my work life is sitting. I sit and read, sit and talk, sit and study, right? But that's not when I feel best. It helps my mood, too.

People are clearly important. But I am not the type that strikes up conversations with strangers. So, when I go to the market, I'm not busy chatting up people. I'm just doing my thing and I respond if people reach out, but I don't initiate. But when I'm running with my friend or eating a bagel, or whatever, then the conversation is constant. It doesn't feel forced or awkward. I enjoy it. I think the value there is maybe some combination of connection and intimacy.

My parents, as I said, are particularly important and so I would say family is a value. But it's also where I feel loved and give love. Yeah, they annoy me at times, but I never doubt their love for me. I guess that's why I like to do things for and with them. It's a way to express my love tangibly—doing something for them.

I like fun, too. When I think about this day, I am smiling and it's kind of how I imagine myself going through that day. There is lots of activity, but it never feels frantic or too busy; I'm just flowing. I see myself smiling, even while cleaning up the apartment. I just feel a peace and happiness having things in order and moving to my own rhythms.

Of course, there is romantic interest. If I'm honest, that's what I hope to find when I am at the club. But I'm too busy to really date or get involved in a relationship, so I'm not really pursuing it. It's more casual. I'm not using any of the dating apps. My mom worries sometimes, right? It's like I want to find someone, but I also recognize I don't have much space for that right now in my life. I don't want to be distracted from my school stuff, but it is something I know that I eventually want. Just not now.

Self-Reflection

We are including Takeshi's self-reflection process here, so you have an opportunity to observe how his self-reflection process has evolved and how it is influencing his thinking. Again, our aim is not to show you the right way, but instead to model one way a person might use this process.

➤ ***There is a deepening process that unfolds as we consider what we like to do on our days off. What did you notice happened for you in this process? What did you observe in your body? What seemed to help you go deeper?***

Here is what I noticed. I started off a little uneasy. My body felt twitchy. I felt restless and I thought, "I never get days off, so how am I supposed to do this activity?" I needed to give myself some space to think about it. So, not giving in to the knee-jerk reaction, but just allowing that space to unfold helped. Then I noticed, it helped to get concrete. To think about a recent time and to start at the beginning. Like, when I get up, what do I want to do?

Then slowly it's like it unfurled. Like I kind of went from this step to the next step. My body relaxed, and I sort of let it flow and asked, "Is that what I'd want to do?" and then let my mind wander to see if there was another answer. If I started to move into tasks, it was good to ask myself, "Is this REALLY what you want to do?" Sometimes, the answer was "yes." Like cleaning up the kitchen does make me happy because my place just feels better to me when it's neat, and it provides a sanctuary from all the business and clutter of my life. So, maybe that's a value, too. Going to my parents' house was another example, where the answer was "yes," and I want boundaries on it. So, it helped me to have space to think, allowing my mind to wander and not closing off an area too quickly, and asking questions, "Is that what I SHOULD want or DO want?," essentially.

Maybe I got a little idyllic with the clubbing. That's not a regular thing for me, but it does sound fun. I'm clearly not a player, but I would like to have some romantic possibilities in my life. It felt good to just sort of let that piece drop in.

➤ ***What feelings drifted up for you, as you thought through this day? What importance does that have? How do these feelings tie into your values?***

I'm surprised at how happy I felt thinking about this day. Like I wanted to make it happen, and it's funny because it felt more real—like I could make it happen. Since I could imagine it, maybe it wasn't so impossible. Like I could carve a day out to do those things, and it really isn't all that farfetched. As I said before, there was also a peacefulness or calmness as I thought about this day, even though I was fully engaged. I wasn't laying in a hammock, lounging around, but when I was thinking about watching the ferries, I could feel that scene, taste that hum bow, smell the salt water, and hear the gulls. I was chilling just thinking about it. It's like "If you build it, they will come" sort of thing. Like by creating it in my mind, I was moving toward making it happen and, perhaps most importantly, wanting to make it happen, feeling capable of it, and not feeling like it was some self-indulgence. Like this fed me in some important way. Looking at everything, I felt more in sync with my values during this day, which led to more positive feelings.

➤ ***What connections do you observe between what you identified as either important or values in this module and the challenge you identified in Module 1? What values do you see underlying your challenge? In what ways are these values in harmony or disharmony with your behavior? What does that mean for you?***

Hmm . . . It seems like this comes at multiple levels. I clearly value action and so my tendency is to get clients active and doing things, then I get frustrated when they do not. It seems I'm pushing my agenda on them, kind of like how I feel when I spend all day at my parents' house weeding. The impulse is there, and I push against it, if I feel like I must do something. It seems like I might be doing that with my clients.

I'm also aware of how self-directed this day felt. I feel in control, which apparently is important to me. So maybe I want to be in control and am not really ceding that to my clients. On the flipside, I'm aware of how motivated I felt when I was self-directed and so my job is to help discover those sources in my clients and not focus on what to do and how to do it so much. Like for me, clients probably have a sense of what fits best for them. It will happen more easily and naturally if they selected it.

Also, I am aware that intimacy and connection are important to me. I know clear boundaries are important and clients are not my friends, but I also wonder if I've been making my boundaries too impermeable. The result is I feel like I'm playing a role rather than being a real person in the room. They feel that and maybe step back, too, and the result is we don't feel as connected as I think would be helpful for them in their work. It's like empathy has become a completely cognitive activity without the emotional component. That's interesting to me.

➤ ***Given these insights, what might need to shift in your work, and how will you do that?***

To begin, I need to slow down. I am too quick to jump to solutions and then to offer specific ideas. It's like I see the problem and I think I know the solution. Oh . . . I just realized this is the fixing reflex in action. Well, that's embarrassing. I totally missed it.

I also need to spend more time finding out what is important to clients. This, of course, is "part and parcel" of what I was just talking about. I see a problem and I decide it's the focus, without taking the time to find out if this is really where clients want to put their focus. I don't think I'm pushy, but I clearly have not been paying attention to the process. So, I need to spend time finding out about what matters before we start working problems. This will require me to NOT jump to providing what clients usually want, which is some relief from their symptoms immediately. I like the day off activity, but I also might try the values card sort—that seems interesting, too.

Having slowed down and found out what is important, I need to provide space for the solutions to emerge. I also need to ask. Like me, I know many will have ideas if I offer that opportunity.

➤ ***What do you think will challenge you in doing this? How might you manage it?***

I get task-focused, and this can make me impatient when I feel like the problem or solution is obvious. I get even more impatient when I know clients have a pressing need for them to act. I want them to avoid the consequences, for example, if they don't act or decide. I think this will require some focused self-talk. I might say things like:

- This is their process, not yours.
- It is their life, they must choose.
- You're the guide, not the driver.
- Provide space for exploration.

Self-Practice

Now it's your turn.

➤ ***Imagine you have a day or at least part of a day to do as you wish, not tasks for work, school, or family. How would you spend your time? You might think back to a time when that happened recently and describe that time.***

➤ ***As you consider this day, what immediately grabs your attention and why?***

➤ *What role do people play in this day?*

➤ *What was an unexpected discovery, as you considered this day?*

➤ *As you sift back through this day, what is important to you and what underlying values do they seem to reflect?*

Self-Reflection

➤ *There is a deepening process that unfolds as we consider what we like to do on our days off. What did you notice happened for you in this process? What did you observe in your body? What seemed to help you to go deeper in connecting with your values?*

➤ *What feelings drifted up for you, as you thought through this day? What importance does that have? How do these feelings tie into your values?*

➤ ***What connections do you observe between what you identified as either important or values in this module and the challenge you identified in Module 1? What values do you see underlying your challenge? In what ways are these values in harmony or disharmony with your behavior? What does that mean for you?***

What If: Applying Skills to My Current Context

Bridging Questions to Practitioner-Self

These questions are designed to help you bring the insights from personal self-practice into your work with clients.

➤ ***Given the insights you gleaned in the last question, how does this help your work with clients? What might need to shift in your work with client values, and how will you do that?***

➤ *What do you think will challenge you in doing this, and how might you manage it?*

➤ *What are your main* takeaway *messages from this SP/SR experience in relation to your understanding of the concept of exploring values in your MI work with clients . . .*

- *From a practical perspective?*

- *From a theoretical perspective?*

➤ *What if you were to apply this process to other areas of your professional practice (e.g., in a role as supervisor or trainer perhaps)? How might you apply your learning to this new context?*

➤ ***How has this exercise influenced your understanding of or personal relationship with MI as a way of being?***

____

____

____

Final Thoughts and Applications to Other Settings

The exploration of values feels as if it might be specific to therapy situations, yet it is an essential element in many change settings. For example, people with Type 1 diabetes must manage multiple things in their lives. While for endocrinologists and diabetes educators the reasons for engaging in all these behaviors might appear straightforward—maintain health and avoid diabetic complications like heart attack, stroke, blindness, amputation—for people living with diabetes, the reasons are much more individualized:

- *I'm an artist, and I need to protect my eyesight so I can do what I love.*
- *I'm the sole breadwinner, and my family counts on me to be here.*
- *I love to hike, and I want to be able to do that.*

Even for things as apparently simple as flossing, dental hygienists and dentists know that it is a challenge for many patients, and simple knowledge is rarely enough to change behavior. Patients need their personally important reasons for engaging in flossing daily.

For supervisors, mentors, and coaches, understanding values may follow a similar track. Why are people engaging in this process? Why does it matter to them? For those who are externally motivated, helping them think through their reasons may aid in developing more internalized motivation and thereby a richer and more engaged learning process.

MODULE 12

Routes of Travel

Module Purpose

This module invites you to experience and explore the ***intentional*** and ***directional aspects of MI*** practice. In this module, we invite you to pay careful attention to your deliberate and intentional practice using skillful questions that are supported by reflective listening and affirmations. By the end of this module, it is our intention that you have a deeper or perhaps re-appreciation of the deliberate and directional aspect of MI, how our skillful and intentional use of MI skills can shape our client's journey, and the critical role of autonomy in this process.

The *Why*: If These Are Clients' Journeys, Then They Must Choose the Route of Travel

Within ***engaging***, we work with clients to help them see other possibilities, and now as we move into ***focusing***, our aim is to help the client decide where they would like to go and how they will get there. Through exploration of values, we began to identity endpoints that provide meaning and motivation to the movement. Now, we work to identify the routes we might take to get there.

This is one of the clear aspects when MI veers away from traditional *Rogerian, nondirective person-centered* work (cf., Grant, 2010). MI is directional and intentional. We actively work with the client to identify what matters to them and then help them determine, *if this is a direction they wish to move*, how they might get there. Toward this end, our role as practitioner is one of guide, respecting the autonomy of the individual to select the route and the means of conveyance. The places they wish to go, how they will get there, and what they will see along the way are theirs to choose.

Or to use our gardening analogy, we are the master gardener who listens to what the gardener hopes to achieve; makes inquiries about soils, sun or shade, climate, and resources; and then offers possibilities based on the client's vision. The gardener will decide what to plant, where, when and in what order, and what help will be needed. Through thoughtful inquiries and listening, the master gardener helps the gardener arrive at the plan that fits them. We are aware of our expertise and experience in this process but remain mindful of not stepping into the ***expert trap*** where we make it our garden. Instead, we support the client's *autonomy* and *competence* in creating the garden that is right for them.

As noted in the prior module, autonomy is an essential part of this process. It is not client independence per se. Many times, clients will be compelled to change in a situation where motivation is extrinsically directed—*I must do this or else*—but it is the perceived ability within that circumstance to choose the direction consistent with a sense of self and values. That is, *I may be required to consider changing this behavior, but I am choosing to act in a way that feels consistent with my values and beliefs.* Using our metaphor, they've been forced to rethink their garden to accommodate the growing conditions (e.g., personal or cultural context), but they choose to replant in a way the reflects the garden they wish, even if some things are required to be a part of it because of the type of soil or climate they live in.

The *What*: Tools for Moving Forward

As is evident, by being directional, the practitioner has influence within this process. This is the point at which we might both introduce our agenda and must be mindful of the client's autonomy. For example, if we work at a depression, anxiety, or pain clinic, it is no surprise that we have an agenda to help clients alleviate those presenting symptoms. We introduce these areas with transparency (*I think looking at how your thoughts might be influencing your depression could be helpful*), while simultaneously respecting that the client must choose (*What do you think about that?*). There is a danger here of the ***fixing reflex*** creeping in, so it requires that we be mindful of how we elicit and reinforce client autonomy as they make *their* choices (see Module 4 for more information on autonomy). Later, we will discuss sharing concerns in Module 16: Sharing Information, as there are times when we may be troubled by the direction of a client choice. For now, we will simply note that it is the client in charge of these choices.

In terms of choosing routes of travel, we will focus particularly on the productive use of questions. It has been our experience that participants arrive at MI training as proficient questioners. They ask many questions—some open and some closed—and often view this as the best and most direct route of travel in their work. Frequently, an accompanying belief is that questions are much less intrusive than listening, which seems presumptive of what clients are thinking, feeling, or believing. It makes sense people would hold this belief as it is what they've had the most experience doing, and they've had success with it along the way. Questions are, in fact, helpful (e.g., Walthers et al., 2019), and research suggests that listening well and intentionally is a powerful influence in the appearance of ***change*** or ***sustain talk*** (e.g., Barnett et al., 2014b), which leaves clients feeling well understood rather than "presumed upon." Thus, questions have important contributions to make when used delicately and intentionally, and not just as the first response when there is a pause in the conversation.

Several factors contribute to improving questions' productivity. To begin with, there is being intentional in the asking of the question. That is, choose it from a host of potential responses—silence, ***affirmations***, ***reflections***, or ***summaries***—rather than make it a habitual response. When choosing, select a direction of travel. Don't make it any question but rather one that points in a direction that based on our prior knowledge of the client, the current discussion, client goals, change or sustain talk, or the dynamics of the issue under consideration will help the client move forward in a productive manner. Unless a simple fact-finding question is needed, make the question open-ended and invite exploration. Instead of *Don't you think these two things are connected?*, we might ask, *I wonder what connections you see between these things?* Sometimes ***open questions*** are too broad to be helpful for clients, *Why do you think you did that?* Consider narrowing your focus, even as you invite exploration, *How do you think your frustration may have fed into what happened?* Tentative words may increase exploration. While we've suggested that open-ended questions are preferred, the truth is the client determines how they will perceive and respond to a question, such that closed questions can act like open questions, and many a beautiful open question has gone nowhere in the shoulder shrug of a put-upon adolescent. On balance then, we believe open questions are more productive and encourage their use. Finally, we encourage spaciousness in questions and the time provided for the client to consider it. In our MI coaching, we have observed beautiful questions being undermined by the asker who, instead of waiting patiently as the client ponders the answer, rushes in with a second or third question. Our suggestion is to be confident in the question and in the client's ability to answer it, to provide clarification if something is not clear, and in our own ability to detect the client's confusion. It is also important to be mindful that skillful open questions (and ***reflective listening statements***) can often evoke emotion in clients they need to process before formulating a response. The practitioner's ability to tolerate silence and sit with the discomfort of the *not knowing position* is a key skill. Yet, there is often a fine line between a helpful and productive silence and one that is perceived to be oppressive. We encourage you to make this a spacious silence that allows clients the room to think and moving on if it becomes clear the client is unable or unwilling to respond.

The *How*: SP/SR on Exploring an Atypical Experience as a Different Route of Travel

Overview of the Exercise

For this activity, we want you to think about or discuss with your limited-practice partner your challenge and specifically, identify and reflect on a day when something different happened regarding that challenge. That is, you encountered the challenging situation, and it did not take its usual course. Take your time in this process so you can get into the details.

Structure of the Exercise

We believe this session is enhanced by your working with a partner. However, if you're doing it as solo work, think about a time when this happened recently and play it back in your head as if it's a movie and observe the experience of that time. Even if you cannot see it, recall the bodily experiences, feelings, and thoughts you had along the way. Then write your answers to the questions.

If you're working in a limited-practice setting, we encourage you to use the self-practice questions as written to elicit specific pieces of information, as well as guide the discussion. Work to deepen this information through careful, curious listening. This is a module focused on being intentional with questions, so as you add to the questions written here, be intentional and directional in the questions you choose. As always, pay attention to what lies underneath the words and activities, and reflect these to your partner. Listen for and notice values. Affirmations are helpful in this practice as well.

Traveling Companion: An Example with Quincy

Quincy will help us illustrate this exercise. Recall Quincy is a 38-year-old, cisgender, straight woman of African descent who works as an AOD counselor. Growing up in a vibrant community, she has strong family ties. She was feeling some burnout with substance use clients and has sought out personal support with an MI-informed therapist.

➤ ***What happened that was different?***

I've been working with this client who has been in and out of treatment. She gets clean for a while, claims she's doing better, and then ends up back doing the same thing. She's on probation and has random UAs [urinalysis for alcohol and drug use]. She came back with a positive UA [indicates drug use], and we had to speak on it. This is one of those points where I tend to get confrontational with my clients because they lie and say, "I don't know how I could be positive. The test is wrong." But instead of getting discouraged or irritable or judgy, I tried some of the things I've been working on. I tried listening and she ended up telling me about some of her struggles and we put together a plan. She felt more invested; it wasn't the attitude I usually get at the end of these encounters.

➤ ***Now, let's back up a little bit and think about the time prior to this happening. What were your thoughts and feelings as this difference or event began to unfold? What was happening in your body?***

I started out thinking "different day, same crap." I could feel my hands and jaw tighten. I didn't feel it so much as just knew my shoulders started to hunch up. But then I caught myself and thought, "Okay, here's a chance to try something different." I realized that I was kind of protecting myself from being manipulated and so I didn't want to listen. I wanted to tell her I was on to her, but I thought about this being part of the process and that she was likely to be scared. She didn't want to go to jail, and she did keep coming back to treatment. So, I took a few deep breaths, relaxed my shoulders, arms, and hands, and then thought about what I wanted to say or ask to begin, and I felt a lot calmer and more at peace.

➤ ***What were the circumstances? Who was around, where were you, when was this occurring, what was happening?***

The experience started outside my office space immediately prior to the session, in the waiting area. This is where I meet her and then escort her back to my office. There were other people in the space. I noticed her fidgeting and looking nervous, but a little defiant. Normally, this is when I'd start to tighten up. But I reminded myself to be cool and be glad to see her. So, I smiled and said hello, and she looked a little surprised. In the office, it was just the two of us. Her in her usual chair. I just started by saying she looked a little worried in the waiting room, and I'd noticed some changes in her. I was wondering how she was doing. She told me about her struggles to make ends meet and troubles at home, and how everything is piling up on her. As we talked, it became clear she was hanging on by a thread but was clinging to that thread like it was a lifeline. I affirmed her determination and she seemed to lighten. Talking about the positive UA was then easy because we both knew she was trying, and I'd already told her I was committed to helping her. I just introduced it as a statement rather than a question, "You're probably not too surprised then your UA is positive," and she admitted that she had been struggling hard to stay off the drugs.

➤ ***How did your body feel as all this was happening? Where specifically in your body did you feel this? How did your body communicate the specific feeling to you?***

I felt relaxed, instead of feeling disconnected and tense. It felt like we were working together so it felt kind of easy. I noticed my shoulders were relaxed, as were my hands. The smile showed my jaw was relaxed. Before I understood her, I felt like I was having to manage my emotions, but when I focused on her, that just kind of went away.

➤ ***What, if any, role did your values or what's important to you play into what happened?***

That's an interesting question. When I was getting myself ready to meet this client, I reminded myself of what addictions are about and that change is hard. I also reminded myself that I got into this work to make a difference. Those two things helped me to focus on her needs, instead of me, which made all the difference.

➤ ***As the situation ended, what was happening in your body? How did this connect with your thoughts and feelings? What thoughts and feelings did you have?***

Well, this is the interesting piece to me. I felt relaxed. My body felt lighter and open. I felt compassion for this client, good about the work we'd done, and more hopeful for her future. I was thinking, "Damn. This MI thing works." I was thinking I need to do more of this with my clients.

➤ ***As you thought about it afterward, what was challenging in this circumstance? Why was it challenging for you?***

I think the biggest challenge for me was before I got into the room getting myself in the right head space. Now, I don't know how it would've gone had she just walled up and said, "I'm cool. Everything is cool." I think I still would've been okay because I wouldn't have taken it personally. I'd just have known this is the process and my job is to help her. The why it is challenging goes back to things I've discussed previously. I've become more self-protective and in the process of that I've closed myself off to clients, which has led me to receive what I expect.

➤ ***What ended up being helpful for you and why?***

I think the time I spent ahead of time, particularly thinking about what makes this important and not just a problem, and that I chose this work because it is important to me. So, getting my head right was the most helpful thing. I'm seeing the beliefs and attitude I am bringing into the room are affecting what is happening.

➤ ***How specifically were you able to bring those helpful things into the event or situation?***

By really paying attention to her, instead of myself. In the waiting room, it was like I really looked at her rather than filtering through my "liar" lenses. Also, by focusing on the relationship and seeing her strengths, it made it easier to introduce the UA. I think also stating my commitment to her helped, but doing it in the context of demonstrating that I cared about her. I have said that at other times, but I don't think people believe it because I was also telling them how they were messing up.

Self-Practice

Now it's your turn.

Think about or discuss with your practice partner your challenge on a day when something different happened. Use the questions to guide your thinking or discussion. If done with a partner, when you are in the practitioner role, pay careful attention to the questions you ask and make liberal use of reflections between questions.

➤ ***What happened that was different?***

➤ ***Now, let's back up a little bit and think about the time prior to this happening. What were your specific thoughts and feelings as this difference or event began to unfold? What was happening in your body?***

➤ ***What were the circumstances? Who was around, where were you, when was this occurring, and what was happening?***

➤ ***How did your body feel as all this was happening? Where specifically in your body did you feel this? How did your body communicate the specific feeling to you?***

➤ ***What, if any, role did your values or what's important to you play into what happened?***

➤ *As the situation ended, what was happening in your body? How did this connect with your thoughts and feelings? What thoughts and feelings did you have?*

➤ *As you thought about it afterward, what was challenging in this circumstance? Why was it challenging for you?*

➤ *What ended up being helpful for you and why?*

➤ *How specifically were you able to bring those helpful things into the event or situation?*

Self-Reflection

➤ *As you step back and consider this whole experience or event, what caught your attention as surprising or important?*

> ***The focus of this module was the intentional use of questions. What did you notice in general about our questions?***

> ***How did particular questions deepen your exploration? Did any seem to get in the way?***

> ***If you had a peer counselor, how did the counselor's listening between questions influence the process? What did you observe in yourself?***

What If: Applying Skills to My Current Context

Bridging Questions to Practitioner-Self

These questions are designed to help you bring the insights from personal self-practice into your work with clients.

- ***How have you tended to use questions in your work with clients?***

- ***What will you need to do to become more intentional in your use of questions?***

- ***How might you incorporate the questions you found helpful in this exercise in your work with clients? Here is something you might consider. Some people have found writing down the questions and trying them out with clients to be helpful. Feel free to write them here, if helpful.***

➤ *What are your main* takeaway *messages from this SP/SR experience in relation to your understanding of the concept of routes of travel in MI . . .*

- *From a practical perspective?*

- *From a theoretical perspective?*

➤ *What if you were to apply this process to other areas of your professional practice (e.g., in a role as supervisor or trainer perhaps)? How might you apply your learning to this new context?*

➤ *How has this exercise influenced your understanding of or personal relationship with MI as a way of being?*

Final Thoughts and Applications to Other Settings

We all have preferred routes of travel. Watch people going about the daily activities of their lives, and it's easy to see that we fall into routines and patterns. The same is true for us as practitioners and the solutions we prefer for the client issues we encounter. We see a problem and the goal, and think we know the best route to get there. As we work in our areas of specialty, it becomes easy for us to develop preferred routes of travel. Of course, we leave the client out of that process and, as we know well, they will ultimately decide.

In some settings, it might be easy to see there are multiple routes of travel. A physical therapist might explore different exercises, settings, times of day, and client tolerances that help the person do rehab after a surgery. A team sports coach might do the same with athletes in the off season, but in-season conditioning may be viewed differently—all participants must do this activity at this point in the practice—so there is one route of travel that all do together. In this instance, paying attention to *autonomy* and *connectedness* becomes important. The coach might communicate that we do this as a team so we can achieve the goals that you've identified and we've embraced together. It's hard work that done in unison helps us get to the finish line as a team.

Finally, there will be times the goal is chosen for us and we simply have no choice. In that instance, we empathize and show compassion. An example of this was when my (D. B. R.) child needed a vaccination to begin school. Shots, never an issue with my daughter before, had suddenly become a source of terror. Exploration of her fear, her desire to attend school, given choices, offered rewards, distractions, all led to the same dead end, "No!," and shrieking and tears when she was approached by medical staff. After another calming period, I placed her on my lap, gently but firmly told her this needed to be done, and held her tightly as the pediatrician administered the shot. Upon completion, my child bounced off my lap, went to where she knew she could get a sticker for going to the doctor, and proudly turned and asked, "Wasn't I brave Daddy?" What would you say? Here's what I wished I'd said, "You were afraid and still you did it."

MODULE 13

Discovering Strengths and Capacities

Module Purpose

The module aims to convey the value and use of ***affirmations*** in MI as a key skill within strength-focused work. By the end of this module, it is our hope the qualitative differences between praise and deeper affirmations will be clear, and you will have a deeper appreciation of how to use affirmations in your work to help clients to identify, embody, and utilize their strengths.

The *Why*: Strength-Focused Work Helps Us and Clients See Capacity

Traditionally, within the helping field, we tend to adopt a *deficit* or *disease view* in working with our clients. In our experience, this is even more prevalent in acute clinical areas of work; particularly in those areas of helping located within a wider medical model context (e.g., clinical psychologists, dietitians, physiotherapists who are working within a physical health setting such as an acute hospital setting). What is the deficit, problem, or diagnosis and how can we help the client fix it? While there have been notable exceptions over the years—William James, Carl Rogers, Abraham Maslow—it wasn't until *positive psychology* began studying the science of thriving that the helping field began to embrace more broadly the value of positive, *strength-focused work*. Chris Peterson (2006) summarizes this view succinctly: "Positive psychology is the scientific study of what goes right in life, from birth to death and all stops in between" (p. 4). This view regards the capacity of change as residing within the individual and asks what we can do to help this individual thrive and what resources—internal and external—are available to assist with that. This stance fits well with MI.

As MI practitioners, we focus on the strengths and capacities of our clients, and their ability to find solutions and choices that fit for them. "Focus" is the correct word as it implies that where we place our attention matters. There is also the matter of expectations. Research—falling under many names including the Pygmalion effect and self-fulfilling prophesies—suggests that our belief as a practitioner, or lack thereof, influences outcomes for clients (cf., Stukas & Snyder, 2016). There are nuances to this phenomenon, and research in leadership suggests that the recipient's view is also essential (Veestraeten et al., 2021). Thus, it is not enough that a practitioner has high expectations, clients must also see a way forward and believe they have the skills and capacity to succeed. This returns us to the concept of *competence*, which we raised earlier in the context of self-determination theory (see Chapter 2).

Competence is viewed as one of the three basic psychological drives that need to be met for us to thrive. Ryan and Deci (2017) view competence in a specific manner, "feeling effective in one's interactions with the social environment—that is, experiencing opportunities and supports for the exercise, expansion, and expression of one's capacities and talents" (p. 86). The belief that we can act in a manner that will influence our environment suggests the competence need is being met, while feeling that our efforts do not matter and/or that someone must do it for us suggests the opposite.

Thus, the competence need leads us back to a question we posed in an earlier module: Who is the gardener in this metaphor? From an MI perspective, it is the clients; they determine the nature of their garden. While they will not have control over all the elements (e.g., rainfall and climate), they will decide the type of garden, its design, and the order of work. They will tend it both while we're working together and after we are no longer on the scene. Our education about tools might be useful, as might our knowledge of what helps and hinders specific plants and garden features. However, as practitioners, we remain mindful this is their garden. Our job is to assist them in being competent in its tending. While all the foundational skills can assist us in this process, including careful listening and thoughtful questions, it is *affirmations* that seem best suited to this task.

The *What*: The Tools of Affirmation

In the latest edition of *Motivational Interviewing*, Miller and Rollnick (2023) indicate there might be two levels of *affirmation*. A basic level might involve a *compliment* or *praise*. It suggests a general appreciation for the person, but it remains superficial, can be overused, and runs the risk of clients making arguments to please the practitioner and gain praise, rather than truly doing it for themselves. This level can feel disingenuous if the practitioner is careless in its use. The deeper level of affirmation, the one that we prefer to teach, goes beyond the surface. It prizes the individual and looks specifically for strengths and capacities. It offers examples to bolster the observation. To illustrate:

You're a good parent who clearly loves your children.—This is praise.

You're a parent who pays careful attention to who each of your children are and then meets their needs based on what you observe and believe will help them the most.—This is an affirmation.

While we see the value in utilizing genuine praise and appreciating clients in an honest and transparent way, we also believe *competence*—the perceived ability to influence the environment and experience mastery—comes from this deeper *prizing*. In this context, we define prizing as being nonjudgmental and accepting the person fully, just as they are. We therefore reserve the term affirmation for that clinical skill. As was obvious in this example, the practitioner anchors the affirmation *in* strengths. It is a statement about the observable and not an opinion. This approach avoids the issue of "supersizing" in affirmations. That is, the affirmation *feels* exaggerated as we try to give it power and emphasis, *You're a fabulous parent!* Truth and genuineness matter in our work and especially so when it comes to orienting clients to their strengths and capacities. Like a wrong note in an otherwise exquisitely played musical piece, our ears immediately hear the falseness and attend to that rather than all the other notes.

There are other considerations in offering affirmations. We avoid the use of "I" and "me" as a lead-in and generally direct our statement directly to the client, *You. . . .* They are matched to the person and cultural context of the client. As authors, we have laughed that a Seattle affirmation would result in raised eyebrows in Scotland. Affirmations may take the form of reflective statements and be difficult to distinguish from deep reflective listening. Sources of affirmations *are* gleaned from careful listening, thoughtful questions, and by probing areas that clients might not view as strengths, for example, an effort the client views as a mistake. Finally, affirmations can be tuned to where a client is within the four processes in MI. This means early in ***engaging***, affirmations may be about general skills and capacities, and the ability to find options and solutions (e.g., *You know from your life experience you can find your way through tough situations*). In ***focusing***, it might be about core values and prioritizing (e.g., *You're clear that it must match what is most important to you, if you're going to do it*). Later in ***evoking***, it might be about self-knowledge and capacity to choose a path (e.g., *Some of those things might work for others, but you know that you must have something you're moving toward and one of those things is music*), and in ***planning*** it might be about specific knowledge and skills in implementing the steps along the path (e.g., *You have some ideas and also know that you need a specific plan—what happens and when—or it will just be put off until later*). These are not dictated by the task, but rather by understanding the task and the client, the practitioner may be better prepared to focus on the right thing at the right time and in the right manner.

The *How*: SP/SR on Using a Mistake to Explore Strengths and Capacity

Overview of the Exercise

For this activity, we will begin in what might seem an odd place—a mistake. We want you to think about or discuss with your practice partner a time when you made a mistake. This should not be a little mistake, but a larger one. We all make mistakes, and this is one you made, admitted, and took responsibility for, though it might have taken a little while, and asked for help. Thinking about this mistake may bring up feelings of shame and/or humiliation. Feeling flooded by these feelings is unhelpful so we will encourage self-compassion, just as we would with clients. If this is a very recent event, it might be difficult to talk about it with perspective. We encourage choosing another example with less immediacy, especially if it feels as if the resulting emotion could be too much. Remember, keep it 3 to 7 on that 10-point difficulty scale.

Structure of the Exercise

We believe this session is enhanced by your working with a partner. This person can assist if the emotions become too strong and/or you begin to feel emotionally overwhelmed. As in all these exercises, preserve your safety, and if this feels like too much, choose a different direction altogether or discuss a time when you struggled to succeed, but were eventually able to do so.

If you're working in a limited-practice setting, use the self-practice questions to guide the discussion. Work to deepen this information through careful, curious listening. Be attentive to your partner's emotions and demonstrate your compassion. Remember, this is an area requiring tenderness. Pay attention to what lies underneath the words and activities and reflect these to your partner. Listen for and notice strengths. Offer affirmations that are grounded in these strengths, as well as general prizing (e.g., *It is moving to watch someone who is so honest and vulnerable with themself, and willing to grow from it*).

If you're doing this as solo work, remember to use self-compassion. Imagine how you might respond to a client describing a similar situation and use that to guide how you replay this back in your mind. Again, if you're able to visualize the experience well, play it back in your head as if it's a movie and you're simply observing. If that is not a strength of yours, simply recall the experience of it and try to fill in the details, like where you were, who was present, how you felt in your body, your emotions, and your thoughts. Then write your answers to the questions.

Traveling Companion: An Example with Sam

Sam will help us illustrate this exercise. To recap, Sam is a White, cisgender, gay woman of European descent, who has been a successful counselor for many years. Ten years ago, she injured her back and because of that experience has shifted her private practice to health-focused care. She had a cancer scare last year, and her wife is encouraging her to retire. Sam is ambivalent about making that change, and this has become a point of contention between them.

> ***We all make mistakes, and some are bigger than others. If you would, please talk about a time when you made a bigger mistake, were able to admit the mistake, take responsibility for it, and ask for help.***

Oh, God. I cringe just thinking about this situation, but it immediately leapt to mind. After I injured my back, we still wanted to get into nature and so Debra suggested we get a little camper for our truck. So, we did, and it was great. We loved that camper and others thought it was cool, too. In fact, Debra's niece wanted to use it for her "honeymoon suite." She and her new husband were going camping across the Rockies, and this would be perfect. The couple was to be married on Saturday, stay a night in a hotel, and leave early on Sunday.

I woke earlier on that glorious Saturday, cleaned the interior of the camper, and had it ready to go. Fresh sheets on the bed and a few goodies for the happy couple completed the interior. I wanted to move the unit from our driveway to a little parking area we have on the side of the house to wash the exterior. Our niece was to pick it up, in a few hours, on her way to the wedding site. This is when I made the mistake—actually, it was a couple of mistakes.

On the side of the camper are support stanchions that stabilize the camper when it's parked. I only raised these a foot since I was going a short distance. Then I relied on my back-up camera that showed me the back of the truck. There is a rock at the entrance to this space that rises about 16 to 18 inches [or 40 to 46 cm]. While I could see the rock on my camera, what I couldn't see was my stanchion, which projected out about 6 inches further than my truck. I clipped that rock and tore the stanchion loose, but not off. Geez!

➤ ***What were the thoughts and feelings when the mistake first happened?***

I was shocked, devastated, and furious with myself. I'd not only ruined the camper, but I had also ruined my niece's plans. I just laid my head on the back of the camper and wanted to cry or blame someone else for the mistakes, but they were all my own.

➤ ***You were able to take responsibility. How did that come about?***

Well, the taking responsibility part was not easy, but it started when I laid my head on the back of the camper. For a moment, I just wanted to give in to all the emotion and self-rebuke—and there was a lot of it—and maybe some self-pity. But then I thought to myself, "You need to fix this," and there are 3 hours until she'll be here to pick it up. So, I told myself to work the problem and I did.

As it was, I didn't think I could fix the stanchion, but the camper would still work as it was. It would be a little less stable, but it could work. The issue was if my niece wanted to take the camper off—leave it at the camp—so she and her husband could take the vehicle into town without having to break camp and repack the camper. This is something we had discussed, and she'd practiced taking it on and off with me. I also needed to tell Debra and I knew she'd be upset, but she wasn't up yet, and I didn't want to waste time in that argument. So, I prioritized and focused on how we could safely get the camper off and on.

➤ ***You asked for help. Sometimes that is against our usual instincts. How were you able to do that? What helped you to do this and why?***

This ran counter to my usual approach, which is—I made the problem, so I need to fix it. I thought through the issue and determined that RVs must have powerful jacks, I'd see if I could get a tongue jack at an RV store. It would be more stable than a scissor jack. I also decided at that point I would just swallow the shame and humiliation and tell people what I'd done to see if they had any better solutions. If I was going to fix this, I needed to set my pride aside. So, I sat in my car and started searching the internet. The closest places were closed on Saturday, and the third wouldn't answer the phone and it was at best a 75-minute drive. I'd just made the decision to go to an auto parts store nearby when my neighbor Sue came by walking her dog.

I'll admit it—Sue was the last person I wanted to see. It's not that she isn't nice because she's lovely. It's just that she's incredibly competent at everything she does and is very handy—her family is full of mechanics—so I've always felt like I don't quite measure up. When she asked how I was, my immediate reaction was to say fine, but instead I said, "Not well." Then I explained to her what happened and the mess I was in.

➤ ***How did the person or people respond when you told them about your mistake? What was the impact on you—in your body, in your feelings, in your thoughts, and in your subsequent behaviors?***

She listened well actually. She didn't laugh either, though she did chuckle at the end just a bit and said, "Girl, I have been there. Let's look and maybe I can help." It's funny because I felt myself releasing this tension. Like I could take a full breath again. When she chuckled, it felt like it was with me and about a common bond we shared in having made a royal mistake. My thought was I don't feel ashamed or humiliated. In fact, I feel sort of liberated and now I have help. All those feelings of jealousy toward Sue were gone and I just felt appreciation.

Later, while I was on the road with Sue to get some materials, I texted Debra about what had happened. I specifically asked her not to be angry now as I was trying to fix the mess. She immediately responded with a note of love and support, and indicated she would reach out to her niece, who, in turn, then responded that if the camper still worked and was road-worthy, they didn't need to take the camper off. Also, they would wait until the morning to get the camper, which would give us more time and relieve one stressor for them. I start tearing up just thinking about this stuff now. I was expecting to be laughed at or berated or humiliated because that was what I did to myself, and instead I was met with love and compassion, and I just felt such gratitude and connection to these people.

➤ ***What was the outcome, and what are your thoughts, feelings, and bodily reactions as you think about it now?***

Well, Sue was a godsend. She initially suggested we could get a screw jack, like they use for lifting the roof on houses and that could easily hold the weight and would allow us to raise and lower the backend gradually, which is what we needed. But then as she inspected the damage, she realized the stanchion was unbent and that using some bonding agents, epoxy, wood glues, and—get this—wooden match sticks, we could do a temporary fix for the stanchion and have it ready by that evening. She, her son, Debra, and I spent the day fixing the camper. Sue put the last of the caulk on as the sun was setting and we made it to the wedding on time.

It's funny because I feel nothing but love, gratitude, and appreciation for all these people. Sue has these remarkable skills, and I was able to witness and appreciate them up close. Wooden match sticks? Really? It was a huge gift to me, and maybe it provided a gift back because she was able to help in such an immediate and tangible way. Her 16-year-old son gave up his Saturday to pitch in. What a remarkable young man. I also felt deep love for Debra and her ability to rise above a natural inclination and to care for me so tenderly when I had made a mess. When I think about our niece and all the stressors on a wedding day and the grace she displayed in her response, it deepened my admiration of her as a person. I still feel a twang about hitting that rock, but the emotion has really been siphoned off. It was a mistake. It was avoidable. I won't do it again. But what an experience I had because of it.

➤ ***What do you think would've happened had you not chosen this path? What feelings or bodily sensations would've accompanied it and why?***

I think I probably would've arrived at a solution that was a temporary fix, which I would've been embarrassed by. The broken stanchion would've been a reminder of my ineptitude and I would've felt ashamed. That feeling probably would've leaked out and eventually been distorted into resentment. I would've looked back on the whole day as one of shame, and every time it was referenced, I would feel humiliated.

➤ ***As you think back over this story, what strengths do you observe in yourself during this process? What helped you to mobilize these strengths? Again, look through that self-compassionate lens of the present.***

I can see several. The first was when I wanted to give myself over to trying to blame someone else—"Who thought it was a good idea to put a rock at the edge of that space?"—or self-pity—"I'm such a screw-up!"—instead I was able to pivot and say to myself you need to fix this for your niece. I was able to control my emotions, after a little meltdown, and focus on the other person and not me.

The second strength was in breaking down the problem. I was able to reengage my critical thinking and start identifying steps, priorities, and solutions. Even though emotion was still high, I was able to make thoughtful choices like not driving at least 2.5 hours, there and back, to a store that might not have what I needed.

The third strength was a willingness to be vulnerable with Sue. It put me at risk for further humiliation, but it also opened the door to all the solutions that followed. Without doing that, none of the rest would've followed. The same was true with Debra.

The final strength was my attitude of gratefulness and appreciation of the skills of others. Instead of being self-castigating, I simply marveled at their capacities, and that was powerful to me and seemed to be for them, too.

➤ ***Why do you think it made such a difference to take responsibility for the mistake and ask for help?***

I know this seems a little obvious, but by taking responsibility, I also took back my agency. I had some control. At least initially, that control was over my emotions, and once I began to regulate those a little more, then I could begin to take some control over my thoughts and start to diagnose, prioritize, and problem-solve. In terms of asking for help, I'm seeing a parallel process. The not asking for help is an emotional decision made from fear and self-protection. It's not made from strength. Being vulnerable is reasserting the thinking part and operating from strength. It also allowed me to use more brains and have more skills, which is usually a good thing. Asking for help provided more resources.

Self-Practice

Now it's your turn.

➤ ***We all make mistakes, and some are bigger than others. If you would, please talk about a time when you made a bigger mistake, were able to admit the mistake, take responsibility for it, and ask for help.***

➤ *What were the thoughts and feelings when the mistake first happened?*

➤ *You were able to take responsibility. How did that come about?*

➤ *You asked for help. Sometimes that is against our usual instincts. How were you able to do that? What helped you to do this and why?*

➤ ***How did the person or people respond when you told them about your mistake? What was the impact on you—in your body, in your feelings, in your thoughts, and in your subsequent behaviors?***

➤ ***What was the outcome, and what are your thoughts, feelings, and bodily reactions as you think about it now?***

➤ *What do you think would've happened had you not chosen this path? What feelings or bodily sensations would've accompanied it and why?*

➤ *As you think back over this story, what strengths do you observe in yourself during this process. What helped you to mobilize these strengths? Again, look through that self-compassionate lens of the present.*

Self-Reflection

➤ *How did you react in your body as you read or heard the question for this exercise? What feelings and thoughts accompanied this response and why?*

➤ ***Why do you think it made such a difference to take responsibility for the mistake and ask for help? What helped you to do this and why?***

➤ ***What were the other essential elements in the structure of this activity for you? That is, in thinking about and reflecting on this mistake, what was helpful to the process? Were there factors that got in the way or were unhelpful?***

➤ ***How does this process of exploration and discovery lead to affirmations of your strengths? How does it feel to do this?***

➤ *How does this process feel different from cheerleading? Where did you experience it in your body? What feelings and thoughts did you notice and why?*

➤ *How has this process helped you to better understand the receipt of a complex affirmation and why this feels different from praise?*

What If: Applying Skills to My Current Context

Bridging Questions to Practitioner-Self

These questions are designed to help you bring the insights from personal self-practice into your work with clients.

➤ *Understanding how you felt in answering this question about a time when you made a mistake, how might you use this experience in exploring difficult areas for clients?*

➤ ***In what ways do you think this activity might be helpful for a client? That is, exploring a mistake for strengths?***

➤ ***Specifically, how will you use this process of discovery and exploration in your clinical work to affirm clients' strengths and capacities? What structures or safeguards might you create and why?***

➤ ***Specifically, how do you believe clients' strengths and capacities might appear differently in the tasks of engaging, focusing, evoking, and planning? Why? What might you be listening for in each of those tasks to assist you?***

- *How will you know if you're slipping into praise versus an affirmation? What will tell you that is happening? How might you course-correct in that situation?*

- *What are your main* takeaway *messages from this SP/SR experience in relation to your understanding of the role of affirmations in discovering strengths and capacities . . .*
  - *From a practical perspective in MI?*
  - *From a theoretical perspective in MI?*

- *What if you were to apply this process to other areas of your professional practice (e.g., in a role as supervisor or trainer perhaps)? How might you apply your learning to this new context?*

- *How has this exercise influenced your understanding of or personal relationship with MI as a way of being?*

Final Thoughts and Applications to Other Settings

Of course, we need not rely on mistakes or partial successes to find sources of affirmations. It's just that these tend to be rich and often overlooked resources. Instead, simply being mindful of what it takes for our clients to navigate their complicated worlds and their corresponding tasks provides little gems if we remind ourselves of the fundamental value in looking for them. A general attitude of prizing and appreciation helps, and we remain steadfast in our assertion this must be *genuine, honest,* and *specific* to have value. An ingenuine affirmation is not benign; it plants a seed of doubt in our client's garden about our role as a partner in this process.

Settings exist where we might be tempted to supersize our affirmations. If working with an athlete who has lost confidence or a patient who is losing hope, our ***fixing reflex*** might pull for us to address these issues with cheerleading. There will be both contextual and cultural variations in how much we get pulled into this temptation. It might be fueled by our relative ability and confidence in sitting with distress, and it comes from a place of concern and that is laudable. In this circumstance, we'd suggest a more straightforward approach as follows:

> *I know you're having doubts, and while it's not certain, I have reasons for feeling confident. I am happy to share these with you if you're interested. Ultimately, it is your thoughts, not mine, that matter.*

In working with supervisees, we often feel a dual pull between wanting to aid in their growth and protecting clients being served by the supervisee. That is, we want people to have a realistic assessment of their skills and capacities, so they operate in a manner consistent with them. Toward this end, we encourage honesty and directness, while viewing feedback as an effort at growth and not a bludgeon. Thus, the target should be the supervisee's zone of proximal development. We don't say to a fifth- grade math student, *This is all basic math and you're not doing any of the hard stuff yet.* Instead, we might say, *You've mastered addition and subtraction, multiplication, and division, and understand the order of operations. You're in the process of learning these operations with decimals and fractions. It will take some more work before that feels comfortable, so this is where I think it makes sense to spend time practicing. Once you're there, we can move onto some other things that build on these ideas.* Such is a more nuanced and longer response, but it also acknowledges progress and maintains learner motivation.

In Module 16, we'll discuss and practice this skill set of ***information exchange*** in greater detail, especially how we offer input on areas of concern.

MODULE 14

Pulling the Pieces Together

Module Purpose

The aim of this module is to help you to gain an appreciation for the role, form, and function of different types of ***summaries*** in MI. By the end of this module, we hope that you will have a deeper understanding and felt sense of the impact of receiving different types of helpful summaries and how you can use them in your own practice with clients for specific purposes both within, and across, the ***four tasks in MI***.

The *Why*: The Value of a Good Story and Narrative in the MI Process

We have described the importance of clients making their own choices as essential to the change process, and we recognize this should be an informed choice. We also know that facts and statistics are rarely enough to change behavior. Therefore, it is useful for us to understand the importance of *story* and *narrative*.

Let's pause for a moment and see how that comes into the structure of this book. Each module begins with an implicit question, *Why am I doing this?* This question involves our need to understand and engage with meaning. This type of learning experience may be encouraged by an interest in people, ideas, and stories; we often process this type of learning with and through other people. Thus, we start each module answering an implicit *Why* question. That is, why is a particular concept, technique, or strategy within MI important? Further learning in this way is supported by the "story" element of the traveling companions in this workbook.

In thinking about story, Halvorson (2011) distinguishes a story as a single-event unit, while a narrative is the stringing together of multiple stories into a coherent meta story. This distinction is important because the stories in a narrative can change, while the narrative remains consistent. Thus, a single story may reinforce or undermine a narrative, or be completely divorced from a narrative to maintain the *through-line* integrity. Merriam Webster defines through line as "a common or a consistent element or theme shared by items in a series or by parts of a whole" (*www.merriam-webster.com/dictionary/through%20line*). Understanding these distinctions helps us understand how story and narrative may influence clients.

Research demonstrates what we know intuitively. We're better able to recall and change attitudes and behavior based on story than isolated facts and figure (Graesser et al., 1980; Niemand, 2018). Story has the power to stimulate our brains, especially in our emotional centers, which also link to values and motivation (Cormick, 2019). But there is an important nuance. Cormick (2019) notes, "[T]he power of stories is not in the shaping of us to values within the story, but how well they can tap into the values that we intrinsically hold already" (p. 5). Therefore, our careful listening to and understanding of client values help us then organize information into a story that supports the client's narrative of who they are and what matters to them.

During our journey through these ideas, we've described client statements and responses as the tip of an iceberg. The things above the waterline are apparent (visible) to us and them, but what is often murkier to both of us is what lies below that waterline and how deep that goes. We've noted that the exploration of these things can have power as they bring new understandings to the client and us. We know that new metaphors can be powerful shapers of how people think about, understand, and respond to issues (Flusberg et al., 2017). We will discuss metaphors more at the end of this module, but for now, at the metacognition level, we—the client and us—are co-creating a new understanding and the shaping of this into a story or, at a deeper level, a coherent narrative that assists the client in moving forward on important decisions and changes.

When we co-create this understanding, the client now has a new map to understand their route of travel. Or in the imagery of our garden, there is now a landscape plan where one didn't exist before; the one in use was no longer functional for the client, or through neglect or worse, by self or others the weeds have overgrown the original garden. This brings us back to Cormick's point that what matters in this plan or map is not the values we think the plan should reflect, but rather that the plan reflects the values the client has. This is client autonomy at its essence. So, how do we help create this narrative? While the other foundational skills all contribute to this process, ***summaries*** have the capacity to do this directly.

The *What*: Tools for Creating Effective Summaries

Summaries are an essential skill in this process and not all summaries are equal. Indeed, we all likely have experience in forming unhelpful summaries. Clients' glazed eyes reflect our run-on sentences back to us. While summaries must capture information, they should not capture all; the best are *organized*. We encourage summaries with a few main focal points well stated. A sharp metaphor can be helpful in this process.

As with any good story, there are points of tension. This comes in the form of *juxtaposing*. Things as we have understood them before and as we understand them now. The reasons why we have not changed, and why we're moved to consider them now. The value that seemed to have ascendancy and the one we recognize now. This *self-reevaluation* and accompanying *emotional arousal* provide powerful *processes of change* (DiClemente, 2018). Our structuring of the summary helps to engage these engines of change for the client.

These ideas of organization and juxtaposition point out our third fundamental of summaries—these are *intentional* always and *directional* sometimes. That is because we pick and choose between elements. We are intentional in what we include and omit. We include only the elements most germane to this client and what matters to them. Early in the process with clients—during engaging and focusing—we might not be directional. That is, we do not know in what direction clients wish to travel, how they want their garden to be set up, or how deep the iceberg goes. . . . There is a risk for a premature focus. Our ***fixing reflex*** might also slip in when we believe that we know the direction in which they should travel. But remember, for the story to have power, it reflects the client's values, not the other way around.

Lastly, did we say this already? *Brevity* matters. Long, elegant summaries are difficult for clients to retain. If they can't retain them, they're not useful. Shorter is better. Less is more.

Together then, strong summaries have four elements. They are organized, juxtaposed, intentional, and brief. When done together, they help us discover, understand, and co-create story and narrative.

The *How*: SP/SR on Exploring Narrative and Summaries through Three Short Stories

Overview of the Exercise

For this activity, we will spend some telling and then delving into our stories and how these form a narrative. This is also an opportunity to practice creating summaries. There are opportunities to describe ourselves in five different story forms.

Structure of the Exercise

This self-practice exercise can be done as either a self-directed activity or an interaction with a practice partner. If working with a partner in a limited practice, when acting as the listener, focus on creating summaries and using the four elements just described. Stay within the story form so your practice partner has an opportunity to experience the different pieces each story gathers and reveals. After each story, there is an opportunity to explore the effects of that story. We encourage you to give space to your partner to sort out their thoughts and feelings and then share these with you, with some exploration before moving on to the next story form. Note that this often begins with a focus on bodily sensations, which, in turn, help us to attend to feelings, and then ends with cognitions. At the end, there are opportunities to think across stories to develop a clearer understanding of the narrative. You can decide if it is best to write and talk about these ideas or simply talk them through. As a result of this structure, we suggest you set aside a longer timeframe to have this discussion.

If working alone, stay focused on the present question and work through this process sequentially. Practice writing summaries where you're prompted to do so.

Traveling Companion: An Example with Quincy

Quincy will help us illustrate this exercise. To recap, Quincy is a 38-year-old, cisgender, straight woman of African descent who works as an AOD counselor. From a vibrant community, she has strong family ties. She was feeling some burnout with AOD clients and has sought personal support with an MI therapist.

> ***In three or four sentences, please describe yourself. Who are you? What matters to you? What should someone know about you and why?***

I am a 38-year-old Black woman, which means strength is required, every day. Hard work has gotten me here, but that doesn't mean the course was straight or the race was fair. I have great friends and a good community around me, and I love spending time with them. But there are problems here. I was raised by the belief "our problems, our solutions." While we'll take help wherever we can find it, don't rely on other folks. They will disappoint you.

> ***Please tell me an important story from your life. One that has great meaning to you. It can be a success, a failure, a point at which something changed, or just something that has always stayed with you and stuck out. Please provide details like where you were and who was with you.***

When I was 11, I remember it because I was in Ms. Anderson's class. We had to do a project about our family and our neighborhood. We had to write a story or draw a picture, do a poem, create a lyric, or make a collage that we would explain to our class. I liked art, so I wanted to get some things from the store and my dad said we could. He told me that I had $10 and could decide how I would spend it. Money was hard to come by so that was a big deal.

When we arrived at the store, I saw one of those guys sitting outside it asking for money. I was old enough that I knew about homeless people and knew that alcohol and drugs were often a problem. In the way of kids, my friends and I were both afraid and kind of mean to them. Like we'd walk around them, and not speak to them, or say something mean as we ran away or into the store.

On this day, there was a homeless guy who called out to us. My dad told me to go in and do my shopping and he'd catch up with me. I peeked back, once I was in the store, and saw my dad kneeling, talking to the man. When he caught up to me in the store, I saw he had a basket with a sandwich, a banana, a small bag of chips, some cookies, and a water. The kind of things he would put in my lunch or his. Meanwhile, I had glitter pens, paper, and some other little things. He smiled and asked if I had what I needed and then we went to the register and checked out.

On our way out, my dad stopped at the man and said, "Be well, Brother" and gave him the bag. He never said a word to me about it, and the whole way home I kept thinking about the two things he'd said, "Be well, Brother" and "Do you have what you need?"

> ***How did you experience this story in your body at the time? How about now as you retell it?***

Not surprisingly, it felt different during the different phases. Nervous tingly energy at the beginning. Then at the end, as I drove home, I felt my chest kind of swell with pride about my dad, and then I felt myself kind of cringe as I thought about my walking by. I hunched and kind of curled in thinking about the last part.

> ***What were you thinking and feeling?***

I kind of went through phases of feelings and thoughts. On the way there, I was excited and thinking about what I would buy with my $10. I also like being with my dad, and we were doing something special.

The second phase was when we went into and came out of the store. I was a little confused. Did my dad know this man? Why was he talking with him? Wasn't he worried that he would get cooties or something? The man smelled and that was gross, so I remember feeling kind of icky. When I saw the stuff in my dad's basket, I thought it was weird that he was buying lunch stuff for himself. Normally, we bought packages of things and made sandwiches ourselves, so it was weird. Then on the way out when he said "Brother," it wasn't like he was greeting someone on the street, but like something he might say to my uncle. It surprised me.

The last phase was the drive home. My dad had the music on and was just being dad. It was like I'd just been through something big. He stopped and spoke to this man, who everyone else avoided. He called him "Brother" and told him to "Be well." He asked me if I had what I needed and I was wondering if he meant art supplies or something bigger. Truthfully, I felt a little embarrassed sitting with my gel pens. I thought about the Good Samaritan story in church and how my dad had been the one who stopped. I felt proud of him. I also realized that I walked by and that was bad.

> ***Please tell us a second important story from your life. Again, it should be one that has great meaning to you. It can be a success, a failure, a point at which something changed, or just something that has always stayed with you and stuck out. Please provide details like where you were and who was with you.***

This story happened when I was in ninth grade. I grew early, so I was big and strong for my age, and I was playing sports on some of the varsity athletics. Some of the ninth graders were small, and we had some upper classmen who liked to pick on the younger kids. They were tough and had bad reputations, so folks tended to stay clear of them.

One day I was walking past this part of the school where the upper classmen congregated, and I saw they had singled out this small, nerdy ninth grader. They were taunting her. Suddenly, this big girl, a junior, shoved her down. The girl's backpack spilled out. The older kids were like hovering around, and the younger ones were trying to get away. My mom always said, "With great gifts, comes great responsibility" and "Those of us who can, need to stand up for those who can't." So, I took off running and arrived just as the older girl went to shove the smaller girl back down again. I blocked her and told her to leave the girl alone. She got right up into my face, and I knew I was about to get a beating. She was pissed off. I could feel her anger as she stared at me. She cussed me out, told me she'd be seeing me after school, and then left with her crew.

At this point, I turned around and the smaller girl was trembling. I asked her if she was okay. She mumbled something, and then said it was stupid of her to come this way and began gathering her things up. I told her what those girls did wasn't right. I helped her pick up her things and then she just mumbled, "Thanks," and took off.

> ***How did you experience this story in your body at the time? How about now as you retell it?***

Fear and anger intermixed, I guess. Initially, it was sort of that feeling of nausea in my stomach. Then feeling a pull to turn away. Then when I decided to turn toward the situation, it was resolve. Set my jaw. Eyes narrowed. Fists clenched. I might have yelled as I was running, I'm not sure if I did, but it would be like me. Then afterward, it's like feeling all this energy just drain from my body. Like I just want to find a place to sit down and recover. I could feel that power and resolve as I ran toward the girl and as we stood face to face. I also feel a bit drained now and my heart hurts for that girl because I didn't help her more.

➤ ***What were you thinking and feeling?***

Well, my first thought was I hate these jerks. It made me mad. Then I thought I have to help and that was followed with a feeling of dread as I thought I was going to get my ass kicked by the older girl. By the time I sprinted over to the trouble, my adrenaline had kicked in. When we were standing nose to nose, it just reminded me of sports where I was always playing against someone bigger and stronger who was trying to intimidate me. I just never backed down from that situation, and while I got my butt kicked more than once, the other person knew they were in a fight.

Afterward, I thought I needed to comfort this girl, but I didn't really know how. I stopped the attack, but I knew it didn't change what had happened. I felt sad and angry for her, but realized I didn't really know what to say to help her. I wished I'd taken her to the counselor or asked her to talk about her feelings. Or at least that's what I think now. As for me, the adrenaline was starting to drop, and I was starting to worry about what would happen after school.

➤ ***Please tell us a third important story from your life. Again, it should be one that has great meaning to you. It can be a success, a failure, a point at which something changed, or just something that has always stayed with you and stuck out. Please provide details like where you were and who was with you.***

This is a shorter story. During the summer of 2020, after the deaths of George Floyd, Breonna Taylor, Ahmaud Arbery, and others, there were protests around the world under the banner of Black Lives Matter. It felt like this great awakening. Like maybe we could finally achieve some justice. White people joined the protests, and it seemed like there was some momentum. Then one day, I was talking with a White colleague I've known for many years. I really like her and she's a very kind, good-hearted woman. Her political beliefs fall at the other end of the continuum to mine, but that has never stopped us from getting along. But on this day, as I was talking about the Black Lives Matter protest I'd gone to, I could see that affected her. So, I asked her about it, and she said, "I've never really understood the purpose of protesting. What if we put that energy toward changing something? I also think that All Lives Matter." I was stunned. She didn't see it or understand it. Until then I kind of thought if the evidence about racism just became clear enough people of goodwill would see it and there would be a shift, but I realized then that would not happen. Black, Brown, Indigenous Peoples—hell, women—would have to fight for everything we wanted and while allies can be helpful, we can't rely on them.

➤ ***What were you thinking and feeling?***

Like I said, I was stunned. My first reaction was "Really? You don't see that Black Lives have been treated differently?" Then I started to get irritated, and I wanted to argue. But I've also learned that getting angry and arguing with White people gets you labeled as a "mad black woman" and then you get ignored. So, instead I thought I need to calm down and just offer the other side. I knew it wouldn't convince her, but I didn't want her to think I agreed either.

➤ ***How did you experience this story in your body at the time? How about now as you retell it?***

This was a time where there was a lot of righteous anger and energy. We were demanding change. So, my body felt energized. When I heard this reaction from this woman, I was discouraged and irritated. I could feel myself disconnect, even as my body tensed, my hands tightened. I also made a concerted effort to breathe and force the tension out before I responded, but I also left shortly after that so I wouldn't say something I'd regret later. Now, I start to feel the tension rise again.

➤ ***Summarize what made Story 1 important to you.***

To begin, I was a good kid, but focused on my own needs and wants. My dad's demonstration of compassion was powerful. It showed me who he was and made me look at my choices and behavior. I didn't like what I saw and decided I needed to change my focus.

➤ ***What values do you see, hear, think, or feel are within this story?***

Compassion—not just toward the man, but to me. My dad didn't lecture me or shame me. In fact, he just loved me, just like that man. Being of service to others. God's will. For me I guess, I saw the tension between self-care—my art project—and other care—this man in need that I would've walked right past. I also saw honesty. I looked at myself hard, even as an 11-year-old.

➤ ***Summarize what made Story 2 important to you.***

Again, there was another person in need. This time, rather than safety, I chose action on behalf of someone else. The action stopped the assault, and I learned there was more that I needed to be able to do if I truly wanted to help.

➤ ***What values do you see, hear, think, or feel are within this story?***

Care and concern for self and others. Compassion. Courage. Honesty.

➤ ***Summarize what made Story 3 important to you.***

Being Black matters. It is the lens through which I see and interact with the world, and it interacts with me. While sometimes I don't want it, it is always there. For me, it provides force and focus to my choices and values.

➤ ***What values do you see, hear, think, or feel are within this story?***

Honesty still matters, but so does thoughtfulness. Community. Social justice. Care for self and others.

➤ ***Summarize the connections you observe between the three stories, including what makes them important, or the values that underlie them.***

I never thought about this. . . . There is a thread running through these stories about caring for others and what that does demand of us. Our actions and inaction matter. They say something about us and our values. While running to the need or the fight is important, it is not the only need. To be effective, we must recognize the nature of the need and learn how to respond to it. Learning is an important part of this process.

> ***What connections do you observe between the things you just wrote, and the initial story you told about who you are in three or four sentences? Take a moment to think about it. Then summarize your three most important connections.***

There is a clear link between that description of who I am and these three stories. The first is that I am a Black woman, and the world isn't fair. Second, I was raised with a set of values that we need to take care of each other. Third, we need to be ready to struggle—with ourselves, with others, and the larger community—to make it a better place for all.

Self-Practice

Now it's your turn.

> ***In three or four sentences, please describe yourself. Who are you? What matters to you? What should someone know about you and why?***

> ***Please tell me an important story from your life. One that has great meaning to you. It can be a success, a failure, a point at which something changed, or just something that has always stayed with you and stuck out. Please provide details like where you were and who was with you.***

➤ *How did you experience this story in your body at the time? How about now as you retell it?*

➤ *What were you thinking and feeling?*

➤ *Please tell us a second important story from your life. Again, it should be one that has great meaning to you. It can be a success, a failure, a point at which something changed, or just something that has always stayed with you and stuck out. Please provide details like where you were and who was with you.*

➤ *How did you experience this story in your body at the time? How about now as you retell it?*

➤ ***What were you thinking and feeling?***

➤ ***Please tell us a third important story from your life. Again, it should be one that has great meaning to you. It can be a success, a failure, a point at which something changed, or just something that has always stayed with you and stuck out. Please provide details like where you were and who was with you.***

➤ ***How did you experience this story in your body at the time? How about now as you retell it?***

➤ ***What were you thinking and feeling?***

> ***Summarize what made Story 1 important to you and why?***

> ***What values do you see, hear, think, or feel are within this story?***

> ***Summarize what made Story 2 important to you and why.***

> ***What values do you see, hear, think, or feel are within this story?***

> ***Summarize what made Story 3 important to you and why?***

➤ ***What values do you see, hear, think, or feel are within this story?***

➤ ***Summarize the connections you observe between the three stories, including what makes them important, or the values that underlie them.***

➤ ***What connections do you observe between the things you just wrote, and the initial story you told about who you are in three or four sentences? Take a moment to think about it. Then summarize your three most important connections.***

Self-Reflection

➤ ***Who we are might reflect our personal narrative and, of course, the stories that we hold onto help to shape and reinforce that narrative. As you step back now and think about the bigger picture of your life, what is your narrative? How does this narrative affect you? Why?***

- ***How does it feel as you consider this narrative? What sensations do you notice in your body? What thoughts do you have?***

- ***What did you discover or rediscover about your narrative as you worked through this process? What was different than you remember?***

- ***Why did the exploration of values matter in understanding your narrative? How did this help you in your understanding and why?***

➤ ***If you worked with a partner, what type of summary, or summaries, did you receive? Where did you feel it? If you had feelings, what were they? What thoughts went through your mind?***

____

____

____

____

____

____

➤ ***To clarify the experience of receiving a summary, how helpful was it, even if you were the one who wrote it? What mattered?***

____

____

____

____

____

____

➤ ***In what ways did the focus on summaries sharpen your focus in considering different areas or ideas?***

____

____

____

____

____

____

What If: Applying Skills to My Current Context

Bridging Questions to Practitioner-Self

These questions are designed to help you bring the insights from personal self-practice into your work with clients.

➤ *How does the experience of your narrative help you to think about your clients' narratives? What did you experience that might be helpful for them? What might get in the way?*

➤ *How might summaries be useful in this process of exploring client narratives?*

➤ *In thinking about your use of summaries with clients, what specifically needs to shift or change and why? Where do you need to get better and why?*

➤ *What specific techniques can you use to assist in refining your skills in offering good-quality summaries to your clients? What will this include and why? What will help you to do this and to know that you are doing it?*

➤ ***How will you obtain feedback in this area as you work to refine these skills? How will you use that to refine your approach?***

____

____

____

____

____

➤ ***What are your main*** takeaway ***messages from this SP/SR experience in relation to your understanding of how using summaries strategically can help pull the pieces together . . .***

- ***From a practical perspective in your MI work?***

____

____

____

- ***From a theoretical perspective in your MI work?***

____

____

____

➤ ***What if you were to apply this process to other areas of your professional practice (e.g., in a role as supervisor or trainer perhaps)? How might you apply your learning to this new context?***

____

____

____

➤ ***How has this exercise influenced your understanding of or personal relationship with MI as a way of being?***

____

____

____

Final Thoughts and Applications to Other Settings

Of course, we do not have just one narrative but multiple narratives in our lives, some of which will take precedence in particular places and settings and points in time. While narratives might be tied to factors like roles or *ego states*, they're not synonymous with them. Narratives might be like the air we breathe. It surrounds and impacts us, but we rarely notice it unless something happens to bring our attention to the air.

It might seem like this idea of narrative only applies to therapy or counseling situations, where we spend more time focusing on the person rather than a specific need; this analysis may miss important factors that influence clients' thoughts, beliefs, and actions. A person whose narrative is that pain is a punishment for life choices will interact differently than a client who views life as a series of choices, including how we respond to pain and changed circumstances, to someone who views themself as unlucky in life and this is one more bit of evidence supporting that view. The narrative, perhaps unnoticed by the client, will influence their connection to the practitioner, their beliefs about the efficacy of the intervention, and their views of their agency and ability to enact changes.

While our clients have narratives, so do we as practitioners, supervisors, coaches in and for our workplace. The nature of our narratives influences how we engage in our work and with the people we serve. It is worthwhile certainly to consider the stories we tell in these areas and the narrative we weave together in such work.

Metaphors add another layer for us to consider here. A metaphor is something that compares, sometimes implicitly, two things that are unrelated, but by virtue of the comparison provides insight into the subject of interest. A metaphor, as in the gardening metaphor used in this book, may form a *through line,* or it may be an observation into a discrete subject area, as in client's putting up deflector shields when they feel attacked. Metaphor, as described by Rosengren (2017), allows "clients to understand their situation in a new way while providing an organizational scheme and/or image for incorporating new data" (p. 77). Thus, metaphors can be used as a specific form of deeper reflective listening, which has great power to co-create understanding of a particular area or to provide organizing schema that aid the practitioner and/or the client in understanding the course of their work together. For example, some MI practitioners use the metaphor of MI practitioners being midwives to change. They work hard, are instrumental in the birthing process, and sometimes their technical skills are critical to success. Yet, the life existed before them, and it is the mother who does the incredibly hard work of carrying and delivering new life into existence.

There is additional nuance to consider here in the form of metaphor: *simile* and *analogy.* To begin with, all similes are metaphors, but not all metaphors are similes. Similes use the word "like" to create the comparison, and this comparison is explicit as a result. Analogies make a comparison as well, but the goal is not comparison but to explain something. A common analogy is *It's like we're rearranging the deck chairs on the Titanic.* The point being made is that we are wasting our time on nonessential actions in a critical situation. An *aphorism* is an observation—typically, a pithy one—that contains a general truth, *Power corrupts, and absolute power corrupts absolutely.* Understanding these nuances can assist us in understanding why we're deploying some skills and in certain situations. Circling back to the airport to land this paragraph—okay, we couldn't resist—the ability to define and distinguish these techniques is not nearly as important that we recognize the value of metaphors and similes in deepening understanding and providing a way forward for us and clients, and that analogies and aphorisms might have great value and can slip into advice giving if we're not attentive.

MODULE 15

Beyond Tipping the Balance

Module Purpose

The aim of this module is to explore the concept of ***ambivalence*** in MI, look at the use of a *decisional balance*, take a deeper dive into ***vertical ambivalence*** for more multifaceted and/or multilayered dilemmas, and consider the role of listening well and tolerating uncertainty as ambivalence emerges. By the end of this module, it is hoped that you will have a clearer and deeper understanding of ambivalence, the purpose of listening well with ambivalence, and the power of sitting with uncertainty when ambivalence goes deeper than the surface level of a specific, concrete behavior.

The *Why*: Ambivalence Doesn't Leave Us

Early MI writings focused on resolving ambivalence as one of the presumed mechanisms of change within the method. However, over time it became clear that this was not quite an accurate depiction. It seems we often don't resolve ambivalence; instead, we tip it enough to allow movement away from a sticking point. Thus, neither we nor clients should expect that the path will be clear and the aim unfettered. Often, we will feel pulls to return to the old behavior even as we make progress. It is only through repeated reassertion of the aim and continued action to obtain and maintain it that the ambivalence begins to recede.

DiClemente (2018) notes a series of shifts in reinforcers, self-efficacy, and temptation that all occur as someone moves from the *action* to *maintenance* to *termination* stages in changing behaviors. Of intrigue in his accounting of the move from maintenance into termination is the individual shifts from being an "ex" (i.e., an ex-user), as this defines someone by what they're not, into freeing that energy into new areas and new ways of being in the world. While DiClemente (2018) writes in the context of addiction and change, a similar process can occur within the context of the uptake of a positive behavior, though the presentation might appear different, and the language of termination may not fit. For example, people who take up meditation as a self-care process don't necessarily terminate a behavior, but rather embrace a new way of seeing themselves in the world. Plain language describes this stage as *The New Me* (Prevention Research Institute, 2008), which captures this sense of new identity and opportunity. At this point, little energy is devoted to the change or residual ambivalence, and if there is, this is a concerning prognostic sign (DiClemente, 2018).

Miller (2022), in *On Second Thought*, describes all the usual forms of ambivalence well known to psychology—a wish for two positive goals or desires, a wish to avoid two negative goals or desires, or a mix of negative and positive goals and desires—but adds a new idea: vertical ambivalence. Here, the ambivalence is between a clear motivation for a positive aim or desire and yet continued engagement in a behavior that prevents such an occurrence. He illustrates this with examples, including clients who consistently chose the same type of problematic intimate partner. The pole that keeps the issue unresolved might be unconscious, an uncommon concept in the MI world but familiar to those coming from psychodynamic traditions, or unknown at present. We might regard this unknown area as the parts of the "iceberg" unexplored by the client or us. However defined, we note an aspect of the client's motivation is obscured for them and for us. Together, we come to understand that unknown part will be essential to understand if the balance is to be tipped.

Miller (2022) adds psychological and social factors that also influence the ambivalence process, though they are not directly causative, an idea like that proposed by the lifestyle risk reduction model (Daugherty & Leukefeld, 1998). This seemingly small idea—psychological and social factors influence but are not causative—is monumental as it leaves client choice as the key ingredient in the change process. It's clear that choices directly influence outcomes. It is also an overstatement to say that social and psychological factors have no direct impact on outcome; they do. It's just we often overstate the case. For example, *adverse childhood events* (ACEs) do NOT cause *substance use disorders*, but they can and do powerfully influence client choices, which, in turn, cause the use disorder. This position recognizes people's agency even in difficult situations. As a result, choice lies at the heart of change.

To be clear, we are neither blaming clients nor asserting they have chosen to experience their problems, challenges, or inability to grow or progress. These influences are extremely powerful. Still, the client's capacity for autonomy remains an essential ingredient in the initiation of change. Using Ryan and Deci's (2017) definition of autonomy, the client is the *locus of causality* for change, not the *locus of control*. They do not control all the factors that influence them, but they can weigh the situation and decide to act in a manner that is consistent with their values and their core identity. To get to that choice, we assist clients in seeing and understanding these factors, and then sorting through them to decide.

Finally, Zuckoff (2023) recently added a wrinkle to these ideas. Specifically, he described research that indicates ambivalence has benefits. For example, within complex problems and decision making, ambivalence can slow us down and lead us to better solutions, allow us to consider new information as it comes to light, reduce our impulsivity, and increase our creativity. These ideas are consistent with information that Pink (2022) addresses in considering the value of regret. Because of its balance of positive and negative emotions, ambivalence may lead to better coping in stressful situations when important goals conflict, which, in turn, leads to a more balanced perspective, along with improved judgment and meaning making. It appears these benefits are not equally distributed across people and may accrue more to people who have less need for cognitive consistency. People who can hold opposing viewpoints—dialectical thinkers and paradoxical thinkers—may be able to also hold in mind the idea that two apparently disparate elements can be true and thereby come to a deeper understanding. Zuckoff (2023) argues that our goal then might not just be tipping the balance but instead, for some people, expanding their capacity to sit with ambivalence before finding their way forward perhaps in a manner they had not anticipated. Moreover, that we might need to shift from a directional model (i.e., ***cultivating change talk*** and ***softening sustain talk***) to considering a conflict resolution model (e.g., Arkowitz et al., 2015; Westra, 2012). In contrast to the directional model, this model holds there is a conflict within the individual between opposing elements, and the exploration of these conflicting sides allows them to become less antagonistic to each other. Resolution occurs when the conflict lessens, and the opposing elements become more integrated. Conversely, failing to explore the opposing sides allows the conflict to remain and undermine efforts at change. It seems ambivalence continues to produce nuances worthy of exploration.

The *What*: Tools for Working with Ambivalence

Given these ideas, it makes sense that a process like a decisional balance activity might be an area of debate within the MI field. We know not all factors weigh the same for clients. Moreover, there may be elements that are essential in the weighting process that are either unknown or unclear to either party. A straightforward tallying of costs and benefits would be puzzling in such a situation. As noted earlier, our elicitation of sustain talk is likely to elicit more sustain talk, which is problematic if our aim is to help the client tip the balance. Of course, we will also elicit change talk, which will lead to more change talk. The issue would seem to come when these things are evenly and intentionally balanced, which leaves the client as ambivalent as when the process began. Miller and Rollnick (2023) suggest a decisional balance might be most useful when there is not a clear direction the client has voiced and our aim, as practitioner, is to stay in balance about the goals (e.g., *Should the client adopt a child or donate a kidney to a loved one*) or when the client has already decided to change, and the decisional balance is a way to strengthen that decision.

We take a slightly different view of this situation. We believe there are at least three considerations, whereby a decisional balance might be helpful. To begin, it can be exceptionally helpful to explore sustain talk to understand what is maintaining a behavior, attitude, belief, or perception of self. This process can be done early, when little readiness to change is evident or late as the person approaches commitment to an action and a plan will soon be developed. In either situation, this opens the door to understanding the *Why* of the behavior, and when change is in the person's plans, what will need to be included. This process builds connection, as well as assists with competence in planning effectively. Westra and Norouzian (2018) reinforce the notion that this type of exploration is helpful early in the intervention process, but only if it focuses on sustain talk; this predicts better outcomes. If the process elicits dissent or discord, this predicts worse outcomes, suggesting such is a benefit of exploring and deeper understanding of opposing forces, which is lost when we engage client defenses by our pressing for change.

The second consideration is moving from sustain talk to change talk. An exploration of sustain talk may build engagement and deepen understanding, while reducing defensiveness, and the concern is that if we leave things at this point, we will have strengthened the reasons not to take a vaccine, to sustain problematic drinking, or to continue finding problematic intimate partners. But this is not our plan, though Zuckoff (2023) suggests that we may benefit from sitting in this space longer, and particularly with some clients (e.g., those who find value in exploring opposing ideas). Still, if we have explicitly and systematically worked through a decisional balance with intention and purpose, the next step is to explore the other side of the ambivalence.

When we've explored the sustain talk well and without pressure, the person often turns without prompting to the change side. Early in the change process, the focus is usually on the problems of the current situation. If this does not happen naturally, using gentle prompts to introduce this side helps us. Terms such as "the downsides," "less good things," or "challenges" may be preferred to "problems," unless that is a term introduced by the client.

The third consideration of ***focusing***, to find out what matters to the client, is important here. It is why we would not recommend a decisional balance activity until ***engaging*** has occurred, though it could be that engaging and focusing emerge together. That is, we start to learn what matters for clients as they articulate their concerns about a particular behavior, attitude, belief, or choice. Our aim is to explore these reasons patiently, respectfully, and curiously, including asking for examples and elaboration, where appropriate. This assumes the direction aligns with the client's values and supports their autonomy.

There are a few issues to be mindful of in this process, including the ***fixing reflex***. As always, clients are the ones articulating change talk, though our reflections may help to focus attention. We also need to be particularly wary of introducing information through the "back-door" by asking a leading question (e.g., *Don't you think . . . , Wouldn't it be . . . , Why wouldn't you . . . , Have you ever thought about . . .*). Direct questions about areas where concerns or issues might be present are appropriate (e.g., *How does your family feel about your choice in partners? What have your friends expressed to you about leaving your job?*), as is asking for elaboration as we work to understand these areas of concern. In the context of vertical ambivalence, we will co-explore the unknown region that seems to be pulling the person away from their apparent goal, but we do not assume that we know what it is. The ability of the practitioner to embrace the *tolerance of uncertainty* is a helpful process skill at lots of stages within a therapeutic encounter and particularly helpful in co-exploring vertical ambivalence. We may offer an idea (i.e., *I wonder if anxiety plays any part in this process. What do you think?*), but it will be the client who decides if this idea fits.

The exploration of a decisional balance is not a simple totaling up of pros and cons, but an attempt to deeply understand the individual, comprehend the important factors and contributing elements, notice how some elements are weightier and more influential than others, understand emotional valance, and consider how value-congruent various elements may be for the client. We then use summaries to highlight and juxtapose these elements. We believe this use of the decisional balance is different than what Miller and Rollnick (2022) express concern about and requires a high degree of skill but can be learned with practice and reflection.

The aim is to tip the balance in favor of the client's change. Thinking about our garden metaphor, we might have thoughts and even aspirations for our client's garden, and ultimately, they will be the one responsible for building and tending it. Clients must choose the *What, Where, When*, and *How*. They will also decide if they have someone (i.e., a who) to help and wish to allow this person to help, and how explicit they want to be about the *Why*.

The tools for our part of this work have already been suggested. We will explore with curiosity our clients' reasons for sustaining things as they are, as well as considering a change. Our listening well becomes the essential tool of this process, especially listening for the unexpressed when it seems there might be vertical ambivalence (e.g., client expresses strong desire

BOX 15.1. An Example of Vertical Ambivalence

L. H. J.: I remember working with a woman a few years ago diagnosed with borderline personality disorder and VERY angry. She needed space to explore her anger toward herself for an issue that had happened 25 years previously. In and out of therapy during those years, she had gained significant weight and relied on a wheelchair at the point of entering our Bariatric Service program. The main decisional balance work was about exploring the anger initially, which allowed her to move toward and into acceptance and forgiveness of herself. Once she had done that exploration, the rest of the *behavioral work* was a breeze. By our fourth session, she was in the pool and back to using sticks [crutches]. She went on to make brilliant behavioral changes with the dietitians and physio staff without much input from me.

to change or add a behavior, but never quite seems able to do it, despite the opportunity to do so). We will be intentional and directional in our reflections, attending to ideas that support their stated goals (e.g., being a good parent, getting out of legal trouble, returning to a more active and engaged lifestyle). We will listen for and elicit information about values. We can work through a decisional balance, either formally or informally, to help the client sort through the different elements in a situation and the seeming influence they have on the decision. We will reinforce their capacity for autonomy, to be the locus of causality, even in situations where their control might be quite limited. Finally, our first task might be not to tip the balance but instead assist the client in expanding their capacity to sit with ambivalence and carefully consider two true but opposing ideas before they find their way forward. Box 15.1 illustrates this experience.

The *How*: SP/SR on Exploring Our Ambivalence about Change

Overview of the Exercise

For this activity, we will spend some time thinking about our areas of dilemma. This is one of the issues that we've chosen to focus on in our book, sorting through some of the elements that might be sustaining things as they are, as well as the reasons why we think that change may be important.

Structure of the Exercise

This self-practice exercise can be done as either a self-directed activity or as an interaction with a partner. As this exercise begins, be mindful of some things. If we are stuck, there is the content we already know. Our thoughts and beliefs, our breathing, are all shallower as we perceive this content. These are patterns we know, and it can be difficult to travel beneath the known. We invite hearing one's usual thoughts and beliefs and then pausing, maybe be a bit empty in thoughts or perceptions, to see if anything else arises. Give space for this emptiness in your self-practice.

New impressions might be slow to surface. Psychologist and writer Candace Crosby notes, "Maybe what will be heard is an accent mark in a different place. In my practice I often found great value with clients, and myself, in hanging out in the blank spot. It takes patience to not rush to [a] story line that makes sense, [that] has action steps" (C. Crosby, personal communication, November 21, 2022). Again, sitting with the *not knowing* position and initially tolerating and then becoming comfortable with uncertainty are key features in learning to listen well.

Consistent with these ideas, if working with a partner in a limited practice, be spacious in this work. When acting as the listener, pose the questions written for the exercise and then give your partner time to "sit in that blank space." Don't rush to fill in silence with questions or reflections. Instead, be attuned to your partner and move more slowly than might be typical. Note that this type of deliberate pace can be anxiety-provoking for practitioner and client, so be prepared for that response. Work on developing your comfort with, and sitting with, the uncertainty and in staying in the curious not knowing position. Use deeper reflections and focused summaries to deepen meaning.

If working alone, stay focused on the present question and work through this process sequentially. Practice writing summaries when you're prompted to do so.

Traveling Companion: An Example with Takeshi

Takeshi will help us illustrate this exercise. Recall he is a 24-year-old, cisgender, straight man of Japanese heritage working on his doctorate in clinical psychology. Stress and high expectations have been ongoing issues. He is a strong student and shows promise as a counselor. He feels some frustration about his clients' lack of change at times. He sought out MI training at the suggestion of his supervisor.

> ***Describe a situation where a pattern in your behavior puzzles you. What do you notice yourself doing?***

As I've talked about previously, it is hard for me to be as direct with clients who are older than me, especially men. I find myself acting in a deferential manner that I think undermines my skills and abilities, and likely reduces these clients' confidence in my ability to help them. It's like I am making myself smaller, physically, and psychologically. I never do this with my friends or professors. Or people out in the world—though it can happen out there, too. It's like I notice myself deferring to their thoughts and opinions, even when I have clear concerns about their correctness.

This might just seem like an extension of Japanese cultural traditions of respecting elders, but I can feel the difference. I know the expectations and customs and can operate fine within those without belittling myself. I can be respectful and not diminish myself.

> ***Where do you experience this dilemma in your body? What do you notice about your thoughts and feelings in this situation?***

This feels a bit muddy to me, as these are intermixed. I am aware of anxiety and tension. My shoulders are hunched, while my arms and hands feel tight. I tend to bend at the neck, like the start of a bow. My thoughts are a bit jumbled, too, because they depend on the situation. Is it a first-time meeting or do I already have a relationship with this person? I'm usually focused on them and what the nature of the encounter is about. I just feel on edge.

➤ ***There seem to be some factors that keep you connected to things as they are in this dilemma. Take a moment to sit with those things. Notice the ones you know well and see if anything else floats into your awareness. When you're ready, tell me what you notice—in your body, feelings, and/or thoughts?***

I think there is an edge of anger here. Like my hands want to ball into fists. I notice an underlying woundedness to these people—these men—and they usually cover it. I feel anger on their behalf and maybe, and I hate admitting this, toward them for not doing something about it. My thought then is, "I don't want to wound them more," so I want to prop them up.

I also think there is something about my own weakness and strength. Like . . . I don't want to embrace my strength because it feels tied to anger and that is dangerous.

➤ ***It seems there is a direction you would like to travel toward in this situation. What is that direction, and why does moving toward it make sense?***

This feels straightforward for me. Clients need me to be at my best—using all my skills and abilities. I am not doing that when I am acting deferential. Now that I consider it, this problem is probably even worse than I thought. It's like I'm treating them as though they're fragile and unable to tolerate or do difficult things. Instead of seeing them as capable, I am subtly communicating, "You're incapable." Ugh. I never thought of it that way.

That is NOT the message I want to communicate. I thought I was being respectful by being protective, but I am being disrespectful and patronizing. This way of acting is not MI-consistent at all. It's inconsistent with all the basic therapy skills I've been taught. Wow.

➤ ***As you move toward this direction, describe what happens in your body. What are your feelings? What thoughts slip through your head?***

Right now, I feel gut-punched. Like, how could I be so wrong? How could I have missed what this was doing to the therapy process? I am embarrassed and a bit ashamed of myself. Writing this down forces me to acknowledge it. I feel drained of energy and in shock, "Have I really been doing this?"

Aside from self-castigation, there's also a curiosity about where this came from. This stance is certainly not how I consciously work with clients. In classes, we've repeatedly had it drilled into us, about viewing people as capable and doing strength-based work, and I am convinced that is right. Something is driving this behavior.

I also feel like there is something about this anger, weakness, strength stuff that is important. Like I don't fully understand what's happening here. Like there is this life force in the anger I need to be able to tap into, but feel in control of, if I'm going to help these men.

➤ ***As you sit with these thoughts, feelings, and sensations, what other images drift into your mind?***

My dad just popped into my head. That's weird. Outwardly, he has all the trappings of a confident man. He's a successful dentist. He's well liked in the community and has many friends. I always respected and looked up to him. It's weird that he would come to mind.

As I think about it, there has always been a bit of reserve around my dad. He's there and always willing to listen, offer his thoughts, laugh—but it always feels like there is a part held back. Like he's protecting himself. Now that I think about it, I could feel that, and while I wanted to see all of him, I didn't want to pry. It wasn't like he would reject me, more like I was afraid I could hurt him. Like to be that open he'd be vulnerable, and then I could hurt him.

➤ ***Even if no images appear, let your mind roam to other times you might have these sensations, feelings, or thoughts. When was that, who was there, and what was happening? What thoughts slip into your head?***

Oh, man. This is getting a bit deep. My mom is there. She is a force to be reckoned with. We always joked she owns the throne, but it is the truth. This is not the exercise of hard power. There is never open warfare with my mom. It is subtle presses, a sharp look, a direct word that makes her wishes known, and my dad and me, we're supposed to fall in line. Like my dad might get up on a Saturday and say, "I'd like to drive over to the arboretum. The leaves are beautiful." My mom would just say, "That would be nice, but those gutters need attention." There were no negotiations. The arboretum was forgotten, and the gutters would be done.

It might seem like that's how couples are, but it was always the gutters, never the arboretum. There was never a complaint, but he seemed smaller and a little sadder. And my mom seemed just a little taller and somehow pleased. I guess I noticed it because I started to argue for my dad. He would jump in and tell me not to worry. There would be other days for the arboretum. But there weren't. As I got older, I found myself digging in when my mom would tell me what needed to be done. Not that I was a rebellious kid, but I wasn't going to be bullied into doing things either.

➤ ***What things are you aware of now that you hadn't noticed before? How do they fit into this picture?***

Bullying. I don't recall ever thinking about that word with my mom before. Like I said, she was all soft power, but now that I think about it, that seems true. She subtly bullied my dad, and I felt protective of him. It seemed like he was incapable of standing up for himself, so I didn't want to hurt him. My aim was to protect him. It was an act of love and caring toward him, done by a boy.

➤ ***What is the emotion as you think about these things? Where do they show up in your body?***

I am surprised. It's like this is something I knew but had never given words to before. It's funny because I would expect anger might be the reaction, but it's changed. Like the understanding dissipated the anger and left the power, the energy. I see a combination of love, caring, and concern—and not just to my dad. My mom had her own sets of fears and frustrations. I mean—this is a highly capable person with an advanced degree, stuck managing a dentist's office and raising me. She's always said that she was happy, but I am guessing that she had hopes and dreams that never saw the light of day. She sacrificed her hopes for my dad and me. That's sad. My dad's responsiveness to her requests was probably not just capitulation but love for her and what she sacrificed. It's like the story of the husband who sold his watch to give a gift of a hairbrush for his wife's beautiful hair and the wife who cut and sold her hair to buy a fob for his beloved watch. It's love given freely and, in the end, bittersweet.

I feel these things in my chest and throughout my body, but it's not like I feel drained. It's more like a release of tension and a settling in and more powerful sort of experience, but power over me.

Self-Practice

Now it's your turn.

➤ ***Describe a situation where a pattern in your behavior puzzles you. What do you notice yourself doing?***

➤ ***Where do you experience this dilemma in your body? What do you notice about your thoughts and feelings in this situation?***

➤ ***There seem to be some factors that keep you connected to things as they are in this dilemma. Take a moment to sit with those things. Notice the ones you know well and see if anything else floats into your awareness. When you're ready, tell me what you notice—in your body, feelings, and/or thoughts?***

- *It seems there is a direction you would like to travel toward in this situation. What is that direction, and why does moving toward it make sense?*

- *As you move toward this direction, describe what happens in your body. What are your feelings? What thoughts slip through your head?*

- *As you sit with these thoughts, feelings, and sensations, what other images drift into your mind?*

➤ ***Even if no images appear, let your mind roam to other times you might have these sensations, feelings, or thoughts. When was that, who was there, and what was happening? What thoughts slip into your head?***

➤ ***What things are you aware of now that you hadn't noticed before? How do they fit into this picture?***

➤ ***What is the emotion as you think about these things? Where do they show up in your body?***

Self-Reflection

- *At the beginning of this exercise, we encouraged you to "hang out in the blank space" and to give some time for things to surface. What was that experience like? What did your body feel like? What happened with your thoughts and feelings as you gave space and time?*

- *What did you uncover about yourself as you sat in this process of less story and fewer aims to provide space for discovery?*

- *If you did this exercise with someone, what helped you to feel comfortable with this person's presence in this process? What got in the way? What helped you to work with or embrace the uncertainty of the not knowing position and to hold the curiosity?*

➤ ***Carrying these things forward, what connections do you observe with your current dilemma or other dilemmas?***

What If: Applying Skills to My Current Context

Bridging Questions to Practitioner-Self

These questions are designed to help you bring the insights from personal self-practice into your work with clients.

➤ ***As you think about your work with clients, how have you observed vertical ambivalence influencing clients?***

➤ *If we used this process of less story and fewer aims to provide space for discovery with clients, why might this be a deeper form of listening?*

➤ *What specifically would be helpful to integrate from this experience into your work with clients and why?*

➤ *How and when will you bring that into your work? What might this look like? What would be different and why?*

➤ *What challenges might you experience in this process? How might you prepare ahead for these things?*

➤ *What are your main* takeaway *messages from this SP/SR experience in relation to your understanding of the concept of working with ambivalence . . .*

- *From a practical perspective?*

- *From a theoretical perspective?*

➤ *What if you were to apply this process to other areas of your professional practice (e.g., in a role as supervisor or trainer perhaps)? How might you apply your learning to this new context?*

➤ *How has this exercise influenced your understanding of or personal relationship with MI as a way of being?*

Final Thoughts and Applications to Other Settings

It might be easy to think that ambivalence is just an issue with psychotherapy situations and there are many other circumstances where this might not apply. This might be true, though as we consider the high level of nonadherence to prescribed practices in medical settings, it suggests that we might be cautious in rejecting the idea of ambivalence as nonessential for other settings. Indeed, personal experience has taught us that ambivalence can play parts large and small in situations like using glaucoma eye drops, exercising regularly, maintaining a healthy diet, choosing our weekend activities, caring for a beloved pet, and selecting our coworkers. It might be that some forms of ambivalence are less prevalent in some situations. We might not feel vertical ambivalence about using eye drops for glaucoma, but instead may experience ambivalence about how to structure our bedtime routine to ensure that we apply these drops daily. We remain attentive for the presence of ambivalence and prepared to respond when evident, but do not expect it in every situation or that it must be resolved before we can move forward. Helping clients tip it in the direction of their desired direction is often enough to begin a change process. Helping a client to explore their ambivalence in a neutral way can often help them to better understand their *stuckness* by giving *airtime* to all four quadrants in a decisional balance (i.e., without an agenda of tipping toward change when the change focus is still unclear).

In circumstances where interactions are brief, and there is pressure to move quickly, it is easy to see addressing ambivalence as a luxury we don't have. Indeed, in some situations it is appropriate. An action must be taken now to avoid a serious consequence (e.g., a police officer acting quickly to move a child out of a busy street, a physical therapist moving to support a client about to experience a fall). The issue arises when we view all situations through those lenses or come to believe that we have the correct answers for our clients' dilemmas. When it becomes a matter of expedience for us, then the pendulum has likely swung too far into our directing clients' lives. The danger here is for a trap to emerge (e.g., premature focus, expert, confrontation–denial, labeling, question–answer), and a common consequence to a process trap in MI is discord or a therapeutic rupture.

This stance, believing we know what is best, may also be a challenge for supervisors who want their supervisees to grow in particular ways. We can tell people this is important, and until they endorse that it is, the behavior will be an externally reinforced one that may not be sustained when that reinforcer is removed. This is where appropriate scaffolding within a supervisee's zone of proximal development and with a strong supervisor alliance is crucial to help the person explore what they don't yet know that they do not know (e.g., Johnston & Milne, 2012). The use of recordings in conjunction with a process of SP/SR can significantly aid this self-discovery process.

Some ideas from this module extend well beyond the scope of this text but are worth mentioning. For example, what are the implications of these ideas for working with those who struggle with holding opposing ideas, such as borderline personality/emotionally unstable personality characteristics? It seems dialectical behavior therapy and MI might be compatible cousins in this work. Kaufman et al. (2021) offer ideas about areas of convergence, divergence, and integration.

It raises these questions: In sitting with ambivalence longer are we building our ability to tolerate or embrace uncertainty, not just the client's? What are the implications of a deeper capacity for us to hold uncertainty? Moreover, the concept of intolerance of uncertainty (IOU) is linked to so many anxiety conditions. Perhaps this is why those individuals with a trauma background struggle to sit with IOU and may either take more time with decision making or act impulsively? For example, many of those with an emotionally unstable personality disorder diagnosis struggle with impulsivity.

How does a conflict resolution model help here? Maybe it is by understanding the importance of resolving the conflicts within the client before they can move forward. Or perhaps it is helping us as practitioners sit with our uncertainty of exploring all four quadrants of the decisional balance in detail, rather than prematurely focusing on elicitation of change talk at the expense of looking at sustain talk. Perhaps a premature focus on eliciting change talk and softening sustain talk is where the therapeutic art of MI is replaced by a *paint-by-numbers* approach to language use. We move into ***chasing change talk***.

These ideas create a strong argument for giving clients enough time and space to fully explore ambivalence without going in with the *tip-the-balance* agenda. Perhaps we need to think beyond using decisional balance at a behavioral level to work at a belief or attitudinal level. For some, perhaps many, clients, it seems this may take them further down the vertical ambivalence pole and allow them to work at a schema or core belief level. This is where *cognitive-behavioral therapy*, *schema therapy*, and MI can interact in more meaningful ways.

Finally, our clinical experience suggests that, at least at times, there may be a link between the length of time the person has been stuck and how long they may need to work through a decisional balance to become "unstuck." While psychodynamic writers are likely to have an opinion on this matter, we are unaware of any research evidence to support its accuracy. It does remind us to be patient and move at the speed of the client.

MODULE 16

Sharing Information

The aim of this module is to think more deeply about how we *share information* with clients in a helpful way. We hope this chapter will help you unpack the process of information-sharing and better understand the danger of when this can be a *fixing response* and unhelpful versus when it may help further scaffold the person in their own understanding about their change processes. By the end of this module, it is our hope that you will have a clearer and deeper understanding of when and how sharing information with clients is helpful in MI and why.

The *Why*: Sharing Information Is Often Essential to Our Work

If we are master gardeners—or tour guides—this means we have knowledge and skills that are potentially helpful to our clients. Yet, we focus our attention on supporting their ***autonomy*** and in the process downplay the value of our offerings. This does not mean we should ignore our experience and expertise in favor of the client following their own, sometimes ill-advised, choices. However, it is not us who will make the decision; the client will. Our aim, then, is to use our expertise skillfully, wisely, and in a helpful manner, so clients can make well-informed decisions.

Let us begin with a straightforward idea you have heard many times before—context matters. The nature, timing, and volume of the information, and crucially, the client's interest in receiving it all matter. Moreover, it is not just what we say, but *How* we say it that makes a difference. Rather than looking for specific rules, we instead offer guidelines that will be influenced by the situation in which we are working.

The overarching principle is simple—the goal of information-sharing is to assist in the process of change, not to deliver advice. Now that might seem obvious and still, at times, we feel pulled by the ***fixing reflex*** to deliver advice. It often begins with a thought like *I can't let them think . . . smoking is safe, six beers are low risk, flossing is unnecessary,* for example. It does not mean we cannot offer this information; the question is how do we deliver it in a manner the client can hear, understand, and use?

This is a point where MI differs from person-centered approaches. While person-centered approaches tend to follow clients wherever they lead, MI is more *directional*. MI practitioners directly address areas of concern, while respecting the client's autonomy and being mindful of what increases and decreases the likelihood of change for the client.

The *What*: Tools for Sharing Information Effectively

The supporting concepts for sharing information are straightforward and have been articulated elsewhere (e.g., Rosengren, 2017). To begin, this is information-sharing, not information provision alone. That is, this should be a conversation where we learn information from the client, too. It is not a surprise then that we start with a question instead of sharing information. These can take the form of either ***asking permission*** or ***asking what they already know*** about a subject area. Then listen, reflect, and summarize. Note that this does not mean sitting quietly and forming counterarguments in our head as the person tells us their thoughts. When we ***offer information***, make it short and digestible—think appetizer rather than a seven-course meal. Then ***ask for their perspective*** on the information. We refer to this strategy as ***ask–offer–ask (AOA)***; previously, this strategy was called ***elicit–provide–elicit***. As we do throughout an MI-consistent conversation, it is important to maintain our genuine curiosity and listen to understand, not to respond. Finally, recognize this is often a pattern done repeatedly as part of an information-sharing *process*. That is, the pattern is *ask, offer, ask, offer, ask, offer,* and so forth, with lots of reflective listening, summarizing, and affirming interspersed between these elements.

Here are a few other ideas that can help information-sharing to be more welcome. Be hesitant to share information. Remember the client is far more convinced by their thoughts and self-talk than they are by ours. Our listening well provides that forum and might reduce or eliminate our need to share. If you are sharing solutions, set these in the context of other clients. People respond better to models that are like themselves. Offer several options together, not just one at a time. Remind ourselves, and perhaps the client, too, there are multiple paths to success, with the most important being the one the client is willing to undertake. If we have a concern, state it directly rather than trying to sneak in through the "back door" disguised as a question (see Box 16.1). Instead of asking, *Wouldn't it be easier if you did one thing at a time?*, we might instead offer, *I am concerned by your decision to do multiple things at once. Would it be okay if I shared why?*

Here is an example of information-sharing that pulls together several of these ideas:

> *"I am a bit worried about your decision to keep using THC [psychoactive ingredient in cannabis that people use for recreational purposes]. Would you be interested in hearing why? THC feels safe as it has not been the challenge that alcohol has been for you. You've also said THC use often puts you in situations where alcohol is available, and people are using alcohol in high-risk ways. You've noticed feeling tempted to drink in those situations, and you've been clear that is something you don't want to do. Stopping drinking is a priority because you have other plans for your life. It is, of course, your call, not mine. What do you think?"*

The example begins with asking permission before stating what the worry is about. There are a couple of other ideas embedded in this example. Namely, offering information in the

BOX 16.1. Information-Sharing Tips

- Information-*sharing*, not *provision*.
- It's a conversation.
- Ask permission.
- Ask what the client already knows.
- Keep it short and digestible.
- Ask their perspective.
- Be curious.
- Listen to understand, not respond.
- Clients are more convinced by their thoughts.
- Use success models like the client.
- Offer a menu of options.
- There *are* multiple paths to success.
- State concerns directly.
- The client draws the conclusion.

context of important goals and values helps clients see connections with what matters most to them. It also supports clients' autonomy in choosing *their* path. Finally, and this can be hard, it avoids investment in our solutions. *We invest in the client, not the solution.* We are therefore prepared to have the client reject all our information and accept that decision with composure and compassion.

Our tools for information-sharing then flow from these principles. To summarize, we use an ask–offer–ask pattern to share information. Curiosity and listening well are intentional and continuous throughout. We support autonomy by asking permission, asking what clients already know, and actively noting the decision is theirs. We use a menu to offer ideas about solutions and ask the client what they think about these. Finally, we keep in mind that *less is more.*

The *How*: SP/SR on Reviewing the Status of Our Change and Receiving Information

Overview of the Exercise

For this activity, a practice partner is recommended, though we will offer an option for self-directed learners. We will explore our dilemmas with attention toward identifying information that might be helpful in moving closer to a decision, solution, or plan. Our partner will use the questions below to guide that process. This conversation branches: That is, there are two different conversations based on our readiness to change. Work through the chosen branch. Partners are encouraged to offer information, using the principles and tools discussed, as opportunities arise. The sequence provides opportunities where information-sharing could be appropriate. If unsure how to do AOA effectively, we recommend looking at examples in Rosengren (2017, Chapter 8) or the companion website.

Structure of the Exercise

As noted, there is a branch in this process after the initial questions, based on your readiness to change. Choose the sequence that fits best at this moment. In Sam's example below, she was not quite ready to make a change and the information-sharing was in that sequence. We removed the alternative branch questions to avoid confusion.

The structure of the self-practice questions is different than in other modules. This self-practice exercise is a dialogue either within yourself or with your limited-practice partner. We labeled the practitioner parts ***PR*** to make that clear. If you are doing this as a self-dialogue, please write those parts as you would state them to a client you're working with. However, in general, we would recommend doing this self-practice with your limited-practice partner. If doing this session in a limited partner practice, the partner should use these prompts as opportunities for information-sharing. However, it is not a rigid script. Allow the interaction to unfold and use reflections and additional information-sharing as the exploration dictates. The questions will provide a general roadmap but modify the questions as needed so they fit the discussion that is unfolding and intersperse them with reflections and affirmations.

If this exercise is done in a self-directed manner, the opportunities to be well listened to and offered information by another will be missed. However, the structure of the exercise will ask you to move into the practitioner role. Offer reflective listening statements and summaries as you would for a client. Also suggest alternatives or information, as you might for a client. This sort of self-distancing process has been found to be helpful in reasoning through personal problems (e.g., Kross & Ayduk, 2017; Pink, 2022). Pause and write in this practitioner mindset. Switching chairs to reflect the different roles—client and practitioner—is something Gestalt therapists recommend, and some people find helpful. When you're the practitioner, try to channel your favorite nonjudgmental mentor, therapist, or listener. The important point is to talk to yourself as you might a client, with compassion and perspective.

When working as the practitioner, we encourage asking questions such as the following before offering any information:

- Would it be okay if I shared a few thoughts?
- I am a little concerned about this direction; would you be interested in hearing why?
- I think there is something important here we might want to consider. Would you be open to hearing about what that is?
- I am curious what you already know about ____________. What have you heard, read, or done in this area before?
- What do you know about ____________?
- How do you feel about ____________?
- I am guessing you have already given this a lot of thought. What are your thoughts about ____________?
- What do you know about what works for you?

There will be a lot of listening and summarizing before offering information. Keep information brief, focused, and in menu form when offering options. Then elicit more of your practice partner's feelings and thoughts about what has been shared. The questions listed will serve as guideposts when we are practitioners.

The nature of this self-practice activity is that there are lots of opportunities to reflect on your work as a practitioner, too. We encourage you when in that role to ask yourself some questions:

- How might I ask permission or query what is already known about the information I'm considering sharing?
- How might I share information I feel is useful at this point?
- How might I check how relevant the information I shared was? What could I ask?

Traveling Companion: An Example with Sam

Sam is a White, cisgender, gay woman of European descent who has been a successful counselor for many years. Fifteen years ago, she injured her back and because of that experience has shifted her private practice to health-focused care. She became interested in MI as part of the learning she did post-injury, engaged in a variety of training and learning, and has recently been considering ways to advance her expertise. She had a cancer scare last year, and her wife is encouraging her to retire. Sam is ambivalent about making that change, and this has become a point of contention between them.

➤ ***Describe where you are now regarding the problem area you are working on as part of this* MI from the inside out *process. Where do you stand on making a decision?***

I'm stuck. I haven't really moved in this process. I've been focused on this book and my work tasks, and haven't yet set up an appointment to see my own therapist. I guess I feel mildly resistant to that, as I feel like it's a step toward making a change I don't necessarily want.

➤ ***What makes it important to do something about this issue?***

That's obvious. It matters a great deal to Debra, and she matters to me. I also had this cancer thing, and it does have me thinking about the future, but I feel like Debra and I look at that differently.

Undecided

Pause and give yourself some information as you would a client in the space below. If working with a limited-practice partner, offer information based on what you've learned about this person over time, not just today.

➤ ***I have some thoughts about your situation. Would you be interested in hearing them?***

It seems clear a change is important to you, and you haven't figured out what the change is you want. Right now, it feels like you and Debra are taking the two sides of the argument instead of you sorting through it. You let her argue for retirement and then—like we talk about in MI - you don't have to deal with the ambivalence. What do you think?

➤ ***Write your response to this information.***

I think you're right. I've been avoiding digging in too deep. I can keep everything at arm's distance and keep my happy life just as it is, even though I know that can't work.

➤ ***Offer a reflective listening statement to yourself (or your partner).***

There is something going on under the surface that you're not sure you want to deal with and yet part of you knows you must.

➤ ***Write a response to your reflective listening statement (or your partner's).***

Truthfully? I think it's facing the cancer head-on and deciding how I want to spend my remaining time, however long that is. I feel so torn there. I am not sure how to proceed.

➤ ***Offer a summary and an observation about what might be keeping yourself (or your partner) stuck.***

You like your life now and don't feel a great need to change it. You're not feeling a great wanderlust. Or like you can't wait to sleep in and wake up when you feel like it. You wake up with purpose and feel like your life has meaning. You are helpful to others and that's rewarding. Your work provides purpose, meaning, and identity. You also dodged a bullet around the cancer, and this is an opportunity to think about the road ahead. I wonder if the focus on work's rewards has you thinking in black-and-white terms—either you are or aren't working. What do you think?

➤ ***Offer a response to this summary and observation.***

These elements—meaning, purpose—are core for me. They are core values. My thinking has been a bit rigid—thinking it has to be one or the other. I've looked at the research about who's happiest in retirement and it's not people who just stop working. It's people who have a plan and sometimes work is part of that plan. Maybe there is another way.

Our life is busy and full, and I love that. I love Debra and her relationship is a core thing for me, too. In fact, it's the most important and so if I had to choose, I would choose her; Debra also doesn't put me in that spot. That's part of why I love her. But I also know Debra feels tension about wanting to travel more, and my job is getting in the way. She also has plans around the house and loves to putter around. I support her in those things and that's her happy spot, not mine.

➤ ***Offer a reflective listening statement or summary.***

These are important values and will need to be built into whatever you do, but Debra is the thing that trumps all. It seems like you might have a little daylight showing here.

➤ ***Provide a response to this reflective listening statement or summary.***

It does feel like a little sunshine is coming in. I feel lighter.

➤ ***What have you thought about doing, or even tried, to help you move forward?***

Well, there is seeing a therapist. The problem is I know everyone I feel good about seeing in the area. I've tried writing up a pros and cons list and that didn't really move the needle. I've talked with Debra, and we just end up taking sides. I've gone for long walks to think about it, but I find my attention just drifting away. I tried ignoring it and that didn't work either.

➤ ***Offer a reflective listening statement and then orient the client to the value of looking at past change. Then ask how they've faced tough changes in the past.***

You've done and thought quite a lot already. I wonder if thinking about how past changes might be helpful. When you have faced other tough changes in your life and been able to make them, how did you accomplish them?

➤ ***Provide a response to this question.***

That is a good question. There have certainly been times when I felt ambivalent and really stuck. Should I stay in my job or risk going out into private practice? In those situations, I could often drill down and identify the thing that I wanted most. It usually wasn't the thing itself, but something underneath the thing.

➤ ***Offer a reflective listening statement and ask a question to prompt continued thought.***

You had to go deeper, something you haven't wanted to do before, but you've been doing now. What has become clearer as you thought this through?

➤ ***Provide a response to the reflective listening statement and/or question.***

How much I have stayed on the surface now and how that has kept me going. I thought I was going deeper, but I wasn't. Finding what it means—"the nugget"—is essential for moving forward, and that requires me to think in a different sort of way. This feels like there is some possibility of movement attached to it and I feel silly for forgetting I know this, but I do.

Self-Practice

Now it's your turn.

➤ ***Describe where you are now regarding the problem area you are working on as part of this*** **MI from the inside out** ***process. Where do you stand on making a decision?***

____

____

____

____

____

➤ ***What makes it important to do something about this issue?***

If you have decided, go to the section marked *Decided.* If you have not decided yet, then go to the section below marked *Undecided.*

Undecided

Begin this part with information-sharing. If self-directed, pause and give yourself some information as you would to a client in the space below. If working with a limited-practice partner, offer information based on what you've learned about this person over time, not just today. Remember to keep the information neutral, brief, and in menu form using MI spirit.

PR: I have some thoughts about your situation. Would you be interested in hearing them? (Pause for response.) Offer the information.

CL: Provide your response to this information.

PR: Offer a reflective listening statement to yourself (or your partner).

CL: Provide a response to this reflective listening statement.

PR: Offer a summary and an observation about what might be keeping yourself (or your partner) stuck.

CL: Provide a response to this summary and observation.

PR: Offer a reflective listening statement or summary.

CL: Provide a response to this reflective listening statement or summary.

PR: What have you thought about doing, or even tried, to help you move forward?

CL: Provide a response to this question.

PR: Offer a reflective listening statement and then orient the client to the value of looking at past change. Then ask how they've faced tough changes in the past.

CL: Provide a response to the reflective listening statement, information, and/or question.

PR: Offer a reflective listening statement and ask a question to prompt continued thought.

CL: Provide a response to the reflective listening statement and/or question.

Decided

If you have decided, answer the following questions:

PR: What was helpful in tipping the balance?

CL: Provide a response.

PR: What have you thought about doing?

CL: Provide a response.

Pause and give yourself some information as you would a client in the space below. If working with a limited-practice partner, offer information based on what you've learned about this person over time, not just today. Remember to keep the information neutral, brief, and in menu form using MI spirit.

PR: I have some thoughts about your situation. Would you be interested in hearing them? (*Pause.*) Offer the information.

CL: Provide your response to this information.

PR: Offer a reflective listening statement to yourself (or your partner).

CL: Provide a response to your reflective listening statement (or your partner's).

PR: What do you think might be barriers?

CL: Provide a response.

PR: What will help you overcome these?

CL: Provide a response.

PR: Offer yourself some information as you would to a client. Provide your lead-in statement as well as additional thoughts.

CL: Provide a response to these suggestions.

PR: Offer a reflective listening statement or summary.

CL: Provide a response to this reflective listening statement or summary.

The rest of the modules will assist with solidifying commitment and formulating a plan or setting the clock if you're not quite ready.

Self-Reflection

If you did this task in a self-directed manner, the questions might be a bit more difficult to answer. We encourage you, regardless of how you did this exercise, to answer these questions focusing on your *experience as the client in this self-practice.*

➤ ***As a client in this practice experience, what do you notice about how your body responded? What feelings did you experience? What thoughts?***

➤ ***When your listener offered information, how did you react internally? Where did you feel it in your body? What was the sensation? What were the accompanying feelings and thoughts?***

➤ ***How did the way the listener shared information influence your reactions? Did the listener's way of doing this make a difference for you? Why? What was it specifically about their interpersonal style that was helpful and why?***

➤ *Was the listener able to communicate investment in you as a person and not in the outcome? How did their sharing of information fit in with your answer and why? What difference did this make in your experience of the exercise?*

➤ *What was the most helpful information your listener shared (or you shared with yourself)? What made it helpful and why?*

➤ *What did you notice about the relationship between information-sharing and further self-exploration? How did this impact on your decision making as a process and why?*

➤ ***Was it helpful or simply covering familiar ground? Why? Was there anything different about it?***

What If: Applying Skills to My Current Context

Bridging Questions to Practitioner-Self

These questions help bring the insights from your personal self-practice into your work as a practitioner with clients.

➤ ***In a word, image, or brief sentence, what is your*** main ***learning from this exercise from a practitioner perspective?***

➤ ***What are you realizing now about yourself as a practitioner in terms of how you share information with clients? Why is this important? What are the implications?***

➤ ***Can you see where you have been invested in the outcome instead of a client in your work and why? Describe what happened and the outcome.***

- ***How do you know when this investment in outcome is happening? What do you experience in your body and why? What is your early warning sign?***

- ***How can you make yourself aware of this when it is happening? How might you shift out of it? What can you do differently in a future situation to avoid a premature focus on an outcome and to shift the balance back to the client?***

- ***What is some information you need to share with a client in an upcoming session, where you can practice shifting this balance? How will you change your approach to sharing this information with your client? How will you evaluate if this approach has been successful?***

- ***Imagine you are trying out your new way of sharing information with a particular client. What might act as a barrier in that moment?***

➤ ***Here is a space for your personal questions as a practitioner in relation to sharing information with clients or colleagues, if you would like to write them down.***

____

____

____

____

____

➤ ***What are your main*** takeaway ***messages from this SP/SR experience in relation to your understanding of the concept of sharing information . . .***

- ***From a practical perspective?***

  ____

  ____

  ____

- ***From a theoretical perspective?***

  ____

  ____

  ____

➤ ***What if you were to apply this process to other areas of your professional practice (e.g., in a role as supervisor or trainer perhaps)? How might you apply your learning to this new context?***

____

____

____

➤ ***How has this exercise influenced your understanding of or personal relationship with MI as a way of being?***

____

____

____

Final Thoughts and Applications to Other Settings

Sharing information is a core function of many roles where MI might be used. For example, a sports coach will obviously have ideas about how a player might navigate a game, match, or race environment. However, opportunities to talk through options with lengthy conversations are limited by the game's constraints. It might be that these ideas are best suited for practice situations, or outside of the practice/training environment. Although even in the game, asking what a player thinks might be fruitful, if time will permit.

Physicians, nurse practitioners, health psychologists, dietitians, cardiologists, surgeons, and the like will also encounter many situations where they possess information for clients to consider. But as we have noted, even in situations where clients are motivated and the change seems straightforward, engaging in conversation seems to be the faster route to change overall as it avoids the nonadherence and repetitive conversations replete in these situations.

Asking permission can be a useful tool if done sparingly and can feel like a gimmicky contrivance if done too often. Also, if we notice that we are introducing the AOA strategy regularly into conversations with clients, it may be an indication that we are simply satisfying our *fixing reflexes*, and this is worth paying attention to. Clearly, in some roles, information-sharing is part of the job and will be done often. A simple reminder would be to ask yourself why does the client need to know this, and might they already know it? A discharge nurse might ask, *What do you know about wound care? You probably want to shower; what do you know about how to do that safely for your wound? What has your doctor told you about your meds?* This would prevent a long recitation of facts a client already knows and permits focusing on areas of information they haven't yet solidified.

As with all things, context also matters in information-sharing. As experienced providers, we are all aware that someone who has just experienced a trauma or come out of surgery is going to have difficulty processing information. A person with high anxiety who is currently agitated or an individual in the throes of a deep depression will also struggle to process complex messages. A senior patient with some cognitive decline will need information presented differently than a senior without those same challenges. Differing cultural contexts will add additional layers of complexity. In sharing across these different areas, we encourage using information that fits the situation and the person, with language that is accessible to the person and that they can easily digest and use. As a reminder to us all, the goal is not to deliver the information, but to encourage thought and change the client endorses.

Finally, think of permission, once granted, as having an expiration time. That is, it is good for a certain period—the exact length we do not know—and we can safely operate within that time without repeatedly renewing it. However, permission is not endless, and it does not extend across either sessions or topic areas. Please do renew it. This can be quite straightforward, *I have a few more thoughts about that. Is it okay if I share them?* Or my all-time favorite shift in permission request was from Dr. Terri Moyers to a colleague after a teaching event, "I don't have any feedback about your teaching, but I do have some about your driving, if you're interested."

MODULE 17

Evolving Focus

Module Purpose

This module explores the experience of the evolution of reasons for change and growth. It is not uncommon that our reasons for starting a journey of change may differ from those that help us to maintain those changes. For practitioners, we may conceptualize this as an ***evolving focus***. By the end of this module, it is our hope that, through reflection on your own experience, you have an enhanced awareness of the evolution of reasons for change, why this is important, and how we might actively explore this during the course of our client's change journey.

The *Why*: The Starting Reason Is Often Not the Ending Reason

It is often true that the reasons we begin a change process are ultimately not the final aim we pursue. A moment's thought provides evidence of why that might be so. We often don't know the full scope of something until we are amid it. We might begin with a goal of losing weight and discover that running brings us great joy and decide to set a goal of running a race—irrespective of weight loss. Or we might set a goal of running to control our weight and discover our knees can no longer tolerate the pounding and shift our aims to non-weight-bearing activities. Or we might go to treatment to satisfy someone else and in the process discover there are things of value for us in this process. For practitioners, this means we recognize where the person starts is just that—a place to begin and we meet them there.

Not surprisingly, we often say meet clients where they are. MINT trainer Stephen Andrew suggests a refinement, *Meet people where they dream*. Andrews asserts that where people are is often neither a nice nor a motivating place. It can be a place devoid of hope for their lives ever being better. By meeting them where they dream—in essence, their aspirations for their own lives—new possibilities open. So, when the angry adolescent says through words or, more often, actions, *I don't want to be here, you can't help me, and I'm just doing this to get ____________ off my back*, we accept this statement. It is where they live presently, and what a difficult, unhappy place that is without autonomy, connection, or competence in at least a few areas. The question we're asking together is *Where would you rather be?* The answer is straightforward, *Anywhere, but here!* To find where people dream, we work together to unfold where *anywhere* is until it becomes *somewhere good for me.*

Finally, it is useful to note that when people have clear goals, these are often *outcome goals*: *I know where I want to get to.* What is often missing are *process goals.* That is, goals for the process of achieving my outcome goals: *I know the methods and steps to get to my ultimate goals.* People often do not have a clear sense of the causal and maintaining processes in their situation, which is why formulation and the ***focusing*** task become such an important endeavor once ***engaging*** has occurred.

The *What*: Tools for An Evolving Focus

There is a danger here—the belief that we know the *true* reason for clients' troubles and the *true* place that would be good for them. The ***fixing reflex*** lurks for us. After all, we can see that a relationship is problematic and our client needs to leave it, or THC is getting in the way of their pursuit of the things that would make them truly happy, or losing 40 pounds would help their heart, energy level, and depression. As we noted in Module 16, it is not a problem for us to have thoughts and concerns; it is how we prioritize and discuss these with our clients that matter. A premature focus on ***ask–offer–ask*** can negatively impact on the relationship if done too frequently, too early, and with a pedantic interpersonal style. It may require that we move back to engaging if this happens.

This brings us back to the concept of ***spaciousness***. In this case, it's about giving clients room to consider new possibilities, identities, and courses of action. To offer ideas, but not to insist on them. A master gardener might suggest what is possible to a gardener, but the gardener decides if this fits the garden they envision. Or a guide might know areas in a city the traveler has neither known nor considered, but the traveler decides if this is of interest and if it feels safe to go there. As either master gardener or guide, we give space to people to consider these possibilities and more to our purpose here, to change their mind once experience gives them additional information to consider.

Of course, MI is not all we do. Again, Miller and Rollnick (2023) describe MI as something we add to the other things we do. For example, we might draw from CBT some behavioral experiments to assist clients in exploring either alternative cognitions or behaviors. Or do a functional behavioral analysis to gain greater insight into how antecedents, behaviors, and consequences are fitting together. Or we might look to understand core conflictual relationship themes that keep appearing, how family systems are acting to keep a system in balance, or how our personal narrative is influencing our understanding of possibilities and capacity. Work in all these domains opens possibilities for new understanding, new foci for our work, and aims for the client's change process. MI can assist in these explorations but does not replace it.

Our tools for working with an evolving focus are straightforward. We begin with *listening with curiosity* and interest and not insistence that we maintain a *direction of travel.* We remain alert to a shift in focus and remark on it; at the same time, we assist clients in *narrowing their focus* enough to use the time effectively, *It feels like we're bouncing around a bit. I'm wondering if things might be changing about what feels most important.* We can return to our simple instruments for agenda mapping. For example, returning to a sheet of labeled circles, with some left empty, or a page of concentric circles, with the most important elements lying at the middle and lower priorities as the circles move outward, can help people articulate a shifting focus. We can also make space by setting aside time to reflect on the progress to date and asking people to consider where they are now in the process and where they would like to go. Related to this, we can create forms to track goals and progress, if that is helpful. There is research that *self-monitoring* assists people in behavior change efforts (e.g., Butryn et al., 2020). Finally, continue to encourage clients to recognize that less is more in terms of our focus. That is, when climbing a rugged peak, it is helpful to focus on the next stretch and what is happening in the present process, rather than continually focusing on how far it is to the summit. Helping clients *focus on smaller, achievable, and positively phrased aims*, as always, aids in their feeling success, even as we know this is not the whole journey. We'll discuss more about goal setting in Module 22.

The *How*: SP/SR on Our Evolving Focus in This Workbook

Overview of the Exercise

For this activity, you will find a limited-practice partner helpful, but not essential. We will explore your progress through the first two-thirds of these modules and help you to assess how your focus has begun to evolve as you've dug into this process.

Structure of the Exercise

This self-practice exercise can be done as either a self-directed activity or as an interaction with a partner. If working with a partner in a limited practice, when acting as the listener, focus on creating spaciousness and using reflective listening and summaries to highlight the talker's work. Use the questions to prompt exploration about how the work has changed, or not.

If working alone, stay focused on the present question and work through this process sequentially. Provide spaciousness for your responses. The goal is not to move through the questions quickly but to let yourself look more deeply at the process that has unfolded for you.

Traveling Companion: An Example with Quincy

Once again, Quincy is a 38-year-old, cisgender, straight woman of African descent who works as an AOD counselor. From a vibrant community, she has strong family ties. She was feeling some burnout with AOD clients and has sought out personal support with an MI therapist.

➤ ***What led you to select this book originally and begin to work through it?***

It was a recommendation by my therapist. I told her I was interested in learning more about MI. She suggested I try this as a complement to our work together. I really didn't know much about it, and I was a little skeptical. Okay, a lot skeptical. I'd never heard of "inside out" or "self-practice and self-reflection" and thought it sounded kind of gimmicky. But my therapist didn't make me. She suggested it, and then I did a little research and signed up. I guess I had enough faith in her to give it a shot.

➤ ***What was your initial problem focus? How was this related to your reason for selecting this book?***

My initial focus was on feeling burned out with my clients. I felt annoyed by their "lying," and I wanted some tools to help motivate them, so I'd feel more encouraged and less frustrated.

I guess my original goal was to satisfy my therapist and learn about MI, so they were kind of consistent. But I thought just by seeing her work I would learn and so I kind of thought this would all happen at an arm's distance. Like I wasn't going to get into my stuff, my junk. I guess it's a bit like going into therapy to get marital tips on how to handle your spouse's behavior and discovering there was crap you had to address.

➤ ***What has happened with that initial focus? As you consider this, what thoughts and feelings do you have? Where do you experience these feelings in your body?***

I'm kind of laughing now. I think that "marital tips" analogy is right on. I came in not to work on myself, but learn MI, and discovered that this process is exactly the opposite. By working on my stuff, I can get better at the therapy stuff. This "inside out" stuff works. I love and hate those self-reflection questions.

The first thought I have is that is sort of embarrassing, like I should have known better. But I think, screw it. I feel better and feel more hopeful and capable, so it's been good. I feel this in my chest and shoulders. I laugh and breathe now. There isn't this weight on my shoulders. I also feel it on my face. I smile more now. I feel less burned out. I think that's the best way to describe what's happened, and it's not because my clients changed, but because I did.

➤ ***In what ways has that initial focus evolved? If it helps, you might review your answers to questions in the book, with particular attention to Module 6: Envisioning, Module 8: Seeing the Big Picture, Module 10: Opening Possibility, and Module 16: Sharing Information.***

Well, this is pretty easy to see in retrospect. I am aware that my thoughts and attitudes have changed, and those have been the focus of my personal work. I can also see where my values and my narrative were causing me to both stick with what I was doing and at times feel frustrated with the process. It had become a very external focus in my work, and now I recognize that my growth needs to be internal and then my skills build on it.

➤ ***Were there small shifts, big evolutions, or something in between as you worked in these areas?***

Big evolutions—I mean I went from "complaining about my spouse" in that marital tips analogy to "I've seen the problem, and it is me." That's as big as it gets.

➤ ***What of your MI work? What shifts or changes have you observed?***

I think I always had the capacity to be a good listener and observer, but that had gotten tucked into my therapeutic purse. Instead, I was a pro confronter, advice giver. I was a baller and sure I had the answers. I also changed my view on clients—they're not liars, they're just doing the best they can. I guess I became less judgy. If I think about what has changed, I'm not just waiting my turn when listening, but instead really listening in a nonjudgmental way. This means I am hearing more and better information from my clients. It just feels like we're making more progress. It's not perfect, but it is better.

➤ ***How has this impacted your clinical work?***

Well, I am much more optimistic and hopeful for my clients, and I think that makes them more hopeful. I smile more and am glad to see people instead of dreading seeing folks. Like that person I described previously, she's hanging in there. It sure hasn't been a straight line, but I look forward to seeing her and I know she feels better about seeing me. I'm rooting for her now, instead of betting against her.

Self-Practice

Now it's your turn.

➤ ***What led you to select this book originally and begin to work through it?***

➤ ***What was your initial problem focus? How was this related to your reason for selecting this book?***

➤ ***What has happened with that initial focus? As you consider this, what thoughts and feelings do you have? Where do you experience these feelings in your body?***

➤ *In what ways has that initial focus evolved? If it helps, you might review your answers to questions in the book, with particular attention to Module 6: Envisioning, Module 8: Seeing the Big Picture, Module 10: Opening Possibility, and Module 16: Sharing Information.*

➤ *Were there small shifts, big evolutions, or something in between as you worked in these areas?*

Self-Reflection

➤ *How did it feel as you looked back over the course of your work in this book? What was your energy like? Where did you feel this? What did you notice and why?*

➤ *This practice experience asked you to think about your own evolving focus in this book. What seemed important in this process for you? What experiences, feelings, or thoughts mattered? How and why did they matter?*

____

____

____

____

____

____

____

____

➤ *In addition to a specific change or growth area identified in this book, there is also an emphasis on our ability to deepen our capacity for self-reflection. What shifts or changes have you observed in how you self-reflect either* after *or* in action *going through this inside out process?*

____

____

____

____

____

____

____

____

➤ *Spaciousness was again a focus in this module. What do you like or dislike about that space? Is it helpful, or does it get in the way of your focus in self-practice?*

____

____

____

____

____

____

____

____

What If: Applying Skills to My Current Context

Bridging Questions to Practitioner-Self

These questions are designed to help you bring the insights from personal self-practice into your work with clients.

- ***What of your MI work? What shifts or changes have you observed?***

- ***How has this impacted your work with clients?***

- ***Where did you put your focus for MI improvement initially? What about now?***

➤ ***As you look forward, in what specific areas do you feel that you need to continue to work and improve your MI practice? Why?***

____

____

____

____

____

➤ ***How will you know if you improve in these areas? Where will you experience it in your body? Your feelings? Your thoughts?***

____

____

____

____

____

____

____

____

➤ ***What's a situation with a client where their focus has evolved?***

____

____

____

____

____

____

____

____

____

____

- ***Might it be useful to them to review how this evolution has unfolded? How would you do that and evaluate if it has been successful?***

- ***What are your main*** takeaway ***messages from this SP/SR experience in relation to your understanding of the concept of evolving focus . . .***
  - ***From a practical perspective?***
  - ***From a theoretical perspective?***

- ***What if you were to apply this process to other areas of your professional practice (e.g., in a role as supervisor or trainer perhaps)? How might you apply your learning to this new context?***

- ***How has this exercise influenced your understanding of or personal relationship with MI as a way of being?***

Final Thoughts and Applications to Other Settings

Let us state the obvious. An evolving focus is dependent on our having an ongoing relationship with a client. While the focus might evolve over the course of a single-session encounter, it is more likely that in such a circumstance it is a process of winnowing to what is most important at that moment. Of course, we would expect that in first encounters clients will have trouble telling us everything or explaining what the links are between *causal* and *co-maintaining* factors in their initial presentation. As the encounter deepens and the client comes to trust us, the focus will also change. Perhaps this is simply another form of evolution, though we do tend to think of evolution as occurring over time.

Health care settings are also quite different in that there might be multiple targets of work depending on the nature of the service and the acuity of a "problem." For example, someone who has knee replacement surgery is often required to walk shortly after the anesthesia subsides, which is quite a different physical therapy task than what will be done in the weeks that follow or the prehabilitation program they have been asked to undertake in advance of their knee replacement. The agenda in those settings for the physical therapist and client will look quite different, though the ultimate goals remain the same—increased range of motion, decreased pain, and increased strength and mobility. Prior to surgery, there might be a focus on reducing BMI. Post surgery, the immediate goal is getting a person up and walking who may be in pain and uncertain of the value of the behavior. In outpatient rehabilitation, it is providing focus to the work and working within the confines of what this client's body can do presently, while later it may be maintaining motivation as the client experiences slow gains and setbacks happen. Physical therapists will likely benefit from using MI in these situations, though their foci will be different.

Similarly, for mentors, supervisors, and MI coaches, there will be a general goal of improving a knowledge base, skill set, and the understanding of how to put these elements together. Early in the process, the focus may be global—fewer questions and more reflective listening. Then it may evolve to offering more nuanced and deeper reflections and, as these skills progress, recognizing and responding to change talk and sustain talk effectively. Then it may move to seeing opportunities for change in small openings. In concert with this, there may be more focus on self-reflection and how the practitioner's internal state is influencing the actions they take or do not take. As they become more aware of both the client process and their own internal process, the practitioner deepens their understanding of *Why* things fit together, *What* to do and what makes them effective, *How* to do them, and how their situation requires *What If* modifications to increase their utility and applicability.

The process part of supervision also evolves. As supervisees trust us more, they are more open in their reflections and less protective of their work. We may be better able to bring in practical examples, particularly through using session recordings in supervision. As the supervisee's focus evolves, the recording can act as scaffolding to aid reflection *on action* to then help them be better able to reflect *in action*.

Finally, it is important to keep in mind that the reasons for change and growth, regardless of the specific setting, evolve throughout the change process. Thus, as we hit the maintenance stage of any change, it is not uncommon to see great differences between the reasons for starting the change and growth journey and those for continuing it. Consequently, it is important that as practitioners, we remain attentive to and potentially explore these shifts and changes throughout the change process.

MODULE 18

Reasons for Changing

Module Purpose

This module explores the role of ***change talk***; that is, anything a client may say that is in favor of change or a shift away from the status quo, how we might intentionally encourage it, and how to respond upon hearing it. By the end of this module, it is our hope that you develop an increased awareness of how to recognize reasons for change communicated through different types of change talk and how it impacts us when another person responds to this kind of talk from us. Then we hope you translate this understanding into when and when not to focus on this language, as well as how to elicit and strengthen such talk.

The *Why*: Change Is Hard

Change is hard; you go first. This quip reminds us of the challenge of change. If it were easy, we wouldn't have jobs and this book wouldn't have been written. We would just have parents, friends, bosses, life coaches, or drill instructors tell us the correct course of action and we'd be on our way. As we discussed earlier (see Chapter 2), information alone is rarely enough to change behavior (e.g., Ferrari et al., 2021).

Indeed, change typically happens within a life course context (Bernardi et al., 2019) where previous, current, and future events influence the process, including developmental tasks and challenges. In addition, there is a dynamic interplay between our biological, psychological, and social factors, and our choices that affect our outcomes (Dykstra et al., 2023). Our biology affects risk for certain issues and our experience influences that biology, both epigenetically, as well as in straightforward ways like preferences. Social context impacts us through many factors as well, including the presence of cues, access to low- or high-risk behaviors, institutional bias (e.g., racism, sexism, classism, homophobia), norms, media, life setting, family, and friends. Psychological factors such as adverse childhood events (ACEs), trauma, depression, anxiety, attitudes, preferences, expectations, our sense of agency, and our values also influence us to think and act in particular ways. Then there are different manners in which we learn and grow, and many steps at which things can go awry. Given this array, we might consider it remarkable that any of us manage individual change via personal agency, and yet we do.

At the center of all these factors is us, and our ability to think about and to choose change (Dykstra et al., 2023). We know that thinking about change in particular ways can increase or decrease the likelihood it will happen. Henry Ford catches part of this wisdom with his statement, "Whether you think you can, or you think you can't—you're right" (Good Reads, n.d.). But, in the case of MI, there is a growing literature that indicates the process of engaging in this thinking changes not only whether you think you can or cannot, but also the likelihood of it occurring (Magill et al., 2018).

Our body responses, emotions, thoughts, and behaviors impact us in a range of ways. For cognitive-behavioral (CB) therapists, this is a very common notion and is the basis of many interventions (Bennett-Levy et al., 2015). Within MI, we attend to not all cognitions, but give greater attention to feelings, behaviors, thoughts, in particular verbalized language statements in favor of change. We call this *change talk*.

There is debate as well as complexity associated with change talk. Miller and Rollnick (2023) parse change talk into seven categories: ***desire, ability, reasons, needs, commitment, activation, and taking steps (DARN-CAT)***. Table 18.1 summarizes these categories and provides examples for each.

These seven categories have been further subdivided into ***preparation*** (i.e., desire, ability, reason, and need) and ***mobilizing*** (i.e., willingness, commitment, and taking steps) categories. While there is utility in understanding that change talk extends beyond linguistic statements of commitment and these different facets of change talk exist, the data are muddy about which forms of change talk are most predictive of change and we may need to be more attentive to

TABLE 18.1. Forms and Examples of Change Talk

Form	Definition	Example for weight loss
Desire	Wishing or desiring change	*I'd really like to lose some weight.*
Ability	Capacity for change	*I was able to lose 30 pounds (2.14 stones) and kept it off for 2 years.*
Reasons	The benefits of changing	*My energy would be better if I wasn't carrying the extra weight.*
Need	Impetus for change	*My doctor is concerned that I am showing signs of prediabetes.*
Activation	A willingness or readiness to try change	*I'm ready to give it another shot.*
Commitment	Firm statement toward change	*I've made up my mind and will start tomorrow.*
Taking steps	Begins movement toward or experimenting with new behavior	*I made up a menu and bought groceries for a week of healthier eating.*

context. Specifically, we urge caution in assuming that change and sustain talk always function in the way they are thought to (Hilton et al., 2016). Change talk appears to serve a broader array of functions than just as an engine of change (Lane, 2012). Moreover, there is little evidence that we need to elicit all forms of change talk or that it must happen in a particular order.

With those considerations in mind, a few things about change talk are clear. First, change talk matters. Second, change talk increasing, rather than overall level, or type of, change talk, is a critical marker. Third, ***sustain talk***—reasons not to change—decreasing also matters. We'll talk more about sustain talk in Module 19. While it's clear that people change without engaging in outward statements of change talk, the research also shows that change talk predicts outcomes and therapist behaviors influence the appearance of change talk (Miller & Moyers, 2021).

Change talk is also simple. It is something we hear every day in our interactions with people and is not something unique to a therapeutic relationship. Indeed, we have done it ourselves. These are, simply put, statements that we're thinking about the possibility of change. Our job, as practitioners, is to listen for these statements and to look for where they might be. Like a person trying to start a fire in a wet forest, we look for the kindling elements in likely places, start with a small flame that we help breathe to life, and then sustain and add as much fuel as the growing fire can tolerate. Or switching to our tour guide metaphor, we might begin with why the person wanted to make this trip: Why here, why now? What is it about this place that spoke to them? What do they hope to see, do, and experience along the way? Why is this important to them? The answers to these questions begin to form a path forward, even though the client's not yet on the tour. This is the kindling and the initial flame.

The *What*: EARS as Tools for Change Talk

The tools are straightforward. We learn to recognize change talk, reinforce it when we hear it, and know how to elicit it. To recognize change talk, we often need to tune our ears differently. The unfortunate truth is our ears are exquisitely attuned to sustain talk. We hear it and immediately feel the press of the ***fixing reflex***. It's like we're in that wet forest, trying to help someone start a fire, and all we see are the rain and the moisture dripping off the trees and plants. They are everywhere and discouraging. The heavier the rain and the wetter the forest, the more discouraged we become. But there are dry elements, often protected from the rain and therefore hidden from easy view; we must train ourselves to uncover and find them. This is where knowing all seven categories of change talk can be helpful. Preparatory forms of change talk (DARN), are more likely to be heard first and in weak forms. These are the small bits of fuel for our client's change fire. If we wait to only hear mobilizing forms of change talk (CAT), we will miss important opportunities for us, and more importantly, clients, to recognize their motivation and capacity for change. Therefore, we tune our listening to all these types, especially DARN, and do not just attend to sustain talk. We need to hear all change talk.

Then we need to know how to respond. In this case, we'll use our metaphorical ***EARS*** (***elaborating***, ***affirming***, ***reflective listening***, ***summarizing***). This is a return to our ***OARS*** mnemonic with a shift in the focus of these skills. We'll now ask questions that invite ***elaboration*** or ***examples of change talk*** or that ***evoke change talk*** directly. Using a weight loss example, *Why* *would you consider making a change in your weight? What makes this important to you? Why now?* With affirmations, the focus is on skills or capacities to change, including prior successful or semi-successful efforts. Or even on attendance. For example, L. H. J. recalls a bariatric service patient in the northeast of England coming to the clinic on a day when the parking lot was like an ice rink, with significant snowfall over it. The affirmation was straightforward. *This is really important to you. You have made a massive effort to get into the clinic today when it may have felt much easier to phone and cancel due to the horrendous snowfall overnight.* Reflections are now focused on strengthening change talk and/or softening sustain talk, *You know this will be hard and you feel hope that it can be done.* Notice how this reflection would be looking for that dry kindling in a wet forest. Hope is something that often accompanies prior success and is not typically at the forefront when someone has returned to old behaviors. Clients, too, often look at all the rain and the wet wood. This might, in part, be because of what they expect the practitioner will do—fixing. Finally, we use summaries to organize and emphasize the change talk and soften the sustain talk, as well as provide a route forward:

> *You feel a bit discouraged because you've slipped into some old habits in response to the uncertainty about your new hip, and the result has been some weight gain. You also know that you've been successful before. You know what to do, how to do it, and how to sustain it. Now you're beginning to think about what the next step might be to reengage those things.*

In terms of eliciting change talk, EARS are often sufficient to make that happen. However, we want to use all the tools available in our toolbox. We'll talk more about other tools and how we might use them in Module 19, including the tools already in your toolbox.

The *How*: SP/SR on Eliciting and Exploring Our Change Talk

Overview of the Exercise

For this activity, you will find a limited-practice partner helpful, but not essential. We will again explore your progress through the first part of this book, but this time we will focus on change talk. Feel free to return to Module 17 and compare the questions and see how they differ and how the answers change as a result.

Structure of the Exercise

This self-practice exercise can be done as either a self-directed activity or as an interaction with a partner. If working with a partner in a limited practice, when acting as the listener, be sure to tune from OARS to EARS to focus on the change talk. Remember, we are not building an argument for change. Instead, we're offering back what the client has said and metaphorically asking, *Is this how you see it?* In this process, we will not just repeat what the client has said, but instead will deepen it, choose the most important elements, and hold things in juxtaposition to provide clarity and deepen meaning. Again, the questions will prompt the exploration, but we do not want to simply ask questions.

If working alone, stay focused on the present question and work through this process sequentially. Provide spaciousness for your responses. The goal is not to move through the questions quickly but to let yourself look more deeply at the process that has unfolded for you.

Traveling Companion: An Example with Quincy

We will stay with Quincy here to illustrate how these questions lead us to a different focus. Again, a brief reminder: Quincy is a 38-year-old, cisgender, straight woman of African descent who works as an AOD counselor. From a vibrant community, she has strong family ties. She was feeling some burnout with AOD clients and has sought out personal support with an MI therapist.

➤ ***What made engaging with this book worthwhile for you? What was driving this for you?***

I was feeling burned out in my job. When I began this work, I wanted to make a difference for people in my community, and I was starting to feel like I didn't want them to show up for appointments. I felt mistrustful, frustrated, discouraged, and irritable at times, though I don't think I wanted to admit how much. So, I framed it as a learning opportunity and about getting some support for me, but I think I was looking for a lifeline. I think if this didn't change, my job would have.

➤ ***What made the initial problem focus important? Why this and why now?***

I don't think there was a single event. It was more a slow accumulation, like a pot where the heat has been slowly turned up. It was simmering now, and I didn't want it to boil over. I guess I was most concerned by my increased drinking after work, and my being discouraged and occasionally quick-triggered. I was getting mad, and I don't do that. It is not me.

➤ ***What made you think you could be successful? What prior experiences did you have with making changes?***

Well, I have a lot of history of succeeding when things were stacked against me. I know if I put my mind to something—and work hard—I can do it. But I guess I also know myself well enough that I need to step back and look at what I'm doing and thinking. That whole incident with my dad and the homeless guy at the store told me that I can let my perspective get in the way. So, I kind of knew I needed to change something. I had to stop working hard at the surface, doing all the same things, and see if there was something else, something deeper, which would provide another way. Knowing that about myself is part of what led me to find a therapist who did MI as part of what they do. I was skeptical, but I know I can be wrong, and I am strong enough to step back and admit it.

➤ ***Where have you observed changes in yourself as you've done this work? As you consider this, what thoughts and feelings do you have? Where do you experience these things in your body?***

The truth is me and my responses have been the problem for me and my clients. Trying to fix things led to pushback. I exacerbated rather than fixed the problem. The harder I tried, the worse it got and the more frustrated and discouraged I became. Now, I am less irritable—something I denied—and am more joyful and optimistic in the work.

In terms of my thoughts, I am aware of being more curious. Instead of judging a client's response—and "ouch" it feels bad to even say that—I am curious about what's driving it. My emotions are quieter and more peaceful. I am less thrown by their anger and frustration and more hopeful. I like seeing my people.

In terms of my body, I feel a release from all those tension points—neck, head, shoulders, and hands. Instead, I feel like I breathe more deeply, so I guess I feel it in my chest.

➤ ***How have you sustained yourself when you felt like you might slip back into old behaviors?***

To begin, I use cues to catch myself. When I start to feel frustrated, discouraged, or burned out, that is the canary in the coal mine. It's an early warning, "Girl, there is trouble." Then, I ask myself if my agenda is getting in the way. Often this is the case, and it leads to the fixing reflex and my negative feelings. Finally, I shift the focus onto the client and their needs and agenda.

➤ ***What makes you proud about this work you've done? Where do you feel that in your body? What do you notice about your thoughts and feelings as you think about being proud?***

I feel like this is a big insight for me. Like I figured out something basic that was out of alignment in my work, and it's made me wiser, not so reactive. That I can see it and respond when it happens. It makes me feel capable. I feel this in my face and shoulders. I smile and laugh more easily, and I feel like my shoulders are not tense or squared for battle, but strong and at ease. I also feel it like a bit of warmth in my chest. My thoughts follow that capability line. Instead of feeling like I'm hanging on by my fingernails, I think we can figure this out together. I feel calm and at peace, but ready. Like I am a well-trained athlete ready to perform.

➤ ***What sorts of practices, if any, have you tried out in your clinical work?***

I have focused on clients much more. I start with them and ask their thoughts. I try to be curious about how they see the world, rather than focusing on incorrect or problematic worldviews or thoughts that get them into trouble. I listen more for their reasons and their values. This last part requires me to really shift away from what comes naturally and that has been harder, but I've been doing it. Most of all, I've just been doing lots of listening and less advice giving.

➤ ***What has shifted for your clients because of your changes in clinical work?***

They are much more talkative. Well, some are. They are a lot less argumentative and more likely to tell me things. They seem to be more optimistic and willing to try things out. They're choosing plans they endorse and so seem more open to the whole process of change and to telling me what did and did not work. Overall, they seem in a better spot—most I should say. Not all. But I don't feel as bothered by those who continue to struggle.

Self-Practice

Now it's your turn.

> ***What made engaging with this book worthwhile for you? What was driving this for you?***

> ***What made the initial problem focus important? Why this and why now?***

> ***What made you think you could be successful? What prior experiences did you have with making changes?***

➤ ***Where have you observed changes in yourself as you've done this work? As you consider this, what thoughts and feelings do you have? Where do you experience these things in your body?***

➤ ***How have you sustained yourself when you felt like you might slip back into old behaviors?***

➤ ***What makes you proud about this work you've done? Where do you feel that in your body? What do you notice about your thoughts and feelings as you think about being proud?***

➤ *What sorts of practices, if any, have you tried out in your clinical work?*

➤ *What has shifted for your clients because of your changes in clinical work?*

Self-Reflection

➤ *What did you observe was different in this exploration of your reasons for change than the material covered in Module 17? What did you notice about your body, feelings, and thoughts as you went through this module and had your reasons elicited and were able to observe and reflect on these reasons.*

➤ ***Was it helpful to go through this process to recognize your reasons? If so, what made it helpful for you? If not, what seemed challenging or problematic for you?***

➤ ***Were there any surprises in this process for exploring your reasons? If so, what made them surprising? If not, what does that tell you about how this process works for you? Why might either of these two answers be important to know?***

➤ ***What have you come to see as your strengths or capacities in this work on your own change that you hadn't observed before?***

What If: Applying Skills to My Current Context

Bridging Questions to Practitioner Self

These questions are designed to help you bring the insights from personal self-practice into your work with clients.

➤ ***How does this experience help you understand your practitioner role in working with change talk and why?***

➤ ***In what ways has your recognition of change talk shifted since you began work in this book?***

➤ ***In what ways has your use of EARS to elicit and respond to change talk shifted since you began work in this book?***

➤ ***What has shifted for your clients because of changes in your clinical work with regard to your use of EARS and/or recognition of change talk?***

➤ *How does your awareness of your strengths generally, as well as specifically in working with change talk, now help in your clinical work? In what other ways might you use it?*

➤ *What is your thinking about when and how you'll integrate these ideas and practices? When do you need to be careful about chasing change talk?*

➤ *How will you assess the impact if you do these practices? How will you use this information to make refinements in your practice?*

➤ *What are your main* takeaway *messages from this SP/SR experience in relation to your understanding of the concept of reasons for changing (e.g., recognizing, reinforcing, and eliciting change talk) . . .*

- *From a practical perspective?*

- *From a theoretical perspective?*

➤ ***What if you were to apply this process to other areas of your professional practice (e.g., in a role as supervisor or trainer perhaps)? How might you apply your learning to this new context?***

➤ ***How has this exercise influenced your understanding of or personal relationship with MI as a way of being?***

Final Thoughts and Applications to Other Settings

There is a real danger for practitioners to begin chasing change talk and moving ahead of a client's readiness to change. We hear change talk and jump into planning. This seems to be another form of two interrelated but unhelpful processes: the fixing reflex (though its better disguised since we are not arguing with clients) and a premature focus trap on moving into planning too early. Both processes focus on the solution, not the client. We always want our eyes and ears on the client. We'll discuss this more in Module 19, including how a willingness to explore sustain talk might set MI apart from some other approaches.

In many settings, including health care, it can seem like the need for change is so obvious there is no point in doing this exploration of the *Why* of change. Indeed, if the client is ready to go and looking for a plan, we might get in the way if we spend lots of time eliciting change talk. Still, it is helpful to understand the client's why—for us and them—for sustaining behavior when the change becomes difficult. For example, understanding that a client is having knee replacement surgery to reduce pain is the starting point, but what do they hope to do that they can't now? For one person, it might be to enjoy golf again. For another, it might be to ride a bike, while for a third, it's to play with their grandchildren or to walk their dogs again. Clients need that fuel when the going gets hard, so eliciting and reinforcing their reasons, even briefly, can help buttress the efforts when change becomes challenging.

Finally, Rollnick et al. (2023) change the word "activation" to ***willingness*** and shift the order so that it appears before commitment in listing forms of change talk. We see the value in the change to willingness. It is more descriptive than activation. Also, the order of the terms makes sense. At the same time, we feel the stickiness of the DARN-CAT acronym warrants its continued use. If you prefer willingness, know that our ambivalent hearts go with you.

MODULE 19

Staying Where We Are

Module Purpose

This module explores how we recognize and respond to ***sustain talk***; that is, anything we hear that is in favor of no change or things staying the same. By the end of this module, our hope is that you will more deeply understand the important role of sustain talk in the change process; how to acknowledge and respond to it skillfully, intentionally, and spaciously; and how and when we might want to soften sustain talk in favor of actively eliciting and responding to change talk. Specifically, to do as MINT member Denise Ernst says, acknowledge sustain talk, but don't cuddle it!

The *Why*: Change Is Hard—Really!

We only need think of our own lives and the imperfect ways in which we live to understand that change is not a straightforward process. Even for people who live a well-disciplined life, there are things done and left undone where we fall short of our goals and our expectations. Sometimes it simply comes down to practicalities—there is not enough time to accomplish all the things that must be done and so we prioritize. But for others, we remain ambivalent. There are reasons to change and reasons not to change.

Generally speaking, *sustain talk* is the language that reflects the reasons not to change (Miller & Rollnick, 2023). It falls into two general categories: the ***benefits of the status quo*** and the ***costs of making a change***. In relationship to ***change talk***, we can think of these as the ***pros of non-change*** and ***cons of change***. Table 19.1 depicts these elements as a 2 × 2 figure.

In this example of rehabbing a knee—be it because of injury or replacement—we can see the costs and benefits fall into different quadrants. The indicated prevention program Prime For Life (Daugherty & O'Bryan, 2022) notes that the benefits of the status quo tend to be short-term, but they are immediately rewarding and might be quite powerful. The costs of the status

TABLE 19.1. Pros and Cons of Change—Rehabbing a Knee

	Change	Status quo
Benefits	(1) Long-term gains • *Knee improves and there is less pain than prior to surgery.* • *Able to do activities that bring me joy.* • *Feelings of accomplishment and agency in my life.* • *I feel good.*	(2) Short-term gains • *Avoid the pain, effort, and soreness.* • *More free time.* • *Don't have to explain my failure to complete my physical therapy home program.* • *Avoid the disappointment of failing to progress.*
Costs	(4) Short-term costs • *There is pain, effort, and soreness in the knee as I begin the process.* • *My day is regimented around doing rehab activities.* • *I'm having to shower and clean up after rehab.* • *Progress can be slow and disappointing at times, and I can feel like I let my physical therapist down.*	(3) Long-term costs • *Knee doesn't improve.* • *Range of motion is restricted.* • *Unable to do the activities I want to do.* • *Feelings of disappointment and failure.* • *Feel like my life is becoming more constricted and I don't have control over it.*

quo tend to be more long-term. That is, we usually experience them after the short-term gain of the status quo and only later feel the full consequence (e.g., the cost of inaction continues to grow over time). Conversely, the costs of a change are felt immediately. There is the discomfort of the new and the loss of the rewards associated with the status quo. The benefits of the change tend to only be experienced after we've experienced the short-term costs and may take significantly longer to unfold. The relationship between these quadrants points out why change can be so hard. Quadrants 2 and 4 are powerful short-term barriers to change—this is where sustain talk is housed. Quadrants 1 and 3 are where change talk lives and requires us to tolerate short-term discomfort to get to the value of change (Daugherty & O'Bryan, 2022).

Given that the cost of inaction so often grows over time, a deeper exploration of the longer-term consequences of quadrant 3 can be extremely powerful. In our experience, some practitioners can feel a little uncomfortable in exploring this in detail because it is where there is likely to be significant emotion (e.g., the long-term consequence of inaction in relation to many lifestyle behavior changes is poor health, and often this is associated with loss of independence in the longer term and the knowledge that the person may be feeling they are a burden on others—such as their loved ones). Exploring this in relation to client values can be extremely motivating.

We can see in this example where ***ambivalence***—an equal number and, more importantly, an equal weighting of these factors—can keep us and our clients stuck. When we add the idea of ***vertical ambivalence*** (see Module 15) to this process (Miller, 2022), there is a third dimension present where the status quo is tied to elements that reside below the surface and are not well explicated to the client or to us. The uncovering of these factors can assist us and sustain talk might have clues about what the nature of these things might be. For example, a narrative that involves why I am the one who always has such bad luck might reveal some long-held beliefs about our inherent worth (*I'm worthless*) or our ability to have effectance (*I'm a failure*) and competency (*I'm not good enough*) within our world. Stepping back then, we can think about sustain talk as representing the benefits—typically, short-term—of maintaining the status quo, the costs—typically, short-term—of making a change, and a link to elements that might be keeping us—we and our clients—stuck in vertical ambivalence.

Dissent or discord is a little different. This describes when we take this normal ambivalence about the change process and put it under pressure (Zuckoff, 2023). It is the active pushing back against this pressure. Now the interesting element is that this pressure might come from us as the practitioner; be a residual from prior experience the person had in helping relationships; or may reside in internal representations (i.e., introjects, beliefs, values) the individual has about general social issues (e.g., economic opportunity), cultural issues (e.g., being a person of color residing in a nation with a history of institutional racism), or developmental issues (e.g., being a teen trying to establish an identity in conjunction with peers and apart from family), or life course issues (e.g., experiencing the loss of loved ones) (Bernardi et al., 2019). People will enter our workspaces with varying levels of dissent and discord because of these things, and we have varying degrees of access to these factors during our interactions with clients. But one thing is clear: The more we respond with pressure on these factors, the more pushback we experience in our relationship with clients (Glynn & Moyers, 2010), and the less likely change is going to happen (Magill et al., 2018).

The *What*: Tools for Responding to Sustain Talk and Discord

Our responses to sustain talk and discord fall into three categories. As with change talk, we must be able to recognize and respond to it. Unlike cultivating and strengthening change talk, we want to acknowledge and move past sustain talk and discord. While Zuckoff (2023) suggests that our ability to sit with ambivalence might also be important, we do not wish to remain unintentionally focused on it because this spotlights and strengthens it, thereby decreasing the likelihood that the client will achieve their aims.

In terms of recognizing sustain talk and discord, there is good news. We are already finely tuned to hearing it. Consider this statement:

> *I am feeling burned out in my job. When I began this work, I wanted to make a difference for people in my community. Now, I don't want them to show up for appointments. I feel mistrustful, frustrated, discouraged, and irritable at times. I am not feeling very hopeful it can change. I'm not sure I want to try. Maybe it's time for a new job.*

This is a statement we might imagine Quincy making before she started her *inside out* work. We can hear the frustration, discouragement, and lack of hope that the nature of the job can change. While there is an explicit statement about change at the end, it is about a different form of job. These are examples of sustain talk about Quincy changing how she works with clients. To respond to these statements, Dr. Joel Porter (personal communication, September 22, 2022) notes that we can use our ***EARS*** skills just like we do for change talk, though he has altered the acronym. Table 19.2 summarizes this new form of EARS.

TABLE 19.2. EARS for Sustain Talk and Dissent

Express, Elaborate, and/or Emphasize

- Express interest in the person's position.
- Elaborate using open questions to better understand the person's point of view.
- Emphasize personal choice and control.

Acknowledge, and/or Apologize and Accept

- Acknowledge the sustain talk or discord, but don't reinforce it.
- Apologize for an error and accept responsibility for it.

Reflect and/or Reframe

- Reflection is the mainstay skill of MI for conveying empathy.
- Reflect directionally and intentionally by undershooting and overshooting.
- Reframe the situation to cast it in a new light.

Share, Summarize, and/or Shift Focus

- Share double-sided reflections.
- Summarize sustain and change talk.
- Shift focus to move away from the stuck or the sore spot.

Note. Adapted from Dr. Joel Porter, personal communication, September 22, 2022.

To begin with, we ***express interest*** in what the person has to say and ask them to ***elaborate*** using open questions. We should note this is unlikely to immediately reduce the sustain talk or discord, but it can help to build the relationship. We can also ***emphasize personal control, autonomy, and responsibility***, all key elements in *self-determination theory*. Responding to the example, we might combine these things and say,

> *It's up to you, Quincy, whether you decide to stay in this job* (Emphasize). *You said you didn't feel very hopeful it could change. What do you mean* (Express interest and elaborate)?

Notice how those three utterances address the key elements. The first emphasizes that this is Quincy's decision to make, not ours. It supports her autonomy. The second is a surface-level reflection designed to acknowledge what has been heard. The question leads to an exploration and elaboration of what some elements of vertical ambivalence might be and by its nature expresses interest.

We ***acknowledge the sustain talk***, but we try not to reinforce it. This is a tricky balance because we don't wish to give this small fire a lot of fuel and oxygen to build it into a roaring blaze, while at the same time genuinely attending to the suffering or challenge being expressed. In addition, if we made an error in our response, we want to ***apologize*** for it and ***accept*** responsibility for it. Returning to Quincy, we might say,

> *It seems like this is a battle you're not sure you want to stay in* (Acknowledge). *I apologize if what I've said makes you feel like I'm pushing you to stay in it* (Apologize); *this was not my intent, but I recognize my impact might have landed that way and I'm sorry for it* (Accept responsibility).

As always, we rely on the main skill of ***reflective listening***. We can use this in a variety of ways to soften the sustain talk or defuse the dissent/discord. It could be a straightforward reflection. We could also under- or overshoot the client's statement to encourage either further discussion (undershoot) or move them away from an absolute position (overshoot). That is, our emphasis adds to or lessens the force in a statement or emotion. Porter (2022) goes on to note that focusing on emotion, concern, or worry can be key to understanding and mending the relationship. We might also ***reframe*** the client's experience through the reflection. To Quincy, our response might be

> *You're feeling battered and bruised* (Reflection, might be an overshoot), *and left to wonder if you should come out of the corner when the bell rings for the next round* (Uses a metaphor to reframe the experience).

Finally, we ***summarize*** in a manner that acknowledges the sustain and the change side of the discussion. ***Sharing a double-sided reflection*** can be very helpful in this regard especially when done concisely, beginning with the sustain side, and using the conjunction "and" to pair the two sides. While "but" is a common word to use in this setting, it also has the unfortunate characteristic of dismissing everything that comes before it. *I like your hair cut, but . . .* We all know what that means, while "and" allows both things to be true. We might also ***shift focus*** away from the sustain or discord element. This is done in a transparent manner that acknowledges being stuck and moving toward an area where progress might be possible:

> *There is a part of you that feels like letting go and moving into a new line of work, and another part, the part that brought you here, says I got into this for my community and I'm not ready to abandon that community* (double-sided reflection). *Some of these things feel painful and hard to make progress on, so I'm wondering if we might shift our attention from those areas* (shifting focus) *onto something where perhaps we can begin to help you feel some control again* (Undershoot).

There are other tools available for responding to sustain talk and discord. We'll talk more about these other tools and how we might use them in Module 20, including the tools already in your toolbox.

The *How*: SP/SR on Exploring the Sustain Side and Moving to the Change Side

Overview of the Exercise

For this activity, you will find a limited-practice partner helpful, though it is not essential. We will use a technique often employed in CBT where we explore underlying assumptions, which cognitive-behavioral practitioners often term *conditional assumptions*, that may keep us stuck. We will reflect on the truth within that assumption (i.e., sustain talk), but then move past it to another truth (change talk).

Structure of the Exercise

Here is the structure. Think about your reasons for keeping things as they are, for staying with the status quo. Try to name seven. Then add a first truth that supports the status quo or notes the challenge with change. Then add a second truth that challenges the status quo or supports the change. Within *Prime Solutions*, an alcohol and drug treatment curriculum developed by Prevention Research Institute, this is referred to as finding the *grain of truth* and offering the *balancing thought* (Prevention Research Institute, 2008). This structure means you will make two trips through the worksheet.

When we're the provider in a limited practice, we will use these two truths to guide us in the discussion. First, have the person write down their seven reasons for not changing. Second, the person can write their grains of truth and balancing thoughts one item at a time, followed by discussion or you can simply discuss them. However, maintain the order of grain of truth followed by balancing thought. While this can be a helpful process in tipping the balance of change and sustain talk, it also gives us an opportunity to practice both acknowledging sustain talk and being directional in moving past it toward the side of change. As the listener in this process, we will want to take time to explore the balancing thought.

If working alone, use the same structure. Write all seven reasons (if there are seven) to begin with, then work through the other two elements on each item, pausing to consider your answers, especially the balancing thought. Take your time before moving on to the next one. You might even practice offering yourself a reflection, using some of the techniques discussed in the prior module about self-distancing.

> *David, lying on the couch, watching your favorite team play, and eating chips would feel good and you're aware that you can still enjoy the game with a cup of tea with a little sweetener and feel better and happier afterward.*

While this is the order we have used with clients, Braga et al. (2019), suggest we might handle the order in the self-practice exercise a little differently. Specifically, they report research that suggests reviewing the reasons for not changing as a set (i.e., the grain of truth statements) followed by the reasons to change as a set (i.e., the balancing thought statements) produces deeper thought and more movement toward resolution of ambivalence and change. Meanwhile, doing one grain of truth thought followed by the other balancing thought might lead to less change. This is one study, but you might consider testing this order in doing this practice exercise.

Traveling Companion: An Example with Sam

Sam, who is a White, cisgender, gay woman of European descent, has been a successful counselor for many years. Ten years ago, she injured her back and because of that experience has shifted her private practice to health-focused care. She had a cancer scare last year, and her wife is encouraging her to retire. Sam is ambivalent about making that change, and this has become a point of contention between them.

➤ ***What are your reasons for keeping things as they are, for staying with the status quo? Try to name seven. Be as explicit as possible.***

- **My first reason for staying with the status quo is**

  My work gives me meaning and purpose.

  - The first truth (grain of truth) is

    My work provides a sense that what I am doing matters in the world; it makes a difference in a positive way.

  - The second truth (balancing thought) is

    My work does matter, and it's not the only way I can make a difference. I have volunteered my time for a variety of causes over the years, and I know that just by being a friend to others and a loving wife to Debra, I make a difference.

- **My second reason for staying with the status quo is**

  My work gives me an identity.

  - The first truth (grain of truth) is

    I do know who I am as a therapist and have been successful over the years. I believe that I am good at it and have developed wisdom about how to work with people in need.

  - The second truth (balancing zthought) is

    I am an excellent therapist and that is not all I am. While there is a technical set of skills and specific wisdom I've developed, it doesn't mean this is the only place I can apply them, or they only matter in that situation. Empathy, compassion, and good communication skills apply beyond therapy.

- **My third reason for staying with the status quo is**

  I am happy with how things are now.

  - The first truth (grain of truth) is

    I do enjoy my blend of activities, and work doesn't feel burdensome.

  - The second truth (balancing thought) is

    Being happy requires me to ignore Debra's concerns for me and her desires, which means this is just a surface-level happiness. There is a stone in my shoe, and if I don't address it, the rub will become a blister and then a limp, etc.

- **My fourth reason for staying with the status quo is**

  I don't need to decide now. I have time.

  - The first truth (grain of truth) is

    This is true. My health is fine. Debra is not pressuring me. Our finances are good. Life is in a good place now.

  - The second truth (balancing thought) is

    The squamous cells let me know that time is ticking and is not infinite. My life is finite, and if I knew I had terminal cancer, I wouldn't choose to spend my last months working. I know that. I'd want to spend it with the people I love, in the places I love, and doing the things I love.

- **My fifth reason for staying with the status quo is**

  I am not like Debra. I don't feel the need to travel or putter.

  - The first truth (grain of truth) is

    I'd feel a little lost if I didn't do some planning about how I will spend my days. I can't spend all day puttering or drinking coffee.

  - The second truth (balancing thought) is

    I am not Debra, so I would need to find other things to do. When I have a free day, I can always fill it up and I do know the things that I enjoy doing. Planning for meals and cooking. Being engaged socially in either planned or unplanned ways. Learning something new. I would need to put a plan together.

- **My sixth reason for staying with the status quo is**

  Research indicates that retiring from work can have a negative effect on health.

  - The first truth (grain of truth) is

    There is research that people who don't remain engaged in life fare poorly after retirement and that maintaining some work connection can be helpful.

  - The second truth (balancing thought) is

    It is not an all-or-nothing proposition. Perhaps I could drop down to a day a week and see how that feels for me and Debra. It might help me decide about whether I want to stop entirely or maintain a much smaller engagement. It would allow us to do more of the things on Debra's bucket list.

- **My seventh reason for staying with the status quo is**

  It's my life. I decide. No one else does.

  - The first truth (grain of truth) is

    It is my life, and I should be the one deciding.

  - The second truth (balancing thought) is

    My life is so much better because of the people I love that are in it, and their opinions are important to me because they're important. To ignore them would be like biting off my nose to spite my face.

➤ ***As you went through the different iterations of this process, what did you observe about your internal balance between the status quo and change?***

I felt pretty stuck at the beginning. Like things were balanced and we're not moving in either direction. But now it felt like things have begun to shift, like a scale that started to tip toward one side.

➤ ***How did you experience that balance in your body? In your thoughts? In your feelings?***

It felt like a release. Like I had been frozen in some way. There was held tension that I wasn't aware of and suddenly that began draining away and now I felt some energy. I can't say exactly where I felt it, but it was sort of all over. Like I felt energized. The feeling was hope or optimism, and maybe that's not entirely a feeling but that was my experience. The thoughts were a combination of "Oh yeah, I know that" or "Okay, I see a path forward."

> ***Which item or items seemed to really stand out to you as important? Why were they important to you?***

I was aware from before that I tended to stay on the surface when I was stuck in the status quo, so the longer second truths as a rule helped me dig deeper. But I think it was the statement that I have time. Thinking about my mortality and if death were imminent, how I would spend my time pushed me beyond the surface level. My answer was clear as a bell in my mind, and so then it became about working back from there. That caused the scale to tip.

> ***Where does this leave you now?***

I feel momentum, and I want to capitalize on it. I don't want to go back to being stuck. I feel the need to talk with Debra and start thinking about a plan. I'm fairly certain that this would mean scaling back, so it will take some time to reduce my client load and refer folks out, but I feel the need to start putting some details together. Like a timeline.

Self-Practice

Now it's your turn.

> ***What are your reasons for keeping things as they are, for staying with the status quo? Try to name seven. For example,* I like my routine *or* It feels too complicated to change. *Be as explicit as possible. Fill in all seven reasons, then return to the first reason and complete the* grain of truth *and* balancing thought.**

- **My first reason for staying with the status quo is**

  ____

  - The first truth (grain of truth) is

    ____

  - The second truth (balancing thought) is

    ____

Remember to offer a reflective listening statement on your second time through the questions. This reflection can be written below or spoken aloud. Refer back to the information on EARS if you need help with scaffolding.

- **My second reason for staying with the status quo is**

  ____

  - The first truth (grain of truth) is

    ____

  - The second truth (balancing thought) is

    ____

Offer a reflective listening statement on your second time through the questions.

- **My third reason for staying with the status quo is**

  ____

  - The first truth (grain of truth) is

    ____

  - The second truth (balancing thought) is

    ____

Offer a reflective listening statement on your second time.

- **My fourth reason for staying with the status quo is**

  ____

  - The first truth (grain of truth) is

    ____

  - The second truth (balancing thought) is

    ____

Offer a reflective listening statement.

- **My fifth reason for staying with the status quo is**

  ____

  - The first truth (grain of truth) is

    ____

  - The second truth (balancing thought) is

    ____

Offer a reflective listening statement.

- **My sixth reason for staying with the status quo is**

  ____

  - The first truth (grain of truth) is

    ____

  - The second truth (balancing thought) is

    ____

Offer a reflective listening statement.

- **My seventh reason for staying with the status quo is**

  ____

  - The first truth (grain of truth) is

    ____

  - The second truth (balancing thought) is

    ____

Offer a reflective listening statement.

➤ ***As you went through the different iterations of this process, what did you observe about your internal balance between the status quo and change?***

____

____

____

____

____

➤ ***How did you experience that balance in your body? In your thoughts? In your feelings?***

____

____

____

____

____

➤ ***Which item or items seemed to really stand out to you as important? Why were they important to you?***

____

____

____

____

____

- *As you look over these* grains of truth *and* balancing thoughts, *are there any places where you feel stuck and you aren't quite sure why? What else might be pulling on that for you? Anything you hadn't noticed before?*

- *How may this be related to something unknown? Might it be vertical ambivalence?*

- *If you had this experience, how will you explore that ambivalence anchor?*

- *Where does this leave you now?*

Self-Reflection

➤ ***As you considered the** grain of truth **and** balancing thought, **what did you notice about the tensions between the two? What about tensions within you as a person exploring a difficult personal issue?***

➤ ***How did the way this exercise is constructed affect your experience of these tensions? Why?***

➤ ***What role did your partner's manner play, and particularly their use of*** EARS ***(see Table 19.2), in the exploration of*** grain of truth ***and the*** balancing thought***? Why did this matter for you? If you examined this on your own, what did you observe about how your reflections affected you? Did they matter? Why or why not?***

What If: Applying Skills to My Current Context

Bridging Questions to Practitioner-Self

These questions help bring the insights from your personal self-practice into your work as a practitioner with clients.

➤ ***What techniques, based on your experience in this session, might help with eliciting and tipping the balance on vertical ambivalence? Why? What is it specifically about these techniques that is helpful?***

➤ ***What would you do with a client who at the end of this sequence remains in the same place? Why?***

➤ ***What is hard for you when a client is stuck? What does it pull for? How might it connect to your own vertical ambivalence and why?***

➤ ***How might your experience in this activity help in managing your*** fixing reflex ***with a client who is stuck and why? How might you now approach this issue in a different way? What could you do differently and why?***

- ***What are your main*** takeaway ***messages from this SP/SR experience in relation to your understanding of the concept of staying where we are . . .***
  - ***From a practical perspective?***

    ____
    ____
    ____
    ____
    ____

  - ***From a theoretical perspective?***

    ____
    ____
    ____
    ____
    ____

- ***What if you were to apply this process to other areas of your professional practice (e.g., in a role as supervisor or trainer perhaps)? How might you apply your learning to this new context?***

  ____
  ____
  ____
  ____
  ____

- ***How has this exercise influenced your understanding of or personal relationship with MI as a way of being?***

  ____
  ____
  ____
  ____
  ____

Final Thoughts and Applications to Other Settings

As with change talk, sustain talk has been divided into seven categories: *desire, ability, reasons, needs, activation, commitment, and taking steps* (Rollnick et al., 2023). While it can be helpful to understand and respond differentially to these categories, it is not a simple *if–then* proposition. Instead, we work to understand the client, the circumstance of the statement, the larger context of the conversation, and to respond in an intentional manner understanding why we opted for that direction.

There may be danger for practitioners to engage in deep exploration of sustain talk and dissent. It can be delicious and unproductive for our clients to complain. It's our job to hear and respond with empathy to grievances and still not become the complaint department. The danger on the other side is that we move into the fixing reflex. This is a delicate dance, where we must be well attuned to our client. Zuckoff's observations suggest we may need to be willing to sit in the ambivalence longer, and especially on the sustain side, to help clients move forward. That pursuit of *change talk* can itself be a form of *fixing reflex*.

One of the features that sets MI apart from related approaches such as *solution-focused therapy* or SFT (e.g., De Shazer et al., 2021) is that MI actively works with ambivalence and reasons for no change that may be expressed as sustain talk. Clients often respond well to the opportunity to talk about *what's good* with regard to problem behaviors. Of course, more expert-driven approaches rarely allow for this exploration, and this may have unintended consequences in client feelings of failure and inadequacy. By contrast then, the acceptance that is offered by a more complete exploration of the reasons to change or not (change and sustain talk) is often well received by clients. Indeed, this can be very empowering for clients who may have experienced long-term expert-driven approaches within complex health and social care systems.

Earlier, we noted that pros and cons of the status quo and change can be put into four quadrants. Moreover, there is typically a short-term and long-term quality to the effects of status quo and change decisions. Remaining with the status quo typically has immediate, positive, short-term effects and long-term consequences, while the reverse is true for change—short-term consequences and long-term benefits. From a practitioner perspective, it is often helpful to ask clients to look at these four quadrants and simply consider the difference between reasons cited from a short- versus long-term perspective.

As noted in Module 18, the presence of time pressures in brief encounters can make the desire to move quickly past sustain talk even more urgent. However, even in very brief settings—1 to 2 minutes—Rollnick et al. (2023) note that a shift away from "Find It. Fix It" to a more nuanced approach that involves, "I hear you and would like to offer some help. Here's where you might go. How do you see the road ahead?" (p. 129), can lead to greater autonomy and improve the likelihood of people engaging in a change process. Even in this situation, listening matters more than telling.

Finally, there is a much broader and deeper literature on decision making than discussed in this module. We encourage the reader to explore it further. Michaelsen and Esch (2023) are an excellent place to begin for *health behavior change*, and Bieleke et al. (2021) is a similarly well-suited place to begin exploring *implementation intentions*. We will return to these ideas in Module 22.

MODULE 20

Strengthening Our Reasons

Module Purpose

This module elaborates further on what we discovered in Module 18 about ***change talk*** by extending our learning to address the importance of context for change talk; that is, when to evoke and when not to. We also explore the dangers of ***chasing change talk*** and introduce—or reintroduce—you to strategies for eliciting change talk. By the end of this module, our hope is that you will have a deeper appreciation for the subtle, intentional, and skillful art of strengthening reasons to change, without chasing change talk in such a way that we risk appeasing our own ***fixing reflex***.

The *Why*: There Is Danger in Chasing Change Talk

Motivational interviewing has been portrayed as a behavioral approach that reinforces change talk. Within this viewpoint, a single-minded pursuit of change talk makes sense as it would elicit and reinforce more of the thought and behavior that will lead to the eventual goal. This mechanistic approach regards change talk as good and more as better. Change talk is flowers and sustain talk weeds. Our goal then is to be a gardener who grows the flowers—elicits and reinforces the change talk—and weeds the garden—softens the sustain talk (Barnett et al., 2014a).

To be clear, there is a grain of truth in this view, and it is not the whole story (cf., Magill et al., 2018). To begin, gardens are more than weeds and flowers. There are often lawns, trees, tree roots, hedges, and rocks that give both form and feature to the garden and its design. Perhaps there is water or paths. Each garden is unique, and we've focused on only one element within this garden to the exclusion of understanding the whole garden.

This approach can also send us in the focused pursuit of weed pulling. Moreover, we're pulling weeds and planting flowers in someone else's garden! What if they keep a secret garden that they have not yet allowed anyone into? At a general level, it can lead us into the *fixing reflex*, where we begin jumping in to solve client problems. In a more nuanced way, this can take the form of a disputatious style where we aim to correct client misperceptions and misunderstandings. Cognitive-behavioral therapy (CBT) has taught us this can be quite helpful in challenging faulty or problematic cognitions. While CBT noted the importance of doing this in a collaborative manner, MI suggests this will be much more powerful if it is done by the client than us. Which brings us to what is the fundamental issue with the flowers and weeds analogy—a mistaken belief about whose garden this is and who the gardener is, and perhaps what constitutes a flower and what is a weed.

It is our assertion that these are the clients' gardens, and they are the gardeners. Each garden is unique, and it is their garden to design and tend. It is our job to help them see the garden as it is, understand what strengths and capacities exist within it, consider what might aid in its health, and help them envision what this garden could be, and they then determine how and where to work. We will have ideas, suggestions, and concerns, but the client will decide. So, when we start planting flowers or pulling weeds, or telling clients what must be done with that tree or rock, we've begun to tend someone else's garden.

Circling back to where we began, chasing change talk leads us to miss the big picture of our client's situation and to understand how the change talk fits in. In terms of the MI processes, it's like we're now ***evoking*** in a differential manner, but we've forgotten the ***MI spirit*** elements, as well as the important ones identified in the ***focusing*** process. More specifically, we've set aside the concept of ***autonomy*** and instead substituted our judgment for what is best in a single-minded pursuit of attention to one element. It is not surprising this pursuit can then feel off-putting for clients.

Rather than enhancing motivation for change, this kind of change talk undermines it. For clients, it begins to feel like a technique that is being done *to* them, rather than something being done *with* them. It feels mechanistic and repetitive and therefore false and forced. ***Partnership*** is now undermined, with the goal further away rather than closer.

The remedy flows from what we've described. First, recognize that it is the client's garden, not ours. Second, see the whole garden and don't be too quick to focus on a single element. Third, move at the client's speed, not our own. Last, wait to move into *evoking* until the work of *focusing* tells us what is important. Metaphorically, don't rush into planting the wrong flowers, or planting when the soil conditions won't support them or it's the wrong time in the season.

The *What*: Tools for Strengthening Reasons

With those cautions in mind, the techniques for strengthening reasons for change are straightforward. To begin, the work is *directional* and *intentional*. We choose to follow certain conversational paths because we believe they will help the client move toward their important elements, and we pay attention to some things along the way and not others. Technically, we'll use our ***EARS***; that is, we'll use our basic MI skills in a more targeted manner. As noted in Module 18, our open questions will ask for ***elaboration*** and ***examples*** of reasons for change, difficulties encountered within the status quo, or illustrations of successful past changes. Affirmations will become more attuned to skills and *abilities* for making a specific change, rather than general skills and capacities. Reflections will become more focused and differential in targeting change talk and softening sustain talk. Summaries will juxtapose change and sustain talk in a manner that highlights change. While this combination, using techniques in a purposeful manner in combination with the MI spirit, is often the primary method for eliciting and strengthening change talk, these are not the only strategies.

Other approaches frequently use a combination of a strategy and focused basic skills. For example, ***looking forward*** allows clients to imagine life changed and unchanged in the future, but is heavily reliant on the practitioner's basic skills to explore this information as it emerges. ***Looking back*** in time also uses imagination, but this time to recall the future they'd already imagined for themselves when younger or before a problem behavior emerged; the client uses this information to build a bridge back to it in the present. Asking how ***important others view*** the situation (e.g., family or friends) requires the person to make a perspective shift. ***Using extremes*** (*What's the worst that could happen? The best? The most likely?*) permits articulation of hopes and fears, and a return to the more proximal and potentially manageable challenges. ***Feedback*** through formal assessments or informal methods like *importance*, *confidence*, or *readiness rulers* provides opportunities to elicit, reinforce, and strengthen change talk. Finally, there is straightforward ***exploration of goals*** as well as ***values*** and ***behaviors***, providing opportunities to discover these sources of client motivation (see Box 20.1). Rosengren (2017) describes such strategies in depth, and the reader is referred to that source for further information and practice if these are new concepts.

There are also other tools available in our toolboxes. For example, the *miracle question* is something that has its origins in solution-focused therapy (SFT; De Shazer et al., 2021), but has been expanded into many other settings. It is quite effective in eliciting and strengthening

BOX 20.1. Strategies for Eliciting Change Talk

- EARS
  - *Elaboration* and *examples* of reasons for change are targets of open questions, as well as difficulties encountered within the status quo, or illustrations of successful past changes.
  - *Affirmations* attuned to skills and *abilities* for making a specific change.
  - *Reflections* differentially target change talk and soften sustain talk.
  - *Summaries* will juxtapose change and sustain talk in a manner that highlights change.
- *Looking forward* allows clients to imagine life changed and unchanged in the future.
- *Looking back* uses imagination to recall the future they'd already imagined when younger or before a problem behavior emerged.
- Asking how *important others view* the situation.
- *Using extremes: What's the worst that could happen? The best? The most likely?*
- *Feedback* from assessment.
- *Exploration of goals* as well as *values* and *behaviors.*
- Using *rulers* (e.g., *importance*, *confidence*, *readiness*) with follow-up prompts.

change talk when done in combination with EARS. Indeed, more generally, this is the wisdom of SFT looking for exceptions, which, in turn, lead to strengths, capacities, and change talk. Visualization techniques done to engage either a situation or practice a behavior can also be strong sources of change talk. Positive psychology has introduced techniques that produce change talk. Asking clients to do *takeaways* or *homework* can be rich sources of change talk, as well as opportunities for sustain talk. Of course, all are done within the larger framework of MI spirit and the MI tasks.

Finally, it is essential we recognize that change talk and sustain talk are often intermixed, and that within sustain talk are frequent hints of change talk. Unsurprisingly, it is not complex strategies but careful listening that allows us to hear what lies within clients.

The *How*: SP/SR on Strengthening My Reasons

Overview of the Exercise

For this activity, you will find a limited-practice partner helpful. We will pick up where we left off in Module 18, while acknowledging that Module 19 may have helped resolve some impediments to moving forward. We do a visualization exercise where we imagine 3 years into the future and a successful change has been made in our lives in the area that we chose to focus on in this workbook. The change is now well established, and it is incorporated into our identity.

Structure of the Exercise

You'll use the script below to help visualize what that circumstance would look like and then address the questions that follow.

Once again, voice matters in this process. Whether it is done live by your partner or recorded by you on your phone and played back, do not use your everyday voice. Instead, allow your voice to be more relaxed, gentle, calm, and paced than usual. Feel free to add your or your partner's name to the script. Work to connect all the senses into this process as part of the script.

Find a quiet place where you will be free of distractions and that helps you calm your mind. Feel free to add small accoutrements to this process if it is helpful, like candles, incense, or soft music. Provide a comfortable place to sit.

Here is the script. Review it now, so you know what it says prior to reading Sam's example. Then come back later when you're ready to use it during the self-practice.

> "Sit comfortably with legs uncrossed and hands resting in your lap. You can close your eyes if you feel comfortable. If not, simply find a place to let your gaze land on gently. Breathe in through your nose and out through your mouth. Breathing slowly and evenly. Focusing your attention on your breath coming in and then flowing out. Continue to do this 5 more times, simply attending to your breath as it comes in and flows out. And then after the fifth breath, just continue to breathe naturally and easily, noticing sensations of relaxation flow over you.
>
> "Now, open a picture in your mind's eye. Visualize it opening in front of you. Eventually, focus on what life would look like 3 years from now if you were successful in making

a change in the area you've been targeting. Just allow the image to form and be surprised by what you see. Take your time, allowing it to come into focus. Breathing easily and comfortably. If you cannot specifically see it, let your mind just relax and think about it. Notice where you are and who is there. Feel your body in that space. Where do you feel these body sensations? What do you smell . . . taste . . . hear . . . feel with your skin? What is happening in this situation? Just notice what is happening. Take your time and breathe easily and comfortably.

"What are the emotions that accompany you in this situation? Know that if these are strong emotions, you can touch them, but don't need to feel all the power they hold unless you wish to. You can simply observe and know they're present. As the situation begins to resolve into a hazy cloud, what is the feeling that you are left with?

"Continue to breathe easily in this warm, comforting place. Notice your breath moving in and out easily. Allow yourself to float here. Any sounds that come in simply drift in and out. And now as you drift in the warm comfort of this moment, know that you take with you these feelings of accomplishment and the strength it took to complete this journey. As you continue to breathe easily in and out, in and out, in and out. When you're ready, you can return to the present time and place, bringing with you all that you wish to bring and leaving behind any of those things you do not care to bring forward. You will feel refreshed and invigorated by recalling this journey and all you accomplished, and are strengthened by the remembrance."

Traveling Companion: An Example with Sam

We'll continue Sam's journey from Module 19, as some things had begun to tip for her during the two "truths" process. Recall that Sam, who is a White, cisgender woman of European descent, has been a successful counselor for many years. Ten years ago, she injured her back and because of that experience has shifted her private practice to health-focused care. She had a cancer scare last year, and her wife is encouraging her to retire. Sam is ambivalent about making that change, and this has become a point of contention between them. She completed the visualization exercise and is now responding to the questions.

➤ ***Describe how your body feels after having made this change successfully. How do you experience it in your legs, torso, chest, shoulders, head? What is your breathing like?***

Last time, I talked about how tension had slipped away as I worked through those grains of truth and balancing thoughts. I feel that, and it's not just the absence of tension but being truly relaxed and at peace. Like I'm fully centered in my life and that is reflected in my body. My hands are even relaxed. My breathing is easy and deep.

➤ ***What feelings are present?***

I feel at peace and calm - content. I feel a little smile on my face and so I'm aware of happiness, though I tend to think of that as a by-product. It's like when I am making a meal for friends. I don't set out to be happy, but the process of sorting through recipes, gathering the ingredients, preparing the food, and anticipating the evening all lead me to being happy.

➤ ***What thoughts?***

This is the harder one for me. These feel a little fuzzy in my mind, but I guess it's a combination of things. Like, I am so glad that I made this decision, and I love the rhythm of my life. Debra and I are in such a good place now. Like any couple, we have our moments, yet I can say without any hesitation, I appreciate her encouragement to not just stay in the groove I was in but ask myself if this was where I wanted to be. Maybe it was a little more forceful than that, but that's what I am thinking now.

➤ ***What is happening at work? What is different here?***

Well, I still have a few clients, but it's all contained on 1 day and that feels like plenty. In fact, I'm down to four clients now, with two alternating every other week, so it feels very contained. I don't feel stressed by it, and it is enough that it keeps my brain energized and engaged. It keeps me learning and thinking, but I don't feel pressure. I do it because it brings pleasure. Billing is easy and manageable, and the business things can be handled on that same day. I'm loving it, and Debra is okay with it, too. I'm also beginning to think about a time when I would let it all go and that feels okay, too, where before that was hard for me to imagine.

➤ ***What is happening at home? What is different here?***

Well, this is the best part. It turns out that I do like having a little more time with my cup of coffee. When the weather is nice, I can sit out on the front porch and greet the day. I get to see the neighborhood kids and talk to them, like Mrs. Haddid did for me. I've even begun to bake some cookies for the kids, with their parents' permission, of course, so they can stop by and grab one on the way home. I decided to do it on Thursdays, and now it's become a routine for all of us. Sometimes they sit and chat on the porch, and sometimes they just grab their treat and are on their way. I did learn early on that it's like Halloween candy—you must set a limit, or some will grab great handfuls.

With Debra, things are great. We have our little adventures, but we just seem to be in balance and rhythm. With the tension about me retiring gone, our squabbles are few and far between. It's a joy to spend time together.

➤ ***How has this impacted your relationships with friends?***

I've made a whole new set of connections with the neighborhood children, and I love that. I also feel more attached to the neighborhood, which is something I always wanted. With friends, we have more time for activities. I am also volunteering 1 day a week and so that has brought in another source of connection.

➤ ***How are you living in relationship to your values? Why is that important?***

Over the last 10 years, I've focused with my clients on self-care and balance; while I thought I was doing that myself, it seems clear now that it wasn't entirely true. Love, health, caring for others, and self-care are all there and feel at the heart of my decisions. I keep coming back to balance, peace, and contentment. My life is a blessing to me. I don't know how long it will last, but I know that I'm living in the manner that will leave me without regrets if something were to suddenly change.

➤ ***As you think back over the 3 years, what were big turning points? How did you accomplish these? Or when you ran into the inevitable tough spots, how did you work your way through them?***

A big turning point was at the beginning, when I decided that it didn't have to be either work or retire, that it could be something in between. I know it sounds stupid, but I was locked into some black-and-white thinking. Then there was the talking to clients.

I decided to make a plan and lay out a timeline, and I had to decide how I would prioritize who I would keep and who I would refer out. I had to think through the words and have a couple of visualization episodes to get myself ready. But I did it. There was also the first time someone called and wanted to return, and my first impulse was to make space. I reminded myself of the goal and found a trusted colleague, and then made a referral. The person wasn't happy, but she did it.

Finally, there was a big house expense. It made me nervous about money and think I should work more hours, but we talked to our financial advisor. He assured us that we'd be okay. The biggest help was not giving in to my first response of fear in all these things.

➤ ***How are you applying this information in new ways in your life?***

In general, I feel like I've been a little bolder. Whenever I've felt afraid, I try to remind myself that is the first response, but it doesn't have to be the last one. It's gotten me out to try some of the new things that Debra always wanted to do, and I was less sure of.

➤ ***What's something you know about yourself now that you didn't know at the beginning of this process? Why is this helpful for you?***

Over time, I'd allow fear to drive more and more of my decision making. That was never me, and I didn't see how it had crept into my life. I'd always been bold, so this was a chance to reconnect with myself. I like it and it reinvigorates me. Doing the cookies with kids just sounds fun and so I'll do it. It seems like I'm paying forward Mrs. Haddid [neighbor when Sam was young], and that just seems right.

➤ ***What are the three best reasons now to have made this change? Why are these important to you?***

I feel like I've recaptured a part of myself that I really loved and valued and somehow lost sight of along the way. My relationship with Debra just feels so good. It's where I want it to be. My life feels in balance and true to myself and who I want to be in the world. These things are important because they're me at my core and me at my best. That's who I want to be. Not someone gritting my teeth and grinding out work for a few more dollars.

➤ ***As you think about your area of challenge, what are you observing that has now changed?***

I feel settled. Like the air has gone out of that balloon. I feel resolved and ready to make a move. The task now is to figure out a plan, including some timelines. I feel excited and energized.

Self-Practice

Now it's your turn.

Imagine 3 years into the future and a successful change has been made in your life in the area that you choose to focus on in this workbook. The change is now well established, and it is incorporated into your identity. Close your eyes and visualize what that would look like and then address the questions that follow.

- ***Describe how your body feels after having made this change successfully. How do you experience it in your legs, torso, chest, shoulders, head? What is your breathing like?***

- ***What feelings are present?***

- ***What thoughts?***

- ***What is happening at work? What is different here?***

➤ ***What is happening at home? What is different here with family, partner, or animal companions?***

➤ ***How has this impacted your relationships with friends?***

➤ ***How are you living in relationship to your values? Why is that important?***

➤ ***As you think back over the 3 years, what were big turning points? How did you accomplish these? When you ran into the inevitable tough spots, how did you work your way through them?***

- ***How are you applying this information in new ways in your life?***

- ***What's something you know about yourself now that you didn't know at the beginning of this process? Why is this helpful for you?***

- ***What are the three best reasons now to have made this change? Why are these important to you?***

- ***As you think about your area of challenge, what are you observing that has now changed?***

Self-Reflection

- ***As you worked your way through these questions, what changes did you observe in your visualization/imagination of your life—including your bodily sensations, feelings, thoughts, attitudes, and beliefs—and why?***

- ***Were you someone who tended to see and feel these things, or did you have an experience that mainly resided in words and thoughts? What was the effect of those experiences on you?***

- ***What role did your practice partner's words and careful listening, including all EARS skills, play in the exploration of these ideas?***

- ***How did your practice partner use the other elements of EARS in the exploration of these ideas? How did this affect you? How did you feel and why? What did you do and why?***

➤ ***What helped you in this process, and what got in the way?***

What If: Applying Skills to My Current Context

Bridging Questions to Practitioner-Self

These questions help bring the insights from your personal self-practice into your work as a practitioner with clients.

➤ ***Based on your experience of visualizing/imagining here, what do you think needs to be emphasized more when you do this work with clients? What needs to be done less? Why?***

➤ ***How can the use of EARS be brought into this process to assist you as a practitioner?***

➤ ***Think about a client in your work who's struggling. In what areas might a focus on listening assist them in strengthening their reasons for change? Why do you believe this approach will matter? How would you go about doing it?***

____

____

____

____

____

➤ ***What are your main*** takeaway ***messages from this SP/SR experience in relation to your understanding of the strengthening of a client's reasons . . .***

- ***From a practical perspective?***

  ____

  ____

  ____

- ***From a theoretical perspective?***

  ____

  ____

  ____

➤ ***What if you were to apply this process to other areas of your professional practice (e.g., in a role as supervisor or trainer perhaps)? How might you apply your learning to this new context?***

____

____

____

➤ ***How has this exercise influenced your understanding of or personal relationship with MI as a way of being?***

____

____

____

Final Thoughts and Applications to Other Settings

We began this module with a focus on why chasing change talk can be an issue. Yet, we've also said it's important to respond differentially when in the process of *evoking*. For new MI practitioners, this can be a confusing and seemingly contradictory set of ideas, like Han Solo telling Chewbacca to "fly casually" in the presence of an Empire ship. Like Han, we want you to see and understand the big picture, to navigate intentionally and directionally, but without hurry or a single-minded focus. Remember, this is about clients finding their internal motivation for objectives they have articulated.

In settings where time and conversation are limited, it might feel as if we need to get down to it and not waste precious time with unimportant details. Yet, these details are the clients' lives, and they matter to them and should to us. Moreover, these details become impediments if we don't understand how they fit into the whole picture of the client's life. We must therefore practice rapid engagement, hear what matters to the client, and then focus on the elements that are most important in that context. Like the plant in the garden, we can help the client determine if it is the right plant, the right location, soil conditions, nutrients, and water for this change, but the plant will grow at the rate it grows. We can, of course, impede that growth by the things either we do or encourage clients to do.

When time is of the essence, there are certain actions that will help, and these are already well known to us. Focus on a single issue rather than multiple issues or a singular focus on an outcome goal (e.g., eating more fruits, instead of losing 25 pounds). Help the client target small steps toward a larger goal (e.g., eating some fruit in the evening instead of a sweet dessert, like a bowl of ice cream). Tie efforts back to values and processes linked to these values, not outcomes (e.g., eating healthier, rather than losing weight). Lend hope when progress falters (e.g., note how change happens in a nonlinear manner typically). Practice patience and equanimity, while maintaining a realistic belief that change can happen (e.g., reviewing progress on small goals and revising as needed). The pull in these circumstances will be the *fixing reflex*, a tendency to cheerlead, and a heavy focus on change talk. We're better off summarizing, acknowledging the grain of truth in sustain talk—change is hard, and the goal remains off in the distance—and reinforcing the progress made and the reasons why the client selected this goal. Remember, ambivalence is not necessarily resolved just tipped enough to allow forward movement.

MODULE 21

Committing (or Not)

Module Purpose

This module aims to extend our learning from the preceding three modules (Modules 18, 19, and 20) whereby we explored *Why*, *How*, and *When* we actively elicit and respond to ***sustain*** and ***change talk*** to working with the client as they either do or do not reach a point of commitment. There are often crosscurrents in *our* motivations as we honor our client's autonomy and work within the structure of practice settings where change is part of the agenda desired by the agency, service, or referring agents. By the end of this module, it is our hope that you will have an enhanced understanding of the role of readiness in the change process and how to reinforce client decisions toward change from a values-based perspective and respond when they do not; in other words, we develop a deeper appreciation, understanding, and ability to manage the crosscurrents.

The *Why*: Committing or Not Committing

One of the interesting pieces of relearning for many practitioners is that wanting to change is part of change talk. It falls under the category of desire, and practitioners are often well attuned to "talking the talk is not the same as walking the walk." Said more simply, wanting or knowing is NOT the same as doing. We see this so often within a health behavior change context whereby most people who smoke are aware of the health consequences (knowledge) and may even want to quit, but this rarely predicts change behavior. We're often skeptical of this sort of talk—*I know I should stop* or *I want to stop*—prior to learning MI, and once we've learned the value of this language, we tend to be more accepting of it. Now we see it as a steppingstone on the path of change.

The fork in that path is when we come to commitment; this makes intuitive sense. We choose change, or not, and we do that by committing, or not. Yet, research suggests that the process is a little more complex and may need to include factors like the strength of client language, in addition to when it occurs (e.g., Magill et al., 2019). There might also be a nuanced but fundamental problem in both the research and in our path model. That is, committing is not a singular act, but rather a recurring process (DiClemente, 2018). Our goal then is to be aware of when the client is ready to commit initially, while recognizing this is one branch on the path and there will be many like it along the way.

Rosengren (2017) articulated signs of possible readiness to commit. There is a lessening of sustain talk, and there may also be a sense of resolve or quiet that falls upon the person. There may be experimentation with new behavior. Questions about change, in combination with envisioning in more practical and concrete terms what that effort requires, might emerge. This is often accompanied by a shift in the energy of the session.

When we observe these elements, it tends to excite us as practitioners and can lead to a sequence of prematurely jumping to action. That is, we see the readiness and want to capitalize on it, so we hop into *problem solving* immediately. We hear the *commitment* and jump to *planning*. It's important for us at this point to stay attuned to our clients, begin with their feelings and thoughts, and not jump ahead.

The What: Tools for Asking for and Responding to Commitment and Noncommitment

Our tools for committing are straightforward and do not take long to use. We begin by noting the shift by using a reflection or summary and then asking the question directly: Have you decided? Now, what's interesting is that the form of this question often varies, but it is the underlying intent that matters. We can then reinforce such commitment using either ***reflections*** or an ***affirmation*** and avoiding praise or cheerleading. We can also help solidify those reasons by gathering in a ***summary*** the ***change talk*** and the values that support this decision. While it does not need to be long, this is an inflection point worth marking. Once the client has clearly chosen, we move into the ***planning*** task.

But what if the client balks or chooses to turn right instead of left, opts for no change rather than change? This is an important time for us to manage our feelings as a practitioner. The client is so close. There is a real temptation at this juncture to give them a push, maybe even a shove. We want to get them into the pool and swimming. Yet, this would be incongruent with ***MI spirit***, especially ***autonomy***, and undermines psychological safety.

In addition to regulating our feelings, we suggest a few concepts to bear in mind in this situation. To begin, consider whether a gentle nudge—not a push—might be in order. This is a simple press on the decision to see if this is indeed what the client wants or if an emotional reaction (e.g., fear) is pushing them toward a "safe" response. This might be done in concert with reviewing the reasons they've articulated for considering change, rather than remaining with the status quo. Again, be attuned to NOT engaging in the *fixing reflex*. We may be tempted to employ their reasons to argue for the change (e.g., *but you said . . .*), essentially using their arguments against them. Empathy and compassion, as well as autonomy support, are important tools, as is acknowledging the reasons to *not* change in this situation. We are simply exploring further. We can think of this as investing in people, not their outcomes. Finally, we can ***set the alarm***—like a clock or phone—to help us wake in the morning or ***plant a seed***. In setting the alarm, our aim is to help them observe that if now is not the right time, *when* might it be and *how* will they know it is the time. We ask them to identify markers and to become active watchers in their own process. When planting a seed, we note the person needs more time to let an idea, a process, or a possibility germinate. They need a chance to see it grow to decide if it is right for them. Here's how these things might look for someone considering a relationship change:

> *You've decided that staying in the relationship is the best option for now. You've told me there are moments with your partner you really appreciate, and it all feels overwhelming to think about how you would disentangle your lives and make ends meet if you split* (acknowledging sustain talk). *Let me be clear this is your decision to make, not mine* (supporting autonomy).
>
> *It is also a difficult spot. There are areas you've been concerned about and that led you to say you're not happy. There has been disconnection, and your attempts to reconnect have not worked. These have made you wonder about your future together.*
>
> *You've also seen yourself take risks and act courageously in the past and contemplated if you could summon those parts of you now* (reasons for and ability to change). *When I hear those things, I wonder if fear might be getting in the way for you now* (gentle nudge). *What do you think?*
>
> *Again, this is your life, and it may be that now is not the right time. Can you imagine a time in your future where that might change? What would need to happen for that to occur* (setting the alarm)*?*

Throughout this sequence, we would expect interaction with the client and lots of reflective listening. The timing of this process would also be dependent on the context and the length of *our* relationship. Shorter connections and less relationship would suggest being more hesitant to give a gentle nudge. We need to be mindful of believing we know what the right solution is for this client and pushing them toward it. We may have ideas and understand what has helped others, but that does not make it the right decision for them.

The *How*: SP/SR on Committing (or Not) to a Change

Overview of the Exercise

For this activity, you will find a limited-practice partner helpful. Your task is straightforward; discuss where you are with respect to making the change you've been working on throughout this book.

Structure of the Exercise

When the practitioner in this practice, use the questions posed here to initiate the conversation, but then recognize it will branch out based on your partner's answers. Employ all the MI skills liberally in addition to the tools discussed in this module. Since this module is not done following the flow of an MI session, the timing for committing may be perfect, off entirely, or somewhere in between. It might be too soon or too late. Nonetheless, practice either the committing or not ready skills, based on your partner's readiness. If your partner has already committed and begun changing, have your partner articulate the reasons for their choice, and reinforce the commitment.

If done as a self-directed activity, work your way through the questions. Stop periodically to offer a reflection, summary, or even an affirmation. Use your name to assist with the self-distancing if it helps and you feel comfortable doing so.

Traveling Companion: An Example with Sam

Sam has been moving toward a choice point. Momentum has been building. We will use her journey to illustrate a person ready to make an initial commitment. Recall that Sam, who is a White, cisgender woman of European descent, has been a successful counselor for many years. Ten years ago, she injured her back and because of that experience has shifted her private practice to health-focused care. She had a cancer scare last year, and her wife is encouraging her to retire. Sam has been ambivalent about making that change, and this has become a point of contention between them.

➤ ***You've been on this journey, exploring your thoughts, feelings, and your body's responses. Where are you sitting right now with that decision, the change you've been contemplating?***

It's interesting. Because last time I talked about feeling peaceful, calm, and content as I imagined the future and that has stuck around. I just feel more settled in my life. Like I've already made the decision, but I just haven't quite said it aloud yet. I think I'm ready.

➤ ***As you offer these things, what do you notice in your body specifically and why?***

This is interesting, too. Just as I say these things, I feel a little jolt. It's both excitement and anxiety. Like "Am I really going to do this?" and "I am really going to do this!" at the same time. I feel both calm and nervous at the same time. Maybe, it's more like anticipation. Like it's something you really want, and you want to have it happen now, but at the same time, you're not quite sure how it will all turn out and so maybe you don't want it right now. So, my hands feel a little fidgety.

➤ ***What emotions are accompanying these sensations?***

Well, I think I started getting into those already. It's like being at the top of a high dive. When you know you're going to jump and you're excited, but still a little afraid. You could back out, but you don't want to. It's the mix of being electrified stirred in with anxious anticipation. Like maybe when the roller coaster begins that slow climb up the first ramp, before you go racing down. I'm screwing my courage up. Reminding myself why I am excited to do this, and at the same time, I have a few negative thoughts slipping in—"It's not too late to pull out."

➤ ***Summarize your thoughts about this decision.***

In terms of retirement, I am just aware that I've been operating out of fear and concern about loss of identity and meaning. But as I've thought through these things, I know they are not mutually exclusive. I also know that I am not someone who's operated out of fear. I'm someone who has always gone "boldly in the direction of my dreams." This is who I am, when I am at my best, and I want to be at my best. I know this will be better for me and Debra—she matters to me. "We" matter to me.

➤ ***Given this, what happens now?***

I jump. I start actively planning my retirement and begin moving toward it. I am not going to just quit everything and walk away, but I will set a target—1 day a week, no more than five clients—by year's end and begin working from there. It's funny even as I write that, there is part of me that thinks, "Yeah, maybe only four."

➤ ***If you're ready to commit, what's your first step?***

I need to tell Debra I've decided and what it will look like. That will cement it. I'll need to figure out plans and a timeline and contingency plans for when things don't go the way I expect them. But the first step is I tell her. She will be thrilled. Although I think she'd like me to step away entirely, that's not my goal. Then we get into the nuts and bolts of planning.

➤ ***What thoughts do you have about when and how you might do this?***

I want to do it soon. I don't want to hang out on top of the high dive. So, I'll do it at dinner tonight. I will make a meal and start to sort through some of the mechanics, as I know Debra will have questions. I may even buy a bottle of champagne to make it special and let her know we're celebrating something. I'm getting excited.

Traveling Companion: A Second Example with Takeshi

Takeshi will help us illustrate the other side of this exercise. Recall he is a 24-year-old graduate student of Japanese descent working on his doctorate in clinical psychology. Stress and high expectations have been ongoing issues. He is a strong student and shows promise as a counselor. He feels some frustration about his clients' lack of change at times. He sought out MI training at the suggestion of his supervisor.

➤ ***You've been on this journey, exploring your thoughts, feelings, and your body's responses. Where are you sitting right now with that decision, the change you've been contemplating?***

Well, that's the problem. As I mentioned before, there are multiple strands here. There's my relationship with my dad, with my mom, with older men, toward older male clients, and in my dating life. So, which change are we talking about? I need to figure out the priority and start there, and I don't feel like I quite have that done. It's more like I had this realization, it provided some tension release, but I haven't figured out where I am going next.

➤ ***As you offer these things, what do you notice in your body specifically and why?***

Well, these realizations brought me relief, but I also experience tension because my focus hasn't landed on any one place. It's sort of like I relaxed and am doing better with my clients in general, but now I'm pinging off all these other things and that makes me feel unsettled. My body feels restless, like I can't figure out where to look, to focus.

➤ ***What emotions are accompanying these sensations or feelings?***

Anxiety pops to mind, but I am unsure if that is right. Unsettled is probably the right term, but I'm not sure that's a feeling. Disquiet? It's like I have this insight, but I am unsure what to do with it and where to go next. Maybe, there is a little frustration within me. I feel a little stuck. I guess, also a little fear. Like now that I know it, I must deal with it and I'm not quite sure I want to.

➤ ***Summarize your thoughts about this decision.***

Which decision? I think that summarizes it well! I can see where multiple areas are both intertwined and need to change. I need to choose one and focus my attention. I haven't quite done that yet. In fact, I've been kind of ignoring it as a way to deal with it. I need to put it back on my list of things to do and decide.

➤ ***Given this, what happens now?***

I need to set aside some time and give this matter attention. School and life have been busy, so it's been easy to ignore. Until I do that, nothing will happen, but that will also bother me.

➤ ***If you're not ready to commit, what might need to happen for you to be ready?***

Well, I'm not ready to commit to a decision, but I do need to make some time for this to occur. I will need to schedule some time. I am thinking it will be good to get myself out of my usual places. A pen and a pad to do some writing is a must. This is not something I want to do on my phone or tablet. While I'd like a coffee shop and they have tables for writing, I'm likely to get distracted, so maybe a park or even the arboretum. I'll also need to set a time and schedule it, or it will just get taken up by something else.

Then I gotta write and decide. I don't think deciding will be hard, though it might be.

➤ ***How will you know when that happens?***

That I've decided? I'll write it down. If you mean when I'm ready to decide, that is the million-dollar question. Typically, when I'm quiet and give myself space, those things kind of bubble to the surface. It's when I'm busy that I don't give myself enough space, so the question remains unresolved. I expect I'll know, but then I'll need to set a date to start, or it might get lost.

Self-Practice

Now it's your turn. Your task is straightforward; discuss where you are with respect to making the change you've been working on throughout this book. Use the branching query, *Given this, what happens now?*, to decide which set of questions to answer.

➤ ***You've been on this journey, exploring your thoughts, feelings, and your body's responses. Where are you sitting right now with that decision, the change you've been contemplating?***

➤ ***As you offer these things, what do you notice in your body specifically and why?***

➤ ***What emotions are accompanying these sensations or feelings?***

➤ ***Summarize your thoughts about this decision.***

➤ ***Given this, what happens now?***

- ***If you're ready to commit, what's your first step and why?***

- ***What thoughts do you have about when or how you might do this?***

- ***If you're not ready to commit, what might need to happen for you to be ready?***

- ***How will you know when that happens? What might be the first signs to look for?***

Self-Reflection

➤ *As you worked your way through these questions, what did you notice about your ambivalence toward the change?*

➤ *What role did your writing or talking play in responding here?*

➤ *If you had a practice partner, what role did your partner's words and careful listening play in this decision-making process?*

➤ *What helped you in this process, and what got in the way? What role did timing play in all of this? Was this important? If "yes," please explain why.*

What If: Applying Skills to My Current Context

Bridging Questions to Practitioner-Self

These questions help bring the insights from your personal self-practice into your work as a practitioner with clients.

➤ ***How might your work with clients be out of rhythm with their timing? Why?***

➤ ***What timing cues in working with commitment can you observe now that you might have missed before in this process?***

➤ ***In what ways are nudging and shoving different for you? Why are these different?***

➤ ***When have you wanted to push people toward change recently? How did you know if it was happening: What were the clues in your body, or in your thoughts or feelings? What might you do differently next time?***

➤ ***How might you do this process of moving to commitment differently? When will you begin?***

➤ ***What are your main*** takeaway ***messages from this SP/SR experience in relation to your understanding of the concept of committing (or not) . . .***

- ***From a practical perspective?***

- ***From a theoretical perspective?***

➤ ***What if you were to apply this process to other areas of your professional practice (e.g., in a role as supervisor or trainer perhaps)? How might you apply your learning to this new context?***

➤ ***How has this exercise influenced your understanding of or personal relationship with MI as a way of being?***

____

____

____

➤ ***What if you were to apply this process to other areas of your professional practice (e.g., in a role as supervisor or trainer perhaps)? How might you apply your learning to this new context?***

____

____

Final Thoughts and Applications to Other Settings

As was suggested by the length of the activities here, this is not a long process. It is a decision point, and if folks linger, that typically means they're not yet ready to commit. We can offer information (with permission) at this point, as part of a gentle nudge, but this again risks a reduction in autonomy. We are not pressing for change, rather asking them to notice what's influencing their thinking and ensuring this is an informed choice.

In situations where time is limited, as we've noted before, the fixing reflex will pull stronger, not less. We feel it strongly—our role is to deliver clear and unequivocal information so clients can make the best choice, which is the one *we recommend*. When we've reached the precipice—when we're standing at the top of that high dive—and the client expresses concern about jumping off, the pull is very strong. But shoving a client off the high dive rarely leads to either a greater trust in us or a sense of autonomy.

For supervisees, the pressures associated with performance expectations will apply pressure to commit to practices the supervisor deems necessary or appropriate. It will be important to recognize this tendency and to offer *autonomy support* not only in trying out skills and accessing opportunities, but also in determining the focus of these areas. Compliance may be an issue in this situation, and we need to be attentive to the signs, like repeated failure to complete expected tasks after promising to do so. L. H. J. finds that asking supervisees to submit audio/video tapes early in the process is crucial and having trainees observe her work as a supervisor right from the start. This process helps trainees be more relaxed about recording their work and more open to feedback.

As with clients, there will be multiple opportunities for supervisees to commit to something new. The focus of this commitment will evolve over time, and ambivalence is likely to reemerge, especially as people move from a recently accomplished competency zone into a new zone of proximal development.

MODULE 22

Building *My* Plan

Module Purpose

This module explores the task of ***planning***, which includes the reappearance of the ***fixing reflex***, *autonomy*, *competence*, and *relatedness*, as well as the values and limitations of *goal setting* and *implementation intentions*. We specifically address how to strengthen change plans through creating ***if–then*** scenarios. By the end of this module, it is our hope that through the experience of integrating practical and evidence-based ideas into a ***change plan*** for your challenge, you have a more nuanced sense of what helps and hinders when working collaboratively with clients in this process.

The *Why*: The Fun Part!

We are now at the point that many practitioners enjoy. Clients begin acting on their change. There is often a sense of excitement for clients and for practitioners as this unfolds. All the hard work has led us here. It's as if we have climbed the hill—or mountain—of change and now we can begin the trip down the other side, with all the momentum that accompanies going downhill. While ***sustain talk*** may appear in this process, too, in general there is a shift to focusing on the actual challenges associated with changing and what will need to be done to address these if the person is to be successful.

It's ironic that the *fixing reflex* can make an appearance here, too. After all, at this moment clients are engaged, motivated, and ready to begin the change; therein lies our challenge. Now that they're ready, we have lots of tools about *how* they can change at our disposal, and we are eager to share them. We have spent our professional careers building this tool chest and we have experience with what works, when it works, and with whom, and how. There is a strong pull to tell clients what to do as they begin building their plan, which makes this a good time to revisit *autonomy*, *competence*, and *relatedness* (e.g., Chapter 2, Modules 3 and 4).

All three basic psychological needs are present in the planning process. Clients must assemble a plan that reflects their aims and values, and fits with their reasons for undertaking this process. Autonomy is reflected not only in choosing the change, but also in how they will bring it about. They must also feel capable of enacting this change and believe the change will lead—eventually—to the outcome they seek. Sometimes they will borrow our hope in this process because they will learn and try something new. But they must believe it *could* impact their environment to act. Thus, competence might be based on prior experience, but it also may result from their sense of connection and trust with us. The idea that they matter to us, and we matter to them, underlies a willingness to consider a suggestion from us. While we can see this connection, along with other factors (e.g., scarcity, perceived expertise) that increase the power of suggestions (Cialdini, 2016), we remain mindful of our client's autonomy.

These plans are for our clients' gardens, not ours. They will be the gardeners, and our job is to assist them in building their garden, so the plan must be one they can execute and that will work for them. Our expertise matters here, but we help them build *their* own plans.

The *What*: Tools for Planning

Our tools are straightforward. We begin by asking them, *What have you thought about doing?* We then explore past successes to see what they can build on. Once this information is available, we *offer* ideas (with permission), as well as concerns. This can be direct, *I'm concerned about this course of action.* Clients will decide if it fits for them or not. In this manner, we co-construct a plan. Once it's been developed, we then review it and again ask for commitment. As noted in Module 20, revisiting and reinforcing commitment will be an ongoing process.

Implementation intentions are important in the planning process. This area arises from *goal-setting theory* (Locke & Latham, 2019), which is a broad and deep tradition of research into areas such as *persistence* and *goal disengagement* (Brandstätter & Bernecker, 2022). Implementation intentions indicate that if we can create plans that use if–then prepositions, we are more likely to be successful in following through on our goals (Bieleke et al., 2021). Essentially, we are saying, *If this thing occurs (X), then I will do this (Y).*

There are several elements that seem to matter here. For implementation intentions, we need to specify the *Where*, *When*, and *How*. To begin, the X part needs to be broad enough to encapsulate the goal, but specific enough to cue the response. For an anxious person, this might be *If you experience a desire to escape, then . . .* For someone who wants to establish a morning exercise routine, it might be *If the alarm goes off in the morning, then . . .*

Next, the second part must be a specific response in line with the person's goal. For the anxious person, it might be *If you experience a desire to escape, then take five focused breaths and decide.* For the morning exercise routine, if getting out bed is difficult, it might be *If the alarm goes off in the morning, then the feet hit the floor.*

When the person works through *change planning* in this manner, the decision is already made *prior* to the event. That is, when emotions and activation are low. They engage in this top-down reasoning in the calm, cold, and clear light, and then use bottom-up responding, cue response, in the agitated, heated, or foggy light of the cue.

The form does seem to matter here. That is, if–then phrasing produces better outcomes than the same information articulated in a less clear form (Gollwitzer, 2014). Rosengren (2017) notes that using implementation intentions helps us to start on goals, maintain effort, disengage when goals become problematic, and avoid fatigue in their pursuit.

Given the apparent value of using implementation intentions, it makes sense that we would discuss their usage with clients. This discussion would be in the form of offering such information and, if the client expresses interest, helping them identify and refine their if–then plans. Further information and a review of this literature can be found in Bieleke et al. (2021).

Finally, while this is a book on MI and not implementation intentions and goal setting, there are a few more elements worth considering. First, there is an important difference between a *process goal* and an *outcome goal* (see Box 22.1). Outcome goals focus on where we want to end up (i.e., the *What*), whereas process goals focus on *Why* and *How* we'll get there. Related to this, clients often come to us focused on the What, and our task is to help them consider the Why and the How. As part of this, we typically encourage more process goals than outcome goals. It

BOX 22.1. Outcome and Process Goals—Weight Loss

Outcome goal

I want to lose 14 pounds (6.35 kg) in 6 months' time.

Process goals

How the person plans to achieve their outcome goal (e.g., behavioral focus)

Dietary example

I will reduce my daily consumption of sugar by 21 teaspoons by replacing 1 liter of regular Coca-Cola with tap water.

Activity example

I will walk 100 minutes per day on each of my workdays per week ×5. This will include:

- 20-minute commute to and from work
- 30-minute dog walk first thing in the morning and after work
- 20-minute walk at lunch time with colleague at work
- Recording my walking on my phone to monitor time, distance, pace, steps completed

Implementation intentions

If–then plans are integrated within process goals.

If thirsty for a coke, *then* fill the water glass. *If* time to leave for work, *then* put on walking shoes.

is also helpful to phrase the goals positively rather than negatively; that is, what I want to do and not what I want to avoid.

The *How*: SP/SR on Completing a Planning Worksheet

Overview of the Exercise

For this activity, a limited-practice partner is helpful. If ready to develop a plan, then go through this area in a straightforward manner. If not quite ready, this is an opportunity to do some experimenting with new behavior. Like going for a test drive in a car, or trying on clothes at a store, we're not committing to buying, just seeing how these things look and feel for us.

Structure of the Exercise

If done in a limited partner practice, when we are the practitioner in this practice, the questions posed here are meant to guide and focus our conversations. While there is clearly value in creating a well-organized blueprint—completing all the elements in SMART goals, for example—the best plan is the one our partners are willing to follow and can easily recall, implement, and consistently recommit to as needed. At this point, our use of MI skills is likely more flexible and integrated into other strategies and thus we can give our focus to the person rather than use of a particular skill. Be willing to offer either ideas or concerns, as needed, through this process.

For self-directed work, simply follow your way through the elements. Take your time to practice putting any goals into the *if–then* format.

Finally, a word about the structure of goal writing. We'll use a slight revision of the SMART (specific, measurable, attainable, relevant, time) heuristic developed by Doran (1981) to help us refine these goals (see Table 22.1). We are cautious about insistence on this format as there are some concerns about the evidence base for the heuristic (e.g., Swann et al., 2022) and what it fails to provide (Müller & Kotte, 2020). As a result, we integrated the SMART plan ideas in the reproducible Sample Planning Worksheet (Form 22.1) below, as well as other factors, such as social support and implementation intentions, that have robust support in the literature (e.g., Bieleke et al., 2021; Taylor, 2011).

TABLE 22.1. SMART Goals

S	Specific	Are the goals specific and narrow?
M	Measurable	How will you evaluate your progress and the change approach when needed?
A	Attainable	Can you reach these goals in the timeframe?
R	Relevant	Do these goals align with what is important to you and larger goals?
T	Time	What is the timeframe for beginning and completing these goals?

FORM 22.1. Sample Planning Worksheet

What is most important to me in this situation?

____

____

____

____

What do I hope to achieve long term?

____

____

____

____

How do the prior two answers connect with my values?

____

____

____

____

Here are my goals I intend to focus on in the next ______ (e.g., 7, 30, 90) days:

1. ____
   ____
2. ____
   ____
3. ____
   ____

What are the specific actions I intend to take?

1. ____
   ____
2. ____
   ____
3. ____
   ____

(continued)

Sample Planning Worksheet *(page 2 of 3)*

Create an *if–then* sentence for each of the specific actions described above:

Specify what will cue your action. ***If . . .***	**Specify your response.** ***Then . . .***
Example: exercising regularly in the morning *If the alarm goes off,*	*Then the feet hit the floor.*
1.	
2.	
3.	

When will you begin each of these goals?

No.	Goal	Day	Date	Time
1				
2				
3				

How will you evaluate progress? When will you reevaluate? What is the goal status: not yet begun, underway, needs to be modified, or complete?

No.	How will I measure progress?	Recheck Date	Progress?
1.			
2.			
3.			

(continued)

Sample Planning Worksheet *(page 3 of 3)*

Who can help me in this process?

Three people who support my change	*How might I use this person's support?*
1.	
2.	
3.	

Two people who've made a similar change	*How might I use this person's support?*
1.	
2.	

One person I can count on if I need help	*How might I use this person's support?*
1.	

What challenges are present in my context?	How can I overcome these?
If this challenge . . .	*Then I will . . .*

Traveling Companion: An Example with Quincy

Quincy has been noticing changes following brief experiments with new behaviors. Through this process of *taking steps*, she sees the benefits of making a change and would like to create a clearer plan about how she will accomplish this process. Once again, Quincy is a 38-year-old, cisgender woman of African descent who works as an AOD counselor. From a vibrant community, she has strong family ties. She was feeling some burnout with AOD clients and has sought personal support with an MI therapist.

> ***If you would, please summarize where you started with this process, what you discovered along the way, and where you see yourself now?***

I was crispier than I was willing to admit. The job, people, the needs—all were burdens, and I was carrying them. The more I carried, the less connected I felt to why I was carrying it. I was just tired and frustrated. Through this process, I realized I was becoming someone who wasn't me and I didn't like this version of me. I need to get this handled because the direction is problematic. I see the changes when I do things differently, so it's time for me to get my act together.

> ***Given where you are, what have you thought about doing? What makes sense to you?***

Work is the thing. It's where the biggest issues are, though I can see they bleed into other parts of my life. I don't think it's big things, but instead paying attention to little things. Like I don't want to start some meditation practice. It's not like that's bad, it's just not me. At least not yet. What I need is to give myself a few little reminders to keep myself focused.

See Form 22.2 for Quincy's completed version of the Planning Worksheet.

Self-Practice

Now it's your turn. Your task is straightforward. Either create a change plan or identify some "test drive" actions you might be willing to try out with regard to the change you've been working on throughout this book. Start by answering these two questions and then fill in the sample worksheet in reproducible Form 22.1.

> ***If you would, please summarize where you started with this process, what you discovered along the way, and where you see yourself now?***

____

____

____

____

____

FORM 22.2. Completed Planning Worksheet: Quincy's Example

What is most important to me in this situation?

I need to be true to myself. I am kind, but also smart, persistent, and hardworking. Someone who supports the Black community and lifts people up.

What do I hope to achieve long term?

My long-term goal is to be happy and engaged, not frustrated and resentful. I want people to look at me and say, "She's nobody's fool, but she's good people and she'll help."

How do the prior two answers connect with my values?

These are core to my values. I am someone who's genuine, dependable, and compassionate. Faith is at my core. Hope and caring for others come from that.

Here are my goals I intend to focus on in the next *30* (e.g., 7, 30, 90) days:

1. *Extending trust to clients*
2. *Regulating my frustration*
3. *Being mindful of my bodily tension*

What are the specific actions I intend to take?

1. *Rather than being skeptical when clients are telling me their story, I will remind myself they're being as honest as they can in this moment and be curious about how they see it.*
2. *I will pay attention to my bodily cues when I am feeling frustrated. I will practice shifting my attention to the client and the client's agenda.*
3. *If I feel tension in my body, I will use it as a cue to engage in an alternative or incompatible behavior.*

Create an *if–then* sentence for each of the specific actions described above:

Specify what will cue your action. ***If . . .***	**Specify your response.** ***Then . . .***
Example: exercising regularly in the morning *If the alarm goes off,*	*Then the feet hit the floor.*
1. *If skeptical,*	*Then be curious.*
2. *If frustrated,*	*Then shift focus to the client and their agenda.*
3. *If tension in shoulders,*	*Then take an intentional breath and smile.*

When will you begin each of these goals?

No.	Goal	Day	Date	Time
1	*Skeptical*	*Monday*	*5/15*	*7:30 A.M.*
2	*Frustrated*	*Monday*	*5/15*	*7:30 A.M.*
3	*Tension*	*Saturday*	*5/13*	*When I wake up*

(continued)

Source: Adapted from Miller and Rollnick (2002) and Rosengren (2017).

Completed Planning Worksheet: Quincy's Example *(page 2 of 2)*

How will you evaluate progress? When will you reevaluate? What is the goal status: not yet begun, underway, needs to be modified, or complete?

No.	How will I measure progress?	Recheck Date	Progress?
1.	*My goal is to shift from skeptical to curious 80% of the time to begin, during work hours. I will review at the end of the workday before leaving the office and keep a log of how often I was skeptical and how often I responded by being curious.*	*Fridays, first one is 5/19*	*Not yet begun*
2.	*My goal is 80% of the time to begin, during work. I will review at the end of the workday before leaving the office and keep a log of how often I was frustrated and how often I responded by shifting focus onto the client.*	*Fridays, first one is 5/19*	*Not yet begun*
3.	*My goal is 80% of the time each day. I will review at the end of the day before going to bed. I will track how often I noticed tension and how often I responded with an intentional breath and a smile.*	*Fridays, first one is 5/19*	*Not yet begun*

Who can help me in this process?

Three people who support my change	*How might I use this person's support?*
1. *My therapist*	*Informing her of my goals and then reviewing my logs, especially around clients.*
2. *My coworker Ja'Michael*	*Tell him what I'm doing and ask him to notice when he sees me being tense and reinforce me when I follow my plan.*
3. *My friend Teisha*	*Same thing as with Ja'Michael. Notice and reinforce.*

Two people who've made a similar change	*How might I use this person's support?*
1. *Teisha has been focusing on being more mindful*	*Get specific about how she stays in the now and doesn't trip.*
2. *Not sure who can be my second person. I'll have to think about it.*	

One person I can count on if I need help	*How might I use this person's support?*
1. *My dad*	*Biggest issue with me is getting frustrated, blowing my goals, and then giving up. Probably should let him know what's up now, so if I call, then he can help by reminding me what I'm doing and why.*

What challenges are present in my context?	How can I overcome these?
If this challenge . . .	*Then I will . . .*
If I feel like quitting,	*Then call Dad.*
If I miss a day of logging,	*Then remind myself it's about improvement, not perfection.*
If I mess up,	*Then remind myself it's about improvement, not perfection.*

➤ ***Given where you are, what have you thought about doing? What makes sense to you?***

Now complete the Sample Planning Worksheet yourself (Form 22.1) .

Self-Reflection

➤ ***How did you find this experience of planning and working through the worksheet? What emotions accompanied this process for you?***

➤ ***How did you experience these feelings in your body?***

➤ ***What thoughts came to mind as you worked through this worksheet and why?***

➤ *How helpful was it to work through this worksheet and why?*

➤ *How helpful was it to work through the* if–then *statements and why?*

➤ *Was there anything challenging about the* if–then *process? What was it, and why was it challenging? How did you respond to the challenge?*

➤ *Is there anything about the worksheet that you did not find helpful or that you would like to change in any way?*

➤ *If working in a practice pair, what role did your partner's words and careful listening play as you moved through this planning process?*

➤ ***What suggestions and concerns were helpful in this process? What was not? Why?***

____

____

____

____

➤ ***What did you discover from this*** client–self ***view about setting SMART goals and about implementation intentions specifically?***

____

____

____

____

____

What If: Applying Skills to My Current Context

Bridging Questions to Practitioner-Self

These questions help bring the insights from your personal self-practice into your work as a practitioner with clients.

➤ ***As you think about how you've partnered in planning with your clients, what have you done well based on your experience in this process?***

____

____

____

____

____

➤ ***As you think about how you've done planning with your clients, what might you want to do differently, based on your experience in this process?***

____

____

____

____

____

➤ *When might the process be challenging? What* if–then *plans might you create to help yourself in these situations?*

➤ *When will you do this, and how will you assess your progress?*

➤ *What are your main* takeaway *messages from this SP/SR experience in relation to your understanding of the concept of building* my *plan . . .*

- *From a practical perspective?*

- *From a theoretical perspective?*

➤ *What if you were to apply this process to other areas of your professional practice (e.g., in a role as supervisor or trainer perhaps)? How might you apply your learning to this new context?*

➤ ***How has this exercise influenced your understanding of or personal relationship with MI as a way of being?***

____

____

____

Finally, you might consider completing a worksheet from the *practitioner-self* view. That is, what are the MI practice–related goals you might have, and how might you go about integrating those into your work. You can find blank worksheets on the companion website, *www.guilford.com/rosengren2-materials*.

Final Thoughts and Applications to Other Settings

An essential part of any planning process is recognizing that the initial plan is never perfect. We do our best to help clients create a strong plan, and inevitably challenges will arise. This means we should plan on revising, rather than being surprised or disappointed when hiccups occur. Attention to our mindset then is an essential part of staying engaged in the planning process.

Relatedly, recommitting is also an essential part of the planning and change process. Commitment is not a one-time event; instead, it's a process marked by both cognitive and behavioral elements. We consciously recommit and then act on that commitment, though *if–then* plans can, perhaps, reverse that order by having us act on the change and in that process reinforce the cognitive processes.

In brief intermittent contact sessions, we will often operate as though each session is an independent unit. Therefore commitment, if appropriate, is sought at the end of the session for that day's goals. However, there can be an overarching commitment—maintaining a healthy lifestyle for diabetics, for example—that is also reinforced.

The fixing reflex can show up in this area, too! Indeed, our experience and training can wire us for that response. It requires extra attentiveness to avoid that well-meaning tendency to help and instead assist the client in finding their solutions first. In health care and other settings, this can be especially strong as time is limited, the focus is not on extended discussions but on brief interactions, and the need for effective solutions may feel particularly potent. When a client has not been using a prescribed medication regularly, instead of reemphasizing the importance and suggesting a plan, a more MI-consistent approach might be reinforcing the client's previously articulated reasons for using the medication, finding out what has been getting in the way, and asking what they've thought about these things or how they tried to address them. We can always add our suggestions later, and the client who feels connected to us, competent, and autonomous is more likely to follow through.

If interested in learning more about the application of SP/SR in other therapeutic modalities in which you are trained, you may find the other texts in Guilford's Inside Out series helpful. Go to *www.guilford.com/search/Inside+Out*.

References

Arkowitz, H., Miller, W. R., & Rollnick, S. (2015). Conclusions and further directions. In H. Arkowitz, W. R. Miller, & S. Rollnick (Eds.), *Motivational interviewing in the treatment of psychological problems* (2nd ed., pp. 365–380). Guilford Press.

Armstrong, T. (2015). The myth of the normal brain: Embracing neurodiversity. *AMA Journal of Ethics, 17*(4), 348–352.

Baer, J. B., Rosengren, D. R., Dunn, C. W., Wells, E. A., Ogle, R. L., & Hartzler, B. (2004). An evaluation of workshop training in motivational interviewing for addiction and mental health clinicians. *Drug and Alcohol Dependence, 73,* 99–106.

Barbour, R. S. (2001). Checklists for improving rigour in qualitative research: A case of the tail wagging the dog? *British Medical Journal, 322*(7294), 1115–1117.

Barnett, E., Moyers, T. B., Sussman, S., Smith, C., Rohrbach, L. A., Sun, P., & Spruijt-Metz, D. (2014a). From counselor skill to decreased marijuana use: Does change talk matter? *Journal of Substance Abuse Treatment, 46*(4), 498–505.

Barnett, E., Spruijt-Metz, D., Moyers, T. B., Smith, C., Rohrbach, L. A., Sun, P., & Sussman, S. (2014b). Bidirectional relationships between client and counselor speech: The importance of reframing. *Psychology of Addictive Behaviors, 28*(4), 1212.

Barrett, S., Begg, S., O'Halloran, P., Breckon, J., Rodda, K., Barrett, G., & Kingsley, M. (2022). Factors influencing adults who participate in a physical activity coaching intervention: A theoretically informed qualitative study. *BMJ Open, 12*(8), e057855.

Bear, M., Connors, B., & Paradiso, M. A. (2020). *Neuroscience: Exploring the brain, enhanced fourth edition.* Jones & Bartlett Learning.

Bellg, A. J., Borrelli, B., Resnick, B., Hecht, J., Minicucci, D. S., Ory, M., . . . Treatment Fidelity Workgroup of the NIH Behavior Change Consortium. (2004, September). Enhancing treatment fidelity in health behavior change studies: Best practices and recommendations from the NIH Behavior Change Consortium. *Health Psychology, 23*(5), 443–451.

Bennett-Levy, J. (2003). Reflection: A blind spot in psychology? *Clinical Psychology, 27,* 16–19.

Bennett-Levy, J. (2006). Therapist skills: A cognitive model of their acquisition and refinement. *Behavioural and Cognitive Psychotherapy, 34,* 57–78.

Bennett-Levy, J. (2019). Why therapists should walk the talk: The theoretical and empirical case for personal practice in therapist training and professional development. *Journal of Behavior Therapy and Experimental Psychiatry, 62,* 133–145.

Bennett-Levy, J., & Finlay-Jones, A. (2018). The role of personal practice in therapist skill development:

A model to guide therapists, educators, supervisors and researchers. *Cognitive Behaviour Therapy, 47*(3), 185–205.

Bennett-Levy, J., & Haarhoff, B. (2019). Why therapists need to take a good look at themselves: Self-practice/self-reflection as an integrative training strategy for evidence-based practices. In S. Dimidjian (Ed.), *Evidence-based practice in action: Bridging clinical science and intervention* (pp. 380–394). Guilford Press.

Bennett-Levy, J., & Lee, N. K. (2014). Self-practice and self-reflection in cognitive behaviour therapy training: What factors influence trainees' engagement and experience of benefit? *Behavioural and Cognitive Psychotherapy, 42*(1), 48–64.

Bennett-Levy, J., Lee, N., Travers, K., Pohlman, S., & Hamernik, E. (2003). Cognitive therapy from the inside: Enhancing therapist skills through practising what we preach. *Behavioural and Cognitive Psychotherapy, 31,* 143–158.

Bennett-Levy, J., & Thwaites, R. (2007). Self and self-reflection in the therapeutic relationship: A conceptual map and practical strategies for the training, supervision and self-supervision of interpersonal skills. In P. Gilbert & R. Leahy (Eds.), *The therapeutic relationship in the cognitive behavioural psychotherapies* (pp. 255–281). Routledge.

Bennett-Levy, J., Thwaites, R., Chaddock, A., & Davis, M. (2009). Reflective practice in cognitive behavioural therapy. In J. Stedmon & R. Dallos (Eds.), *Reflective practice in psychotherapy and counselling* (pp. 115–135). Open University Press.

Bennett-Levy, J., Thwaites, R., Haarhoff, B., & Perry, H. (2015). *Experiencing CBT from the inside out: A self-practice/self-reflection workbook for therapists.* Guilford Press.

Bennett-Levy, J., Turner, F., Beaty, T., Smith, M., Paterson, B., & Farmer, S. (2001). The value of self-practice of cognitive therapy techniques and self-reflection in the training of cognitive therapists. *Behavioural and Cognitive Psychotherapy, 29,* 203–220.

Bernardi, L., Huinink, J., & Settersten Jr., R. A. (2019). The life course cube: A tool for studying lives. *Advances in Life Course Research, 41,* 100258.

Bhola, P., Duggal, C., & Isaac, R. (2022). *Reflective practice and professional development in psychotherapy.* SAGE.

Bibeau, M., Dionne, F., & Leblanc, J. (2016). Can compassion meditation contribute to the development of psychotherapists' empathy? A review. *Mindfulness, 7,* 255–263.

Bieleke, M., Keller, L., & Gollwitzer, P. M. (2021). If-then planning. *European Review of Social Psychology, 32*(1), 88–122.

Blackburn, I.-M., James, I. A., Milne, D. L., Baker, C., Standart, S., Garland, A., & Reichelt, F. K. (2001). The revised Cognitive Therapy Scale (CTS-R): Psychometric properties. *Behavioural and Cognitive Psychotherapy, 29*(4), 431–446.

Braga, C., Ribeiro, A. P., Sousa, I., & Goncalves, M. M. (2019). Ambivalence predicts symptomatology in cognitive-behavioral and narrative therapies: An exploratory study. *Frontiers in Psychology, 10,* Article 1244.

Brandstätter, V., & Bernecker, K. (2022). Persistence and disengagement in personal goal pursuit. *Annual Review of Psychology, 73,* 271–299.

Butryn, M. L., Godfrey, K. M., Martinelli, M. K., Roberts, S. R., Forman, E. M., & Zhang, F. (2020). Digital self-monitoring: Does adherence or association with outcomes differ by self-monitoring target? *Obesity Science & Practice, 6*(2), 126–133.

Cave, D., Pearson, H., Whitehead, P., & Rahim-Jamal, S. (2016). CENTRE: Creating psychological safety in groups. *The Clinical Teacher, 13*(6), 427–431.

Chang, E. C., Jiang, X., Tian, W., Yi, S., Liu, J., Liang, P., . . . Hirsch, J. K. (2021). Hope as a process in understanding positive mood and suicide protection: A test of the broaden-and-build model. *Crisis: The Journal of Crisis Intervention and Suicide Prevention, 43*(2), 1–8.

Chigwedere, C. (2019). Writing the "self" into self-practice/self-reflection (SP/SR) in CBT: Learning from autoethnography. *The Cognitive Behaviour Therapist, 12,* e38.

Cialdini, R. (2016). *Pre-suasion. A revolutionary way to influence and persuade.* Simon & Schuster.

Cormick, C. (2019). Who doesn't love a good story? What neuroscience tells about how we respond to narratives. *Journal of Science Communication, 18*(5), Y01.

Dallos, R. (2023). Attachment narrative therapy. In R. Dallos (Ed.), *Attachment narrative therapy: Applications and developments* (pp. 1–31). Springer International.

Daugherty, R. P., & Leukefeld, C. (1998). *Reducing the risks for substance abuse. A lifestyle approach.* Springer.

Daugherty, R., & O'Bryan, T. (2022). *Prime for life Version 9.5 e-manual.* Prevention Research Institute. *www.primeforlife.org.*

Davis, M. L., Thwaites, R., Freeston, M. H., & Bennett-Levy, J. (2015). A measurable impact of a self-practice/self-reflection programme on the therapeutic skills of experienced cognitive-behavioural therapists. *Clinical Psychology & Psychotherapy, 22*(2), 176–184.

DeShaw, K. J., Ellingson, L. D., Lansing, J. E., Perez, M. L., Wolff, M., & Welk, G. J. (2024). Process and impact evaluation of a practicum in motivational interviewing. *International Journal of Health Promotion and Education, 62*(3), 1–11.

De Shazer, S., Dolan, Y., Korman, H., Trepper, T., McCollum, E., & Berg, I. K. (2021). *More than miracles: The state of the art of solution-focused brief therapy.* Routledge.

DiClemente, C. C. (2018). *Addiction and change: How addictions develop and addicted people recover.* Guilford Press.

Doran, G. T. (1981). There's a SMART way to write management's goals and objectives. *Management Review, 70*(11), 35–36.

Duke, P., Grosseman, S., Novack, D. H., & Rosenzweig, S. (2015). Preserving third year medical students' empathy and enhancing self-reflection using small group "virtual hangout" technology. *Medical Teacher, 37*(6), 566–571.

Dykstra, R., Beadnell, B., Rosengren, D. B., Schumacher, J., & Daugherty, R. (2023). A lifestyle risk reduction model for preventing high risk substance use across the lifespan. *Prevention Science, 24*(5), 863–875.

Farrand, P., Perry, J., & Linsley, S. (2010). Enhancing self-practice/self-reflection (SP/SR) approach to cognitive behaviour training through the use of reflective blogs. *Behavioural and Cognitive Psychotherapy, 38,* 473–477.

Farrell, J. M., & Shaw, I. A. (2018). *Experiencing schema therapy from the inside out: A self-practice/self-reflection workbook for therapists.* Guilford Press.

Ferguson, H. (2018). How social workers reflect in action and when and why they don't: The possibilities and limits to reflective practice in social work. *Social Work Education, 37*(4), 415–427.

Ferrari, M., Speight, J., Beath, A., Browne, J. L., & Mosely, K. (2021). The information–motivation–behavioral skills model explains physical activity levels for adults with type 2 diabetes across all weight classes. *Psychology, Health & Medicine, 26*(3), 381–394.

Fixsen, D. L., Naoom, S. F., Blase, K. A., Friedman, R. M., & Wallace, F. (2005). *Implementation research: A synthesis of the literature* (FMHI Publication No. 231). University of South Florida, Louis de la Parte Florida Mental Health Institute, National Implementation Research Network.

Flückiger, C., Del Re, A. C., Wampold, B. E., & Horvath, A. O. (2018). The alliance in adult psychotherapy: A meta-analytic synthesis. *Psychotherapy, 55*(4), 316–340.

Flusberg, S. J., Matlock, T., & Thibodeau, P. H. (2017). Metaphors for the war (or race) against climate change. *Environmental Communication, 11*(6), 769–783.

Fraser, N., & Wilson, J. (2011). Students' stories of challenges and gains in learning cognitive therapy. *New Zealand Journal of Counselling, 31,* 79–95.

Fredrickson, B. L. (2001). The role of positive emotions in positive psychology: The broaden-and-build theory of positive emotions. *American Psychologist, 56*(3), 218.

Fredrickson, B. (2009). *Positivity: Top-notch research reveals the 3-to-1 ratio that will change your life.* Harmony.

Fredrickson, B. L. (2013a). *Love 2.0: How our supreme emotion affects everything we feel, think, do and become.* Hudson Street Press.

Fredrickson, B. L. (2013b). Positive emotions broaden and build. In *Advances in experimental social psychology* (Vol. 47, pp. 1–53). Academic Press.

Freeston, M. H., Thwaites, R., & Bennett-Levy, J. (2019). "Courses for Horses": Designing, adapting and implementing self practice/self-reflection programmes. *The Cognitive Behaviour Therapist, 12,* Article e28.

Frey, J., & Hall, A. (2021). *Motivational interviewing for mental health clinicians: A toolkit for skills enhancement.* PESI Press.

Gale, C., & Schröder, T. (2014). Experiences of self-practice/self-reflection in cognitive behavioural therapy: A meta-synthesis of qualitative studies. *Psychology and Psychotherapy, 87*(4), 373–392.

Gill, I., Oster, C., & Lawn, S. (2020). Assessing competence in health professionals' use of motivational interviewing: A systematic review of training and supervision tools. *Patient Education and Counseling, 103*(3), 473–483.

Glynn, L., & Moyers, T. B. (2010). Chasing change talk: The clinician's role in evoking client language about change. *Journal of Substance Abuse Treatment, 39*(1), 65–70.

Gollwitzer, P. M. (2014). Weakness of the will: Is a quick fix possible? *Motivation and Emotion, 38,* 305–322.

Gonzalez-Liencres, C., Shamay-Tsoory, S. G., & Brüne, M. (2013). Towards a neuroscience of empathy: Ontogeny, phylogeny, brain mechanisms and psychopathology. *Neuroscience and Biobehavioral Reviews, 37,* 1537–1548.

Good Reads. (n.d.). Retrieved January 7, 2023, from *www.goodreads.com/quotes/978-whether-you-think-you-can-or-you-think-you-can-t--you-re.*

Graesser, A. C., Hauft-Smith, K., Cohen, A. D., & Pyles, L. D. (1980). Advanced outlines, familiarity and text genre on retention of prose. *Journal of Experimental Education, 48*(4), 281–290.

Grant, B. (2010). Getting the point: Empathic understanding in nondirective client-centered therapy. *Person-Centered and Experiential Psychotherapies, 9*(3), 220–235.

Green, D. (2003). Organizing and evaluating supervisor training. In I. Fleming & L. Steen (Eds.), *Supervision and clinical psychology: Theory, practice and perspectives* (pp. 93–107). Brunner-Routledge.

Guy, J. D., Poelstra, P. L., & Stark, M. J. (1989). Personal distress and therapeutic effectiveness: National survey of psychologists practicing psychotherapy. *Professional Psychology: Research and Practice, 20,* 48–50.

Haarhoff, B., & Farrand, P. (2012). Reflective and self-evaluative practice in CBT. In W. Dryden & R. Branch (Eds.), *The CBT handbook* (pp. 475–492). Sage.

Haarhoff, B., & Thwaites, R. (2016). *Reflection in CBT.* Sage.

Hackmann, A., Bennett-Levy, J., & Holmes, E. A. (Eds.). (2011). *Oxford guide to imagery in cognitive therapy.* Oxford University Press.

Halverson, J. R. (2011, December 8). Why story is not narrative. *Centre for Strategic Communications.* Retrieved September 30, 2022, from *https://csc.asu.edu/2011/12/08/why-story-is-not-narrative.*

Hamilton, L. G., & Petty, S. (2023). Compassionate pedagogy for neurodiversity in higher education: A conceptual analysis. *Frontiers in Psychology, 14.*

Hilton, C. E., & Johnston, L. H. (2017). Health psychology: It's not what you do, it's the way that you do it. *Health Psychology Open, 4*(2), 2055102917714910.

Hilton, C. E., Lane, C., & Johnston, L. H. (2016). Has motivational interviewing fallen into its own premature focus trap? *International Journal for the Advancement of Counselling, 38*(2), 145–158.

Hilton, C. E., & Murphy, B. (2023). How to pretest non-psychometric tools: A field research example of exploring the acceptability, face validity and utility of Emotioncubes: A novel tool to support therapeutic working with emotions. *Methods in Psychology, 9,* 100128.

Hinds, G., & Kaplan, S. (Hosts). (2022, November 28). Transtheoretical model stages of change in MI (No. 62) [Audio podcast episode]. *Talking to Change. www.glennhinds.com/podcast/ep-62-transtheoretical-model-stages-of-change-mi.*

Hohman, M. (2021). *Motivational interviewing in social work practice* (2nd ed.). Guilford Press.

Ho-Wai, S., Bennett-Levy, J., Perry, H., Wood, D., & Wong, C. (2018). The Self-Reflective Writing Scale (SRWS): A new measure to assess self-reflection following self-experiential cognitive behaviour therapy training. *Reflective Practice, 19*(4), 505–521.

Hutchison, A. J., Breckon, J., & Johnston, L. H. (2009). Physical activity behaviour change interventions based on the transtheoretical model: A systematic review. *Health Education and Behaviour, 36*(5), 829–884.

Jasper, M. A. (2005). Using reflective writing within research. *Journal of Research in Nursing, 10*(3), 247–260.

Jefferis, S., Fantarrow, Z., & Johnston, L. (2021). The torchlight model of mapping in cognitive analytic therapy (CAT) reformulation: A qualitative investigation. *Psychology and Psychotherapy: Theory, Research and Practice, 94,* 137–150.

Johanson, D. L., Ahn, H. S., Lim, J., Lee, C., Sebaratnam, G., MacDonald, B. A., & Broadbent, E. (2020). Use of humor by a healthcare robot positively affects user perceptions and behavior. *Technology, Mind, and Behavior, 1*(2).

Johnston, L. H., McMaster, F., & Hilton, C. (2015). *How can QSR NVivo software help people to reflect on their clinical practice and supervision?* Presentation to the Motivational Interviewing Network of Trainers, Berlin, October 15–17, 2015.

Johnston, L. H., & Milne, D. L. (2012). How do supervisees learn during supervision? A grounded theory study of the perceived developmental process. *The Cognitive Behaviour Therapist, 5*(1), 1–23.

Jona, C. M. H., Sheen, J. A., & O'Shea, M. (2022a). Self-disclosure in a self-practice/self-reflection CBT group in professional psychology training. *Training and Education in Professional Psychology.*

Jona, C. M. H., Sheen, J. A., & O'Shea, M. (2022b). Benefits and challenges of an online CBT group, utilizing self-practice/self-reflection paradigm for psychology trainees. *Training and Education in Professional Psychology.*

Kaufman, E. A., Douaihy, A., & Goldstein, T. R. (2021). Dialectical behavior therapy and motivational interviewing: Conceptual convergence, compatibility, and strategies for integration. *Cognitive and Behavioral Practice, 28*(1), 53–65.

Kellerman, G. R., & Seligman, M. E. (2023). *Tomorrowmind: Thriving at work with resilience, creativity, and connection—Now and in an uncertain future.* Simon & Schuster.

Kolb, D. (1984). *Experiential learning: Experience as the source of learning and development.* Prentice-Hall.

Kolts, R. L., Bell, T., Bennett-Levy, J., & Irons, C. (2018). *Experiencing compassion-focused therapy from the inside out.* Guilford Press.

Kross, E., & Ayduk, O. (2017). Self-distancing: Theory, research, and current directions. In J. M. Olson (Ed.), *Advances in experimental social psychology* (Vol. 55, pp. 81–136). Academic Press.

Lane, C. (2012). *A discourse analysis of client and practitioner talk during motivational interviewing sessions.* ClinPsyD thesis (Vol. 1), University of Birmingham. *http://etheses.bhamac.uk/3708/1/Lane12ClinPsyD1.pdf.*

Leake, G. J., & King, A. S. (1977). Effect of counselor expectations on alcoholic recovery. *Alcohol Health and Research World, 1*(3), 16–22.

Li, M., Gu, Y., Ma, Y., Liu, M., & Tang, Y. (2021). Positive emotions, hope, and life satisfaction in Chinese college students: How useful is the broaden-and-build model in studying well-being in victims of intimate partner violence? *Journal of Interpersonal Violence, 37*(13–14).

Locke, E. A., & Latham, G. P. (2019). The development of goal setting theory: A half century retrospective. *Motivation Science, 5*(2), 93.

Luft, J., & Ingham, H. (1961). The Johari window. *Human Relations Training News, 5*(1), 6–7.

Madson, M. B., Villarosa-Hurlocker, M. C., Schumacher, J. A., Williams, D. C., & Gauthier, J. M. (2019). Motivational interviewing training of substance use treatment professionals: A systematic review. *Substance Abuse, 40*(1), 43–51.

Magill, M., Apodaca, T. R., Borsari, B., Gaume, J., Hoadley, A., Gordon, R. E., . . . Moyers, T. (2018). A meta-analysis of motivational interviewing process: Technical, relational, and conditional process models of change. *Journal of Consulting and Clinical Psychology, 86*(2), 140.

Magill, M., Bernstein, M. H., Hoadley, A., Borsari, B., Apodaca, T. R., Gaume, J., & Tonigan, J. S. (2019). Do what you say and say what you are going to do: A preliminary meta-analysis of client change and sustain talk subtypes in motivational interviewing. *Psychotherapy Research, 29*(7), 860–869.

Manuel, J. K., Ernst, D., Vaz, A., & Rousmaniere, T. (2022). *Deliberate practice in motivational interviewing.* American Psychological Association.

Markland, D., Ryan, R. R., Tobin, V. J., & Rollnick, S. (2005). Motivational interviewing and self-determination theory. *Journal of Social and Clinical Psychology, 24*(6), 811–831.

Marshall, C., & Søgaard Nielsen, A. (2020). *Motivational interviewing for leaders in the helping professions: Facilitating change in organizations.* Guilford Press.

Martino, S., Ball, S. A., Gallon, S. L., Hall, D., Garcia, M., Ceperich, S., . . . Hausotter, W. (2006). *Supervisory tools for enhancing proficiency.* Motivational Interviewing Assessment 246. Northwest Frontier Addiction Technology Transfer Center, Oregon Health and Science University.

Martino, S., Ball, S. A., Nich, C., Frankforter, T. L., & Carroll, K. M. (2008). Community program therapist adherence and competence in motivational interviewing. *Drug and Alcohol Dependence, 96,* 37–48.

McCarthy, B., & McCarthy, D. (2005). *Teaching around the 4MAT cycle: Designing instruction for diverse learners with diverse learning styles.* Corwin Press.

McConnaughy, E. A., Prochaska, J. O., & Velicer, W. F. (1983). Stages of change in psychotherapy: Measurement and sample profiles. *Psychotherapy, 20*(3).

McDermott, F. (2020). *Inside group work: A guide to reflective practice.* Routledge.

McGillivray, J., Gurtman, C., Boganin, C., & Sheen, J. (2015). Self-practice and self-reflection in training of psychological interventions and therapist skills development: A qualitative meta-synthesis review. *Australian Psychologist, 50*(6), 434–444.

Mentha, H. (2020). *Someone good to talk to: Reflections on motivational interviewing in practice.* Author.

Michaelsen, M. M., & Esch, T. (2023). Understanding health behavior change by motivation and reward mechanisms: A review of the literature. *Frontiers in Behavioral Neuroscience, 17,* 1151918.

Michie, S., Van Stralen, M. M., & West, R. (2011). The behaviour change wheel: A new method for characterising and designing behaviour change interventions. *Implementation Science, 6*(1), 1–12.

Miller, W. R. (1983). Motivational interviewing with problem drinkers. *Behavioural Psychotherapy, 11,* 147–172.

Miller, W. R. (2018). *Listening well. The art of empathetic listening.* Wipf and Stock.

Miller, W. R. (2022). *On second thought: How ambivalence shapes your life.* Guilford Press.

Miller, W. R. (2023). The evolution of motivational interviewing. *Behavioural and Cognitive Psychotherapy, 51*(6), 616–632.

Miller, W. R., & Moyers, T. B. (2006). Eight stages in learning motivational interviewing. *Journal of Teaching in the Addictions, 5,* 3–17.

Miller, W. R., & Moyers, T. B. (2015). The forest and the trees: Relational and specific factors in addiction treatment. *Addiction, 110*(3), 401–413.

Miller, W. R., & Moyers, T. B. (2021). *Effective psychotherapists.* Guilford Press.

Miller, W. R., & Rollnick, S. (1991). *Motivational interviewing. Preparing people to change addictive behaviors.* Guilford Press.

Miller, W. R., & Rollnick, S. (2002). *Motivational interviewing: Preparing people for change* (2nd ed.). Guilford Press.

Miller, W. R., & Rollnick, S. (2009). Ten things that motivational interviewing is not. *Behavioural and Cognitive Psychotherapy, 37*(2), 129–140.

Miller, W. R., & Rollnick, S. (2013). *Motivational interviewing: Helping people change* (3rd ed.). Guilford Press.

Miller, W. R., & Rollnick, S. (2023). *Motivational interviewing: Helping people change and grow* (4th ed.). Guilford Press.

Miller, W. R., & Rose, G. S. (2009). Toward a theory of motivational interviewing. *American Psychologist, 64*(6), 527.

Miller, W. R., & Tonigan, J. S. (1996). Assessing drinkers' motivation for change: The Stages of Change Readiness and Treatment Eagerness Scale (SOCRATES). *Psychology of Addictive Behaviors, 10*(2), 81–89.

Miller, W. R., Yahne, C. E., Moyers, T. B., Martinez, J., & Pirritano, M. (2004). A randomized trial of methods to help clinicians learn motivational interviewing. *Journal of Counseling and Clinical Psychology, 72*(6), 1050–1062.

Monk, G. E., Winslade, J. E., Crocket, K. E., & Epston, D. E. (1997). *Narrative therapy in practice: The archaeology of hope.* Jossey-Bass.

Moyers, T. B., & Miller, W. R. (2013). Is low therapist empathy toxic? *Psychology of Addictive Behavior, 27*(3), 878–884.

Moyers, T. B., Rowell, L. N., Manuel, J. K., Ernst, D., & Houck, J. M. (2016). The Motivational Interviewing Treatment Integrity code (MITI 4): Rationale, preliminary reliability, and validity. *Journal of Substance Abuse Treatment, 65*, 36–42.

Müller, A. A., & Kotte, S. (2020). Of SMART, GROW and goals gone wild: A systematic literature review on the relevance of goal activities in workplace coaching. *International Coaching Psychology Review, 15*(2), 69–97.

Niemand, A. (2018, May 7). How to tell stories about complex issues. *Stanford Social Innovation Review.* Retrieved September 30, 2022, from *https://ssir.org/articles/entry/how_to_tell_stories_about_complex_issues.*

Patrick, H., & Williams, G. C. (2012). Self-determination theory: Its application to health behavior and complementarity with motivational interviewing. *The International Journal of Behavioral Nutrition and Physical Activity, 9*, 18.

Peterson, C. (2006). *A primer in positive psychology.* Oxford University Press.

Pink, D. H. (2022). *The power of regret: How looking backward moves us forward.* Riverhead Books.

Prevention Research Institute. (2008). *Prime solutions participant workbook.* Author.

Prochaska, J. O. (1979). *Systems of psychotherapy: A transactional process.* Dorsey Press.

Prochaska, J. O., & DiClemente, C. C. (1983). Stages and processes of self-change of smoking: toward an integrative model of change. *Journal of Consulting and Clinical Psychology, 51*(3), 390.

QSR International Pty Ltd. (2020, March). NVivo. *www.qsrinternational.com/nvivo-qualitative-data-analysis-software/home.*

Quigley, K. S., Kanoski, S., Grill, W. M., Barrett, L. F., & Tsakiris, M. (2021). Functions of interoception: From energy regulation to experience of the self. *Trends in Neurosciences, 44*(1), 29–38.

Ritchie, M. J., Parker, L. E., & Kirchner, J. E. (2020). From novice to expert: A qualitative study of implementation facilitation skills. *Implementation Science Communications, 1*(1), 25–25.

Robichaux, A. (2024, April 9–10). *The human side of transformation* [Conference session]. Uplift by BetterUp, San Francisco, CA. *www.betterup.com/uplift.*

Rogers, C. R. (1961). *On becoming a person.* Houghton Mifflin.

Rogers, C. R. (1980). *A way of being.* Houghton Mifflin.

Rollnick, S., Fader, J., Breckon, J., & Moyers, T. B. (2019). *Coaching athletes to be their best: Motivational interviewing in sports.* Guilford Press.

Rollnick, S., Mason, P., & Butler, C. (1999). *Health behavior change: A guide for practitioners.* Churchill Livingstone.

Rollnick, S., Miller, W. R., & Butler, C. C. (2023). *Motivational interviewing in health care: Helping patients change behavior* (2nd ed.). Guilford Press.

Rosengren, D. B. (2017). *Building motivational interviewing skills: A practitioner workbook.* Guilford Press.

Rousmaniere, T. (2017). *Deliberate practice for psychotherapists: A guide to improving clinical effectiveness.* Routledge.

Ruano, A., García-Torres, F., Gálvez-Lara, M., & Moriana, J. A. (2022). Psychological and non-pharmacologic treatments for pain in cancer patients: A systematic review and meta-analysis. *Journal of Pain and Symptom Management, 63*(5), e505–e520.

Ryan, R. M., & Deci, E. L. (2000). Self-determination theory and the facilitation of intrinsic motivation, social development, and well-being. *American Psychologist, 55*(1), 68–78.

Ryan, R. M., & Deci, E. L. (2017). *Self-determination theory: Basic psychological needs in motivation, development, and wellness.* Guilford Press.

Safran, J. D., & Muran, J. C. (2000). *Negotiating the therapeutic alliance: A relational treatment guide.* Guilford Press.

Sandell, R., Lazar, A., Grant, J., Carlsson, J., Schubert, J., & Broberg, J. (2006). Therapist attitudes and patient outcomes. III. A latent class analysis of therapists. *Psychology and psychotherapy: Theory, research and practice, 79*(4), 629–647.

Sarink, F. S., & García-Montes, J. M. (2023). Humor interventions in psychotherapy and their effect on levels of depression and anxiety in adult clients, a systematic review. *Frontiers in Psychiatry, 13,* 1049476.

Schön, D. A. (2017). *The reflective practitioner: How professionals think in action.* Routledge.

Schwalbe, C. S., Oh, H. Y., & Zweben, A. (2014). Sustaining motivational interviewing: A meta-analysis of training studies. *Addiction, 109*(8), 1287–1294.

Schwartz, S. H., & Sortheix, F. (2018). Values and subjective well-being. In E. Diener, S. Oishi, & L. Tay (Eds.), *Handbook of well-being* (pp. 1–25). Noba Scholar.

Sherman, D. A. K., Nelson, L. D., & Steele, C. M. (2000). Do messages about health risks threaten the self? Increasing the acceptance of threatening health messages via self-affirmation. *Personality and Social Psychology Bulletin, 26,* 1046–1058.

Steindl, S. (2020). *The gifts of compassion. How to understand and overcome suffering.* Australian Academic Press.

Stifter, C., Augustine, M., & Dollar, J. (2020). The role of positive emotions in child development: A developmental treatment of the broaden and build theory. *Journal of Positive Psychology, 15*(1), 89–94.

Stukas, A. A., & Snyder, M. (2016). Self-fulfilling prophecies. *Encyclopedia of Mental Health, 4,* 92–100.

Swann, C., Jackman, P. C., Lawrence, A., Hawkins, R. M., Goddard, S. G., Williamson, O., . . . Ekkekakis, P. (2022). The (over) use of SMART goals for physical activity promotion: A narrative review and critique. *Health Psychology Review, 17*(2), 1–16.

Taylor, S. E. (2011). Social support: A review. In *The Oxford handbook of health psychology* (Vol. 1, pp. 189–214). Oxford University Press.

Thomas, G., & Thorpe, S. (2019). Enhancing the facilitation of online groups in higher education: A review of the literature on face-to-face and online group-facilitation. *Interactive Learning Environments, 27*(1), 62–71.

Thwaites, R., Bennett-Levy, J., Davis, M., & Chaddock, A. (2014). Using self-practice and self-reflection (SP/SR) to enhance CBT competence and meta-competence. In A. Whittington & N. Grey (Eds.),

How to become a more effective CBT therapist: Mastering metacompetence in clinical practice (pp. 241–254). Wiley-Blackwell.

Tirch, D., Silberstein-Tirch, L. R., Codd, T., III, Brock, M. J., & Wright, M. J. (2019). *Experiencing ACT from the inside out: A self-practice/self-reflection workbook for therapists.* Guilford Press.

Veestraeten, M., Johnson, S. K., Leroy, H., Sy, T., & Sels, L. (2021). Exploring the bounds of Pygmalion effects: Congruence of implicit followership theories drives and binds leader performance expectations and follower work engagement. *Journal of Leadership & Organizational Studies, 28*(2), 137–153.

Vygotsky, L. S. (1978). *Mind in society: The development of higher psychological processes.* Harvard University Press.

Wagner, B. C., & Petty, R. E. (2022). The elaboration likelihood model of persuasion: Thoughtful and non-thoughtful social influence. In D. Chadee (Ed.), *Theories in social psychology* (2nd ed., pp. 120–142). Wiley.

Wagner, C. C., & Ingersoll, K. S. (2012). *Motivational interviewing in groups.* Guilford Press.

Walthers, J., Janssen, T., Mastroleo, N. R., Hoadley, A., Barnett, N. P., Colby, S. M., & Magill, M. (2019). A sequential analysis of clinician skills and client change statements in a brief motivational intervention for young adult heavy drinking. *Behavior Therapy, 50*(4), 732–742.

Westra, H. A. (2012). *Motivational interviewing in the treatment of anxiety.* Guilford Press.

Westra, H. A., & Norouzian, N. (2018). Using motivational interviewing to manage process markers of ambivalence and resistance in cognitive behavioral therapy. *Cognitive Therapy Research, 42,* 193–203.

Zaki, J. (2020). *The war for kindness. Building empathy in a fractured world.* Broadway Books.

Zuckoff, A. (2023, November). *Building the capacity for ambivalence through motivational interviewing.* Plenary presentation at the 2023 MINT Virtual Forum.

Index

Note. *t*, *f*, or *b* following a page number indicates a table, a figure, or a box.

G

H

I

J

K

L

M

N

O

Q

R

S

T

U

V

W

Y

Z